CARDIOLOGY RESEARCH AND CLINICAL DEVELOPMENTS

CARDIOVASCULAR DISEASES AND LIVER TRANSPLANTATION

CARDIOLOGY RESEARCH AND CLINICAL DEVELOPMENTS

Additional books in this series can be found on Nova's website under the Series tab.

Additional E-books in this series can be found on Nova's website under the E-books tab.

CARDIOLOGY RESEARCH AND CLINICAL DEVELOPMENTS

CARDIOVASCULAR DISEASES AND LIVER TRANSPLANTATION

ZOKA MILAN
EDITOR

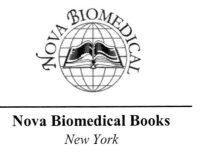

Nova Biomedical Books
New York

Copyright ©2011 by Nova Science Publishers, Inc.

All rights reserved. No part of this book may be reproduced, stored in a retrieval system or transmitted in any form or by any means: electronic, electrostatic, magnetic, tape, mechanical photocopying, recording or otherwise without the written permission of the Publisher.

For permission to use material from this book please contact us:
Telephone 631-231-7269; Fax 631-231-8175
Web Site: http://www.novapublishers.com

NOTICE TO THE READER

The Publisher has taken reasonable care in the preparation of this book, but makes no expressed or implied warranty of any kind and assumes no responsibility for any errors or omissions. No liability is assumed for incidental or consequential damages in connection with or arising out of information contained in this book. The Publisher shall not be liable for any special, consequential, or exemplary damages resulting, in whole or in part, from the readers' use of, or reliance upon, this material. Any parts of this book based on government reports are so indicated and copyright is claimed for those parts to the extent applicable to compilations of such works.

Independent verification should be sought for any data, advice or recommendations contained in this book. In addition, no responsibility is assumed by the publisher for any injury and/or damage to persons or property arising from any methods, products, instructions, ideas or otherwise contained in this publication.

This publication is designed to provide accurate and authoritative information with regard to the subject matter covered herein. It is sold with the clear understanding that the Publisher is not engaged in rendering legal or any other professional services. If legal or any other expert assistance is required, the services of a competent person should be sought. FROM A DECLARATION OF PARTICIPANTS JOINTLY ADOPTED BY A COMMITTEE OF THE AMERICAN BAR ASSOCIATION AND A COMMITTEE OF PUBLISHERS.

Additional color graphics may be available in the e-book version of this book.

Library of Congress Cataloging-in-Publication Data

Cardiovascular diseases and liver transplantation / [edited by] Zoka Milan.
   p. ; cm. -- (Cardiology research and clinical developments)
 Includes bibliographical references and index.
 ISBN 978-1-61122-910-3 (hardcover : alk. paper)
 1. Liver--Failure--Complications. 2.
Liver--Transplantation--Complications. 3. Cardiological manifestations of
general diseases. 4. Cardiovascular system--Diseases--Complications. I.
Milan, Zoka. II. Series: Cardiology research and clinical developments
series.
  [DNLM: 1. Cardiovascular Diseases--complications. 2. Liver
Diseases--complications. 3. Liver Transplantation. 4. Risk Factors. WG
120]
 RC848.F27C37 2011
 617.5'562--dc22
                           2010044749

Published by Nova Science Publishers, Inc. ✦ New York

Contents

Contributors		vii
Preface		xi
Abbreviations		xix
Chapter I	Haemodynamic Profile of Patients with End-Stage Liver Disease *Søren Møller, and Jens H. Henriksen*	1
Chapter II	Coronary Artery Disease and Liver Transplantation *James Y. Findlay*	31
Chapter III	Cardiac Arrhythmias and Liver Transplantation *Andrea Vannucci and Ivan Kangrga*	49
Chapter IV	Valvular Heart Disease and Liver Transplantation *Andrew I. Gardner and Neville M. Gibbs*	67
Chapter V	Pulmonary Hypertension and Liver Transplantation *Michael Ramsay*	83
Chapter VI	Hypertrophic Obstructive Cardiomypathy in Liver Transplant Patients *Paco E. Bravo and Fadi G. Hage*	99
Chapter VII	Obesity and Liver Transplantation *Paul J. Thuluvath*	113
Chapter VIII	Liver Disease and Chronic Advanced Heart Failure *Jill M. Gellow and Askay S. Dessai*	125
Chapter IX	Combined Cardiac Surgery and Liver Transplantation *Eugenia Raichlin, Charles B. Rosen, Ioana Dumitru, Richard C. Daly and Sudhir S. Kushwaha*	139
Chapter X	Previous Chemotherapy and Cardiac Function *Wafaa Abdel-Haidi*	157

Chapter XI	Cardiopulmonary Consequences of Transjugular Intrahepatic Portosystemic Shunts *Florence Wong*	**169**
Chapter XII	Hepatopulmonary Syndrome *Pascal Fauconnet, Vincent Ho, Catherine Pastor and Eduardo Schiffer*	**179**
Chapter XIII	Pre-Operative Assessment of Cardiovascular Function before Liver Transplantation: A Practical Approach *James Y. Findlay*	**193**
Chapter XIV	A Role of Cardiopulmonary Exercise Testing (CPET) in Defining Cardiopulmonary Function before Liver Transplantation *James Prentis and Chris Snowden*	**201**
Chapter XV	Pharmacotherapy of Cardiac Dysfunction in Liver Transplant Patients *Dina Jankovic*	**217**
Chapter XVI	Cardiovascular Monitoring During Liver Transplantation *Giorgio Della Rocca, Maria Gabriella Costa and Zoka Milan*	**239**
Chapter XVII	Cardiovascular Profile and Cardiac Complications Following Liver Transplantation *Aileen R Smith, George Therapondos, Tamer R Fouad and Samuel S. Lee*	**259**
Acknowledgments		**275**
Index		**277**

Contributors

Dr Wafaa Abdel-Haidi, MSc
Consultant Oncologist, Department of Clinical Oncology, Faculty of Medicine, Cairo, Egypt
Paco E Bravo
Department of Radiology and Radiological Sciences, Johns Hopkins University, Baltimore , USA
Maria Gabriella Costa
Department of Anaesthesia and Intensive Care Medicine, Medical School of the University of Udine, Udine, Italy
Richard C. Daly MD
Departments of Cardiothoracic Surgery, Mayo Clinic, Rochester, MN 55905, USA
Giorgio Della Rocca
Department of Anaesthesia and Intensive Care Medicine, Medical School of the University of Udine, Udine, Italy
Askay S Dessai MD
Division of Cardiology, Brigham and Women's Hospital, Boston, Massachusetts, USA
Ioana Dumitru, MD
Department of Internal Medicine, Section of Cardiology, UNMC, Omaha, NE 68198, USA
Pascal Fauconnet
Service of Anaesthesiology, Department APSI, Hospitaux Universitaires Geneve
Rue Gabrielle-Perret-Gentil 4, 1211 Geneve 14, Switzerland
James Y. Findlay, MB, ChB, FRCA
Consultant, Department of Anesthesiology and Critical Care Medicine,
Mayo Clinic, First St S.W, Rochester MN 55905, USA
Tamer R Fouad
Division of Gastroenterology/Hepatology, Menofiya University, Menofiya, Egypt
Andrew I Gardner
Department of Anaesthesia, Sir Charles Gairdner Hospital, Nedlands, Australia
Jill M. Gelow, MD MPH
Oregon Health and Science University, Division of Cardiology, 3181 SW Sam Jackson Park Road, UHN 62, Portland, Oregon 97239, USA

Neville M Gibbs
Department of Anaesthesia, Sir Charles Gairdner Hospital, Hospital Avenue, Nedlands WA 6009

Fadi G. Hage, MD
Zeigler Research Building 1024, 1530 3rd AVE S, Birmingham AL 35294-0006, USA

Jens H. Henriksen, MD, Dr MSc
Professor, Department of Clinical Physiology, 239, Hvidovre Hospital, DK-2650 Hvidovre, Denmark

Vincent Ho
Senior lecturer, School of Medicine, James Cook University Hospital, Department of Gastroenterology, Townsville Hospital, Douglas Queensland 4810, Australia

Dina Jankovic
Department of Pharmacy, Chelsea and Westminster Hospital, 369 Fulham Road London, SW10 9NH, UK

Ivan Kangrga, MD, PhD
Chief, Vascular, Hepatobiliary and Liver Transplant Anesthesia, Washington University School of Medicine, 660 S. Euclid Ave, Box 8054, St. Louis, MO 63110

Sudhir S. Kushwaha, MD
William J. Von Liebig Transplant Center, Mayo Clinic, Rochester, MN 55905, USA

Samuel S. Lee
University of Calgary Liver Unit, Calgary, Canada

Zoka Milan, MD, PhD
Department of Anaesthesia, St James's University Hospital, Leeds, UK

Søren Møller, MD
Associate Professor, Chief Physician, Department of Clinical Physiology, 239, Hvidovre Hospital, DK-2650 Hvidovre, Denmark

Catherine Pastor
Service of Anaesthesiology, Department APSI, Hospitaux Universitaires Geneve
Rue Gabrielle-Perret-Gentil 4, 1211 Geneve 14, Switzerland

James Prentis MRCP, FRCA
Department of Anaesthesia, Freeman Hospital, Newcastle Upon Tyne, UK

Eugenia Raichlin
Assistant Professor, Department of Internal Medicine, Section of Cardiology
982265 UNMC, Omaha, NE 68198-2265, USA

Michael Ramsey, MD, FRCA
Chairman Department of Anesthesiology, Baylor University Medical Centre, Dallas Texas 75240, USA

Charles B. Rosen, MD
William J. Von Liebig Transplant Center, [3]Department of liver transplantation, Mayo Clinic, Rochester, MN 55905, USA

Aileen R Smith
Multiorgan Transplant Program, University of Toronto and University Health Network, Toronto General Hospital, Canada

Eduardo Schiffer MD
Service of Anaesthesiology, Department APSI, Hospitaux Universitaires Geneve
Rue Gabrielle-Perret-Gentil 4, 1211 Geneve 14, Switzerland

Chris Snowden FRCA MD
Department of Anaesthesia, Freeman Hospital, Newcastle Upon Tyne, UK

George Therapondos BSc, MB, ChB
Director, Clinical Trials Unit, Assistant Professor of Medicine, Multiorgan Transplant Program, University of Toronto and University Health Network, Toronto General Hospital, Toronto, Ontario M5G 2N2

Paul J. Thuluvath, MD, FRCP
Institute for Digestive Health and Liver Diseases, Mercy Medical Center, #718, 301 St. Paul's Street, Baltimore, MD 21202, USA

Andrea Vannucci
Washington University School of Medicine, 660 S. Euclid Ave, Box 8054, St. Louis, MO 63110

Florence Wong MB, BS, MD, FRACP, FRCPC
Department of Medicine, Toronto General Hospital, Toronto, Ontario, Canada

Preface

With approximately 8,000 liver transplant operations per year worldwide, this surgical procedure has become relatively routine. Improvements in surgical and anesthetic techniques and immunosuppression have resulted in improved outcomes, but cardiovascular events and sepsis remain the principal obstacles to further lowering morbidity and mortality rates. Consequently, cardiovascular assessment and optimization are of increased interest to anesthetists and other professionals involved in liver transplant programs. This book summarizes the current knowledge on preoperative hemodynamic profiling and cardiovascular assessment of patients awaiting liver transplantation

Chapter 1 - Patients with cirrhosis and portal hypertension exhibit characteristic haemodynamic changes. A vasodilatatory state and a hyperdynamic circulation affect various functions, resulting in multi-organ failure. Thus, the circulation of the lungs, kidneys, brain, gastrointestinal tract and periphery is disturbed. The recently defined cirrhotic cardiomyopathy affects systolic and diastolic functions of the heart and implies electromechanical abnormalities. In addition, baroreceptor response and regulation of circulatory homoeostasis are impaired, and reduced cardiac reserve may also play a role in the development of hepatorenal syndrome. Pulmonary dysfunction involves diffusing abnormalities, with development of hepatopulmonary syndrome and portopulmonary hypertension in some patients with cirrhosis. Recent research has focused on the assertion that haemodynamic and neurohumoral dysregulation are of major importance for the development of many of the organ-related complications in cirrhosis. This aspect is important to take into account in the management of these patients.

Chapter 2 - Coronary artery disease (CAD) is common in patients undergoing evaluation for liver transplantation and its prevalence in this population will likely increase as liver transplantation is offered to a wider range of candidates, particularly older patients. A significant percentage of this CAD is previously undiagnosed. Cardiovascular events are one of the leading causes of mortality and morbidity after liver transplantation and patients with CAD who undergo liver transplantation have a higher morbidity and mortality than controls. Identification of CAD in the transplant candidate is problematic as the symptoms of liver disease confound clinical suspicion and conventional non-invasive screening tests are reported as having poor diagnostic accuracy in this population when used as part of typical screening algorithms. The optimum management of the patient with CAD prior to liver transplantation is currently unknown, current practice suggests correcting identifiable significant lesions percutaneously where possible and providing optimum medical management as per current guidelines. Acceleration of known CAD and the development of CAD are significant issues in the post-transplant population. Modifiable cardiovascular risk factor identification and risk reduction management should be actively undertaken.

Chapter 3 - Pre-existing or perioperative arrhythmias are common in OLT but their incidence and impact on outcomes have not been systematically addressed.

Prolonged QT interval is a manifestation of cirrhotic cardiomyopathy but there is no consensus on its prognostic value or best management. Reperfusion arrhythmias are common intraoperative complications of possible prognostic value for long-term outcomes. Preventative and best treatment strategies have not been defined.

Other serious arrhythmias, such as atrial fibrillation or ventricular arrhythmias, are not specifically related to ESLD or OLT but are prevalent in general population, particularly perioperatively. The aim of this Chapter is to summarize reports of arrhythmias in OLT literature and to provide suggestions for perioperative management based on current knowledge of arrhythmias and clinical challenges of OLT.

Chapter 4 - The implications of valvular heart disease for the liver transplant candidate depend on the valvular lesion, its severity, and its natural history if untreated. There is extensive overlap in the symptoms and signs of both diseases, making clinical estimation of the severity of valvular disease difficult. Moreover, the presence of one of these diseases may influence the symptomatology and progression of the other. There is little information available on the risks of transplantation in patients with valvular heart disease, so most decisions must be based on first principles. This chapter outlines the aetiology, pathophysiology, and natural history of the most common valvular lesions, and describes the medical and surgical options that must be considered prior to liver transplantation. An algorithm for triage of patients with valvular heart disease is presented, and strategies for perioperative management are described.

Chapter 5 - Portopulmonary hypertension is found in 5-6% of patients with portal hypertension. This may or may not be associated with liver cirrhosis. If cirrhosis is present the severity of the liver cirrhosis does not correlate with the degree of pulmonary hypertension. The diagnosis of portopulmonary hypertension includes a mean pulmonary artery pressure of greater than 25 mm Hg at rest and a pulmonary vascular resistance of greater than 240 dynes.s.cm^{-5} and the presence of portal hypertension. Approximately 20% of patients with liver cirrhosis presenting for liver transplantation will have increased pulmonary artery pressures, but in the majority of patients this is the result of intravascular volume overload, together with a high flow state that is typically seen in patients with liver cirrhosis and this may be further affected by the presence of a cirrhotic cardiomyopathy. However the key differentiator of these causes of pulmonary hypertension from true portopulmonary hypertension is that in this group the pulmonary vascular resistance is normal or low.

The etiology of portopulmonary hypertension is not well understood. Initially endothelial dysfunction in the pulmonary arterioles may occur as the result of sheer stress forces from the high velocity circulation and the toxic effects of inflammatory molecules that are either not cleared by the liver or are released by the diseased liver.

The clinical symptoms may be minimal in the early phases of the disease but as it progresses shortness of breath, chest pain, fatigue, palpitations and syncope may present. However these symptoms are not distinct from those of progressive liver disease, therefore all liver transplant candidates should be screened for portopulmonary hypertension. The current screening tool is the trans-thoracic Doppler echocardiogram. If the right ventricular systolic pressure is 50 mm Hg or greater a right heart catheterization should be performed and the pulmonary vascular resistance calculated. Once the diagnosis of portopulmonary hypertension has been made a careful assessment of right ventricular function is required by echocardiography. Liver transplantation will treat many of these patients but not all, and it cannot be predicted which patients will respond to transplantation. The risks of liver transplantation increase with the severity of the pulmonary hypertension and those patients with evidence of right heart dysfunction should undergo pulmonary vasodilator therapy prior to consideration for transplant.

Chapter 6 - Hypertrophic obstructive cardiomyopathy (HOCM) is a complex cardiovascular disorder affecting patients with varying degrees of cardiac manifestations. The optimal treatment strategy for patients with HOCM and end-stage liver disease (ESLD) undergoing evaluation for orthotopic liver transplantation (OLT) is not well defined. Although medical management is the accepted first-line treatment, symptomatic patients with severe left ventricular outflow tract (LVOT) obstruction unresponsive to medications may require further interventions prior to surgery. Perioperative cardiovascular adverse effects in HOCM patients during non-cardiac surgery are relatively high. The anesthetic management of HOCM patients can be challenging and involves understanding the many factors that can be expected to aggravate the dynamic LVOT obstruction during OLT.

Chapter 7 - Obesity is common among liver transplant recipients, and about 10% of liver transplant recipients have severe or morbid obesity. Registry data indicate that there was more than 40% increase in severe or morbid obesity in the past decade among liver transplant recipients. Patients with severe or morbid obesity often have many there co-morbidities including occult cardiovascular diseases, diabetes, hyperlipidemia, cancer and restrictive lung disease. Severe or morbid obesity increases both short and long-term post-transplant morbidity and mortality. Infections, wound dehiscence, increased ventilator dependency and increased intensive care stay are the most common complications in morbidly obese patients, and these complications increase the transplant costs significantly. Cardiovascular complications are the main causes of increased mortality. Patients with preexisting diabetes or coronary artery disease are approximately 40% more likely to die within 5 years from transplantation compared to non-diabetics or those without coronary artery disease with an additive effect with more than one risk factor. Severely or morbidly obese patients, if considered for liver transplantation, should undergo more rigorous cardiovascular screening. Patients with diffuse coronary artery disease or those with significant coronary artery disease that is not amenable to coronary stenting should not be waitlisted. Other contraindications include patients with renal failure who are not eligible for combined liver/kidney transplantation, and those with one or more other serious co-morbidities such as uncontrolled hypertension and micro and macro vascular complications including stroke. To improve outcomes, patients with severe or morbid obesity should undergo careful surveillance and health maintenance programs before and after liver transplantation.

Chapter 8 - Chronic liver injury is common in patients with chronic heart failure. In this population, hepatic fibrosis and cirrhosis are thought to develop as a result of increased venous pressure, hypoxia and hepatocellular necrosis. In addition, advanced heart failure is associated with the up regulation of pro-inflammatory cytokines and increased oxidative stress, both of which may contribute to the development of hepatic fibrosis. The development of irreversible liver injury may be insidious in patients with advanced heart failure, given considerable overlap in the clinical presentations of advanced heart and liver disease. However, the presence of chronic liver disease has important implications for the management and prognosis of patients with heart failure, particularly patients with advanced heart failure undergoing evaluation for heart transplantation or mechanical circulatory support (MCS). The authors review here the clinico-pathologic spectrum of liver disease in heart failure patients, emphasizing the approach to diagnosis and prognostic implications.

Chapter 9 - Liver transplantation (LT) is a viable treatment option for patients with end-stage liver disease (ESLD). However, the high incidence of advanced coronary atherosclerosis or severe valvular disease presents clinical dilemma in the treatment of liver transplant candidates. Combined simultaneous cardiac surgery and liver transplantation has been cautiously explored in this difficult patient population. Several small studies demonstrated that this is a feasible surgical option which can be performed safely, and morbidity is not prohibitive for success. Moreover, simultaneous combined heart and liver transplantation (CHLT) may be a lifesaving procedure for patients suffering from end-stage heart and liver diseases or several metabolic disorders.

Chapter 10 - The past few years have seen remarkable progress in the development of anticancer treatment. Advances have led to better cure rates, median overall survival rates, and time to progression. New chemotherapeutic agents, targeted therapies, and even radioactively labeled molecules are being engineered to match the unique diagnosis and needs of each patient with as few side effects as possible. These measures often result in a better quality of life for patients. Each chemotherapeutic agent has a known spectrum of side effects affecting different parts of the body. One of the main side effects of chemotherapeutic agents is cardiotoxicity. It can occur either acutely or during or long after the course of treatment with certain drugs. Sometimes cardiotoxicity can be the limiting factor in giving the optimal chemotherapeutic dose and can act as an obstacle to a patient's hope for a cure. Chemotherapy-induced cardiotoxicity is extremely difficult both to treat and to manage; therefore, cardiac function should be given priority whenever a cardiotoxic agent is included in the course of treatment and should be monitored carefully with baseline, intercyclic, and posttreatment assessments. Certain chemotherapeutic agents should be avoided in patients with a prior history of cardiac disease so as not to worsen the condition. If necessary, certain prophylactic measures and cardioprotective agents should be used with a very close follow-up of the cardiac functions.

Chemotherapy can be given prior to liver transplantation to control tumor growth and prevent progression, especially if the patient is expected to stay on the waiting list for surgery for more than six months. Some liver transplant patients have undergone chemotherapy before liver transplantation.

Chapter 11 - A transjugular intrahepatic portosystemic stent shunt (TIPS) is a radiological procedure designed to reduce portal pressure. It has been used for the management of complications of portal hypertension. The creation of the shunt transfers a large volume of blood from the splanchnic circulation to the systemic circulation, and therefore significant hemodynamic changes occur with TIPS insertion. The pulmonary circulation responds to the insertion of TIPS with and increase in mean pulmonary arterial pressure, which persists for at least 1 month. This post-TIPS pulmonary hypertension is partly related to an increase in pulmonary circulatory volume, and partly related to pulmonary vasoconstriction, leading to an increase in pulmonary vascular resistance. The systemic circulation responds to the TIPS insertion with systemic vasodilatation, which persists for at least 1 year post-TIPS.

Vasodilatation rather than vasoconstriction occurs in the systemic circulation, related to hyporesponsiveness of the systemic circulation to various vasoconstrictors that are being channeled from the splanchnic to the systemic circulation. The volume overload presented to the heart, together with the high circulating vasoconstrictor levels, can lead to an increased left ventricular mass, with consequent diastolic dysfunction. This diastolic dysfunction, if present pre-TIPS, is associated with a decreased survival and reduced clearance of ascites post-TIPS. Diastolic dysfunction that is still detected at 1 month post-TIPS is also associated with a poor patient outcome. Therefore, patients who receive TIPS should undergo careful cardiovascular investigations prior to TIPS insertion. Patients who have received TIPS should also be followed carefully for the detection of cardiopulmonary complications.

Chapter 12 - Hepatopulmonary syndrome (HPS) is a pulmonary complication observed in patients with chronic liver disease and/or portal hypertension. HPS is attributable to an intrapulmonary vascular dilatation that induces severe hypoxemia. Considering the favorable long-term survival of HPS patients as well as the reversal of the syndrome with a functional liver graft, HPS is now an indication for liver transplantation (LT).

Both patients with mild cirrhosis who present with shortness of breath and all patients with end stage liver disease who are candidates for liver transplantation should undergo screening for HPS. Blood gas analysis and contrast-enhanced echocardiography are two main screening tools, together with lung function tests that can also detect additional pulmonary diseases that can contribute to impaired oxygenation.

If the partial pressure of oxygen in arterial blood (PaO_2) is > 80 mmHg, HPS can be excluded and no other investigation is needed. However, when PaO_2 is ≤ 80 mmHg, contrast-enhanced echocardiography should be performed to obtain evidence of or to exclude pulmonary vascular dilatation.

When the contrast-enhanced echocardiography is negative, HPS is excluded and no follow-up is needed. When the contrast-enhanced echocardiography is positive and PaO_2 < 60 mmHg, patients should obtain a severity score that provides them with a reasonable probability of being transplanted within 3 months. In mild-to-moderate HPS (60 mm Hg ≤ PaO_2 < 80 mmHg), periodic follow-up is recommended every 3 months to detect deterioration of PaO_2.

Although no intra-operative death has been directly attributed to HPS, the immediate post-LT oxygenation worsens in relation to the volume overload, and infections are commonly observed after LT surgery. Mechanical ventilation is often prolonged and the stay in the Intensive Care Unit is extended. A high postoperative mortality (mostly within 6 months) is observed in this group of patients in comparison with non-HPS patients. However, the recovery of an adequate PaO_2 within 12 months after LT explains the similar outcomes of HPS and non-HPS patients following LT.

Chapter 13 - Liver transplantation surgery presents a considerable cardiovascular challenge, and cardiovascular complications are one of the most frequent causes of both early and late transplant-related morbidity and mortality. Coronary artery disease is common; the identification of this and specific cirrhosis-related entities such as cirrhotic cardiomyopathy, portopulmonary hypertension and hepatopulmonary syndrome can result in significant alterations in management. Thus, cardiovascular assessment should be part of the routine evaluation of liver transplant candidates. All patients should have an appropriate history and physical examination, a 12-lead electrocardiogram and a resting echocardiogram. Evaluation for coronary artery disease should be in a protocolized, step-wise manner with non-invasive testing for selected at-risk patients and angiographic confirmation of positive studies. Currently, there is controversy between different published guidelines regarding which patients should undergo non-invasive testing; until further research clarifies the optimum strategy, transplant teams should make reasoned decisions regarding their own practice.

Chapter 14 - Cardiorespiratory assessment is an important component of overall risk assessment in liver transplant candidates, especially in asymptomatic patients. Current investigative methods, often lack specificity and isolate cardiac and respiratory function rather than applying an integrative approach to assessment. Cardiopulmonary exercise testing gives an indication of the combined reserve of the cardiorespiratory system when under stress. In the peri-operative period, similar demands are placed on these organ systems to support an increase in metabolic rate. In this chapter, the authors review the evidence for the use of cardiopulmonary exercise testing in the assessment of patients planned to undergo liver transplantation.

Chapter 15 - Liver transplant patients often present with cardiac dysfunction both independent and as a direct result of the liver disease, which can present a great challenge to anesthesiologists. Anesthesiologists need to be aware of the drug therapy available to treat cardiovascular complications that could arise during or shortly after surgery. Furthermore, they must be aware of the therapy for cardiovascular conditions initiated before surgery and how it could increase perioperative risk.

Cirrhotic cardiomyopathy is fairly common in patients with cirrhosis, but is usually latent unless the patient experiences significant physiological stress such as surgery. Heart failure is the third most common cause of death after liver transplant, following organ rejection and infection. Treatment for symptomatic cirrhotic cardiomyopathy involves the same therapy as treatment for noncirrhotic patients and includes diuretics, angiotensin-converting enzyme inhibitors, beta blockers, and aldosterone antagonists. Interactions between these and immunosuppressive agents must be taken into account. Portopulmonary hypertension can be treated with calcium channel blockers, prostanoids, endothelin receptor antagonists, and phosphodiesterase type 5 antagonists or combination therapy. The choice of therapy depends on the vasoreactivity of the patient and the severity of the disease. Oxygen, inhaled nitric oxide, diuretics, digoxin, and oral anticoagulants can be used as supportive therapy or in acute hypertensive episodes. Nitrates are not suitable vasodilators because of the risk of severe systemic hypotension. Surgery should be delayed in patients with cardiac stents who are taking dual antiplatelet therapy wherever possible until the dual therapy is completed. Where this is not possible, a decision about whether to continue or to withdraw the antiplatelet agents should be made, taking into account the risk of bleeding and stent thrombosis.

Immunosuppressants used to prevent organ rejection can lead to or increase the risk of cardiovascular complications after surgery. Prednisolone, ciclosporin, tacrolimus, and mycophenolate mofetil have all been associated with hypertension in posttransplant patients. Calcium channel blockers are usually the agent of choice in the treatment of immunosuppressant-induced hypertension, along with beta blockers. Diuretics are not recommended. Tacrolimus has been known to cause cardiomyopathy in liver graft recipients, and where this occurs, the dose should be reduced, or the agent completely withdrawn. The risk of posttransplant heart failure does not appear to be greater when tacrolimus is the agent of choice. Increased incidence of hyperlipidemia has been reported in patients taking ciclosporin, tacrolimus, sirolimus, and azathioprine. This condition is treated with lipid-reducing agents as for nontransplant patients.

Chapter 16 - The authors understanding of the cardiovascular changes in end stage liver disease is increasing. Accurate presentation of the changes that occur during liver transplantation (LT) is vital to good anaesthetic management, and the speed at which they take place makes effective monitoring essential. To date perioperative haemodynamic monitoring has been largely based on thermodilution techniques. New developments in this field offer opportunities to monitor preload using variables such as right ventricular ejection fraction (RVEF) and right ventricular end diastolic volume (RVEDV) that seem preferable to those derived from pressures. Trans-oesophageal echocardiography (TEE) is receiving more attention because it is non invasive and can visualise heart structures, filling and dynamic function, but results are operator dependent and prolonged training is needed. Currently other less invasive techniques that provide continuous cardiac output monitoring are being evaluated but different levels of accuracy have been reported in LT recipients. The trend in intraoperative haemodynamic monitoring, a key feature of anaesthetic practice in LT, is towards systems that provide continuous information and are less invasive. A balance is needed between the hazards of an invasive approach and the desire for a continuous stream of accurate information that is robust enough to withstand the surgical and physiological challenges of LT. Despite its importance for anaesthetists, there is no consensus as to which system is best. In this chapter the authors shall examine recent developments in haemodynamic monitoring during LT.

Chapter 17 - Cardiac events in the early post-operative period are common and may influence longer-term cardiac morbidity and even indicate potential mortality. Immunosuppressive therapy may have short-term cardiotoxic effects but is more likely to adversely affect cardiovascular risk factors such as hypertension, diabetes mellitus and dyslipidemia in the longer-term. This chapter will discuss hemodynamic profile post-liver transplant (LT), the early- and late-postoperative cardiovascular complications following LT, the cardiac problems associated with immunosuppression and prediction of post-operative cardiac complications.

Abbreviations

AaPO$_2$	Aalveolar (A)-arterial (a) pressure gradient for O$_2$
ACE	Angiotensin-converting enzyme
ACC/AHA	American College of Cardiology/American Heart Association
ANP	Atrial natriuretic peptide
AS	Aortic stenosis
ASA	Alcohol septal ablation
AT	Anaerobic threshold
AUC	Area under the cure
BMI	Body Mass Index
BMS	Bare metal stents
BNP	Brain atrial natriuretic peptide
BNP/NT-proBNP	BNP/N-terminal (NT)-proBNT
CABG	Coronary artery bypass grafting
CAD	Coronary artery disease
CCB	Calcium channel blockers
CCO	Continuous cardiac output
cGMP	Cyclic guanosine monophosphate
CGRP	Calcitonin gene-related peptide
CHF	Congestive heart failure
CHLT	Combined liver and heart transplantation
CO	Cardiac output
COPD	Chronic obstructive pulmonary disease
CPB	Cardio-pulmonary bypass
CPET	Cardiopulmonary exercise testing
CV	Cardiovascular
CVP	Central venous pressure
DES	Drug eluted stent
DLCO	Diffusing lung capacity
DM	Diabetes mellitus
DSE	Dobutamine stress echocardiography
ESLD	End-stage liver disease
ERA	Endothelin receptor antagonist

ESA	European Society of Anaesthesiology
ESC	European Society of Cardiology
ESLD	End-stage liver disease
ET	Endothelin
EVLVI	Extra vascular lung water index
EVLW	Extravascular lung water
FH	Family history
FIO$_2$	Fraction of inspired oxygen in gas mixture
GEDV	Global end diastolic volume
GEDVI	Global end diastolic volume index
GI	Gastrointestinal
HCM	Hypertrophic cardiomyopathy
HF	Heart Failure
HOCM	Hypertrophic obstructive cardiomyopathy
HTN	Hypertension
HR	Heart rate
HRS	Hepatorenal syndrome
IHT	Isolated heart transplantation
iNOS	Indusible Nitrix Oxide Synthasa
ILT	Isolated liver transplantation
IPAH	Idiopathic pulmonary arterial hypertension
ITBV	Intrathoracic blood volume
ITBVI	Intrathoracic blood volume index
LT	Liver transplantation
LVEF	Left ventricular ejection fraction
LVOT	Left ventricular outflow tract
LQT	Prolonged QT interval
MELD	Model for End-Stage Liver Disease
MET	Metabolic equivalent
MI	Myocardial infarction
mPAP	Mean pulmonary artery pressure
OLT	Orthotopic liver transplantation
OPTN	Organ Procurement Transplant Network
P$_{A-a}$O$_2$	Alveolar-arterial oxygen gradient
PaO$_2$	Partial Pressure of Oxygen in Arterial Blood
PAH	Pulmonary arterial hypertension
PAC	Pulmonary artery catheter
PAP	Pulmonary artery pressure
PAOP	Pulmonary artery occlusion pressure
PB	Atmospheric pressure
PCI	Percutaneous coronary intervention
PDE5	Phosphodiesterase type 5
Peak VO$_2$	Oxygen consumption at peak exercise
POPH	Portopulmonary hypertension
PPV	Pulse pressure variation
PRA	Panel-reactive antibody

PRS	Post-reperfusion syndrome
PTCA	Transluminal coronary angioplasty
PVD	Peripheral vascular disease
PVR	Pulmonary vascular resistance
QTc	Heart rate-corrected QT interval
QTd	QT dispersion
RAAS	Renin-angiotesin-aldosterone system
RAP	Right atrial pressure
ROC	Receiver Operating Characteristic curve
RV	Right heart ventricle
RVEF	Right ventricular ejection fraction
RVEDV	Right ventricular end diastolic volume
RVEDVI	Right ventricular end diastolic volume index
RVSP	Right ventricular systolic pressure
RWMA	Regional wall motion abnormalities
SAM	Systolic anterior motion
SaO_2	Saturation of Oxygen (arterial blood)
$ScvO_2$	Central venous oxygen saturation
SNS	Sympathetic nervous system
SPECT	Single proton emission computed tomography
SRTR	Scientific Registry of Transplant Recipients
SVI	Stroke volume index
SvO_2	Mixed venous oxygen saturation
SVR	Systemic vascular resistance
SVV	Stroke volume variation
STEMI	ST-segment elevation myocardial infarction
TCPID	Trans-cardiopulmonary thermodilution
TdP	Torsade de pointes
TEE	Trans-esophageal echocardiography
TIPS	Transjugular intrahepatic portosystemic shunt
TNF-α	Tumor necrosis factor alfa
TPG	Transpulmonary gradient
TRV	Tricuspid regurgitant jet velocity
TTE	Trans-thoracic echocardiography
UKELD	United Kingdom Model for End-Stage Liver Disease
UNOS	United Network for Organ Sharing
VO_2	Oxygen consumption
VCO_2	Carbon dioxide production
V_D/V_T	Dead space/tidal volume ratio
VE/ VO_2	Ventilatory equivalent for oxygen
VE/ VCO_2	Ventilatory equivalent for carbon dioxide
V_E/ VCO_2	Ventilatory efficiency
VKA	Vitamin K antagonist
VQ	Ventilation perfusion
WHO FC	World Health Organization functional class

Chapter I

Haemodynamic Profile of Patients with End-Stage Liver Disease

Søren Møller[*], *and Jens H. Henriksen*
Department of Clinical Physiology, 239, Hvidovre Hospital,
University of Copenhagen, DK-2650 Hvidovre, Denmark

Abstract

Patients with cirrhosis and portal hypertension exhibit characteristic haemodynamic changes. A vasodilatatory state and a hyperdynamic circulation affect various functions, resulting in multi-organ failure. Thus, the circulation of the lungs, kidneys, brain, gastrointestinal tract and periphery is disturbed. The recently defined cirrhotic cardiomyopathy affects systolic and diastolic functions of the heart and implies electromechanical abnormalities. In addition, baroreceptor response and regulation of circulatory homoeostasis are impaired, and reduced cardiac reserve may also play a role in the development of hepatorenal syndrome. Pulmonary dysfunction involves diffusing abnormalities, with development of hepatopulmonary syndrome and portopulmonary hypertension in some patients with cirrhosis. Recent research has focused on the assertion that haemodynamic and neurohumoral dysregulation are of major importance for the development of many of the organ-related complications in cirrhosis. This aspect is important to take into account in the management of these patients.

Introduction

Patients with end-stage liver disease present with clinical signs of haemodynamic abnormalities. A brief look often reveals a reddish skin and signs of cutaneous vasodilatation

---

[*] Correspondence: Søren Møller, MD, Associate Professor, Chief Physician Dept. of Clinical Physiology, 239, Hvidovre Hospital, DK-2650 Hvidovre, Denmark Tel: +45 3632 3568, Fax: +45 3632 3750, E-mail:soeren.moeller@hvh.regionh.dk.

with presence of spider naevi. Moreover, patients may present with palmar erythema, and a raised and bounding pulse. When taking a closer look, many of these patients often have ascites and peripheral oedema, a characteristic hyperdynamic circulation with increased cardiac output and heart rate, and low or low normal arterial blood pressure [1,2]. The combination of low systemic vascular resistance, abnormal blood volume distribution, and increased activity of vasoconstrictor systems such as the renin-angiotensin-aldosterone system (RAAS) and the sympathetic nervous system (SNS) has lent support to the assumption that these pathophysiological circulatory changes are based on a primary peripheral arterial vasodilatation [3–6]. At present, the forward-flow theory, which is based on the peripheral vasodilatation hypothesis, is favoured [7]. Portal and sinusoidal hypertension induces systemic vasodilatation and reduces systemic vascular resistance, leading to a forward increase in filtration across the hepatosplanchnic capillaries [8,9]. However, the haemodynamic profile of patients with end-stage liver disease is not only restricted to the hepatosplanchnic vascular system, but seems ubiquitously to affect most of the organ systems in the body as multi-organ failure (Figure 1) [2]. In the kidneys, systemic hyperdynamic syndrome restricts renal perfusion and glomerular filtration, leading to hepatorenal syndrome (HRS) [9]. The function of the heart is compromised, leading to cardiac dysfunction, which in turn also may affect the kidneys as part of a cardiorenal syndrome [2,10,11]. The circulation and function of the lungs are disturbed and some patients may develop a hepatopulmonary syndrome [12]. In addition, the perfusion of the brain becomes abnormal, particularly in patients with hepatic encephalopathy, and the reactivity of the peripheral circulation is affected, with increased arterial compliance [13].

This chapter seeks to outline some basic elements in the haemodynamic profile of patients with end-stage liver disease, focusing on vascular and organ-specific dysfunction and neurohumoral abnormalities. Particular attention is paid to changes in bioactive substances that may affect the vasodilatation–vasoconstriction balance and to the effects on the pathophysiology of circulatory homoeostasis and dysregulation in advanced cirrhosis.

Systemic Circulation in End-Stage Liver Disease

Patients with less advanced stages of cirrhosis and portal hypertension may present with normal systemic circulation. But with progression of the disease from the portal hypertensive, preascitic stage to the decompensated, portal hypertensive, ascitic stage, there is an overall direct relationship between the severity of cirrhosis (e.g. reflected by the Child score or the Model for End-Stage Liver Disease (MELD) score) and the degree of hyperdynamic circulation [14–17]. Figure 2 shows cardiac output, mean arterial blood pressure, systemic vascular resistance and heart rate in 396 patients with cirrhosis in relation to severity of liver disease as assessed using the Child-Turcotte score [18].

In general, an increase in cardiac output can be attributed to an increase in venous return, heart rate and myocardial contractility, all of which are controlled by the autonomic nervous system. Arteriolar dilatation, the presence of arteriovenous communications, expanded blood volume and increased sympathetic nervous activity may further raise the cardiac output; most of these pathophysiological mechanisms may operate in advanced cirrhosis [1,19]. In early cirrhosis, the presence of a hyperdynamic circulation is often not apparent.

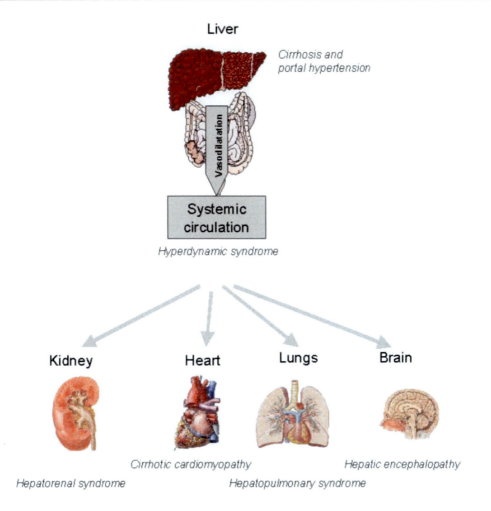

Figure 1. The haemodynamic consequences of portal hypertension and splanchnic arterial vasodilatation in cirrhosis. The circulation is affected in multiple organs including kidneys, heart, lungs and possibly the brain. Thus, 'hyperdynamic syndrome' refers to universal haemodynamic alterations that may be involved in hepatorenal syndrome, cirrhotic cardiomyopathy, hepatopulmonary syndrome and hepatic encephalopathy.

But with progression of the liver disease, there is an overall association with the degree of hyperdynamic circulation (Figure 2). Studies on circulatory changes with posture suggest that these patients are mostly hyperdynamic in the supine position [20–23]. Blood and plasma volumes are raised in advanced cirrhosis, but the distribution between central and non-central vascular areas is unbalanced [24,25]. Thus, the use of different techniques has established that central and arterial blood volume is most often decreased, whereas non-central blood volume, in particular splanchnic blood volume, is increased in animals and patients with cirrhosis [1,24,26,27]. Effective arterial blood volume and central circulation time (i.e. central blood volume relative to cardiac output) are substantially reduced and bear a significant relation to poorer survival in advanced cirrhosis [28]. The haemodynamic changes pertaining to specific vascular beds are shown in Table 1.

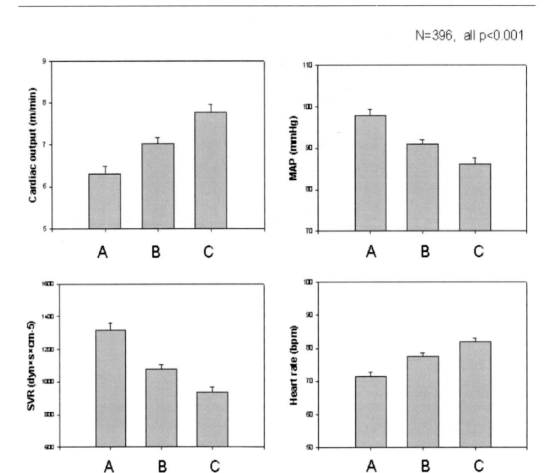

Figure 2. Values of cardiac output, mean arterial blood pressure (MAP), systemic vascular resistance (SVR) and heart rate in 396 patients with cirrhosis: Child class A: n=103; Child class B: n=175; Child class C: n=118. The increase in cardiac output and heart rate are most pronounced in patients with advanced disease. MAP and SVR are lowest in patients with advanced cirrhosis. Reproduced from [18] with permission.

During volume expansion, most cirrhotic patients respond with a further reduction in systemic vascular resistance rather than an increase in arterial blood pressure [24,26]. Infusion of hyperosmotic solutions or albumin in cirrhosis results initially in a shift of fluid from the interstitial space into the plasma volume, with expansion of the latter [24,26]. When considering volume expansion in terms of the severity of the disease, certain differences become clear. Irrespective of severity, volume expansion produces a rise in stroke volume and cardiac output. Whereas in early cirrhosis there is a proportional expansion of the central and non-central parts of the blood volume, in late cirrhosis expansion is mainly confined to the non-central part, with a proportionally smaller increase in cardiac output, probably because of cardiac dysfunction and abnormal vascular compliance [26,29]. The increased plasma volume in cirrhosis should be considered secondary to the activation of neurohumoral mechanisms consequent on mainly splanchnic vasodilatation, low arterial blood pressure and reduced central and arterial blood volume.

Table 1. Circulatory changes in specific vascular beds in cirrhosis

Systemic circulation
Plasma volume ↑
Total blood volume ↑
Non-central blood volume ↑
Central and arterial blood volume ↑(→)
Cardiac output ↑
Arterial blood pressure ↑(→)
Heart rate ↑
Systemic vascular resistance ↓
Arterial and total vascular compliance ↑
Heart
left arterial volume ↑
left ventricle volume →(↑)
Right arterial volume → ↑↓
Right ventricle volume →↑↓
Right arterial pressure→↑
right ventricle end-diastolic pressure →
Pulmonary artery pressure→↑
Left ventricular end-diastolic pressure →
Hepatic and splanchnic circulation
Hepatic blood flow ↓→(↑)
Hepatic venous pressure gradient ↑
Post-sinusoidal resistance ↑
Renal circulation
renal blood flow ↓
Glomerular filtration rate ↓→
Pulmonary circulation
Pulmonary blood flow ↑
Pulmonary vascular resistance ↓(↑)*
Cutaneous and skeletal muscular circulation
Skeletal muscular blood flow ↑→↓
Cutaneous blood flow ↑→↓

↑ → ↓ : increased, unchanged or decreased, respectively. Parentheses denote less frequent changes.
* : portopulmonary syndrome.

In clinical practice, however, the pattern may be more complex and some patients with early cirrhosis may exhibit a hyperdynamic circulatory state, and a few patients with decompensated cirrhosis with considerable fluid retention may present a relatively normal circulation [15].

Moreover, pharmacological treatment, e.g. with beta-blockers, may attenuate a hyperdynamic circulatory state [15,30]. On the whole, however, there is a direct relationship between systemic circulatory derangement, progression of liver disease, and the state of vasodilatation.

Splanchnic Arterial Vasodilatation

Peripheral and splanchnic vasodilatation in cirrhosis may be brought about either by overproduction of vasodilators of intestinal or systemic origin, or by vasodilators that escape degradation in the diseased liver or bypass the liver through portosystemic collaterals [31]. A predominantly splanchnic vasodilatation precedes renal sodium and water retention and plasma volume expansion, which follows activated counter-regulatory vasoconstrictor systems [31,32]. In 1988, Schrier et al. proposed the 'peripheral arterial vasodilatation hypothesis' [3]. According to this theory, primary splanchnic arteriolar vasodilatation leads to a reduction in overall systemic vascular resistance, and to avid arterial underfilling with low arterial blood pressure in advanced disease. A modification of this, the 'forward theory of ascites formation', combines arterial underfilling with a forward increase in hepatosplanchnic capillary pressure and filtration with increased lymph formation [32]. A reduced effective blood volume, which is that part of the blood volume where baroreceptors are located, leads to activation of vasoconstrictor systems and secondary sodium-water retention [3,32–34]. Thus, most of the haemodynamic changes seen in cirrhosis can be explained by this theory, as shown in Figure 3.

Vasodilators

In recent years, research has focused on a number of candidates for splanchnic vasodilatation, as summarized in Table 2. Particular focus has been given to nitric oxide (NO), calcitonin gene related peptide (CGRP) and adrenomedullin. These substances will therefore be discussed in more detail. Other implicated substances with vasodilating properties are natriuretic peptides, tumour necrosis factor alpha (TNF-α), interleukins, substance P and cannabinoids [35–42].

NO is synthesized in the vascular endothelium from L-arginine by NO synthase (NOS) [43], of which three isoforms have been identified: inducible NOS (iNOS), constitutive endothelial NOS (ecNOS) and neuronal NOS (ncNOS) [36,44]. In portal hypertension, there seems to be a diminished release of NO from sinusoidal endothelial cells in the cirrhotic liver [44,45], whereas in the systemic circulation there is evidence of increased ecNOS up-regulation, which is probably related to shear stress [35,43,46]. Exhaled air from cirrhotic patients contains higher NO levels than that of controls and correlates with the severity of disease and degree of hyperdynamic circulation [47–49]. Taken together, there is a growing body of evidence that systemic NO production is increased and precedes the development of the hyperdynamic circulation, thereby playing a major role in arteriolar and splanchnic vasodilatation and vascular hyporeactivity [36,50].

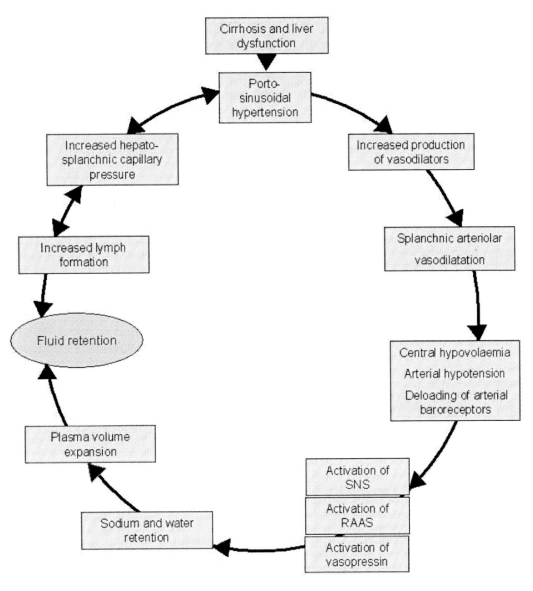

Figure 3. Pathophysiology of splanchnic and peripheral arteriolar vasodilatation and systemic haemodynamic changes in cirrhosis. According to this theory, endogenous vasodilators escape hepatic degradation due to portosystemic shunting and/or hepatocellular damage and induce vasodilatation preferentially in the splanchnic vascular area. Reduced systemic vascular resistance leads to reduced effective arterial blood volume and hence activation of different vasoconstrictor systems. The haemodynamic and clinical consequences are increased cardiac output, heart rate and plasma volume and decreased renal blood flow, low arterial blood pressure, and fluid and sodium retention. RAAS: renin-angiotensin-aldosterone system; SNS: sympathetic nervous system.

In addition, vascular endothelial growth factor (VEGF) seems to stimulate angiogenesis and the development of portosystemic collaterals, and blockade of the VEGF receptor-2 has been shown recently to inhibit this process [51].

Table 2. Vasodilating and vasoconstricting forces involved in disturbed haemodynamics in cirrhosis

Vasodilator systems
Adenosine
Adrenomedullin
Arterial natriuretic peptide (ANP)
Bradykinin
Brain natriuretic peptide (BNP)
Calcitonin gene related peptide (CGRP)
Carbon monoxide (CO)
Endocannabinoids
Endothelin-3 (ET-3)
Endotoxin
Enkephalins
Glucagon
Histamine
Hydrogen sulphide
Interleukins
Natriuretic peptide of type C (CNP)
Nitric oxide (NO)
Prostacyclin (PGI^2)
Substance P
Tumour necrosis factor-? (TNF-?)
Vasoactive intestinal polypeptide
Vasoconstrictor systems
Angiotensin II
Adrenaline and noradrenaline
Endothelin-1 (ET-1)
Neuropeptide Y
Renin-angiotensin-aldosterone system (RAAS)
Sympathetic nervous system (SNS)
Vasopressin

CGRP, a 37-amino-acid peptide with a neurotransmitter function, is on a molar basis the most powerful vasodilating peptide known [52]. It is elevated in cirrhosis, especially in those patients with ascites and HRS [52,53], and correlates to haemodynamic markers of vasodilatation and central hypovolaemia, such as cardiac output, systemic vascular resistance, arterial compliance and central blood volume [37,54–56]. Adrenomedullin is a vasodilating peptide with a sequence similar to that of CGRP, is primarily released from the adrenal medulla and induces relaxation of smooth muscle cells [57]. The circulating levels of adrenomedullin seem to be higher in decompensated patients with cirrhosis and correlate with circulating pressor substances, such as endothelin (ET), renin, vasopressin and catecholamines [39,58,59].

Desensitization to Vasoconstrictors

It has previously been suggested that increased resistance to pressor hormones may also play a role in arterial vasodilatation [60–62]. Thus, it has been observed that patients with cirrhosis are hyporesponsive to the pressor effects of potent vasoconstrictors such as norepinephrine, angiotensin II and vasopressin [50]. There may be an upward shift in the pressor concentration giving 50% effect as well as a reduced maximal effect [62,63]. This may be brought about by a change in receptor affinity, a decrease in the numbers of receptors, and a variety of post-receptor defects [63,64]. Most likely all mechanisms are present in patients with cirrhosis [65]. Thus, Gerbes et al. showed that leucocytes from patients with cirrhosis have a decreased number of β-adrenoceptors [66], and Lee and coworkers have brought substantial evidence that cardiac dysfunction in experimental cirrhosis is in part brought about by both a receptor defect and post-receptor defects in the heart [67]. Helmy et al. have reported hyporesponsiveness to angiotensin II and ET-1 and demonstrated that the reduced vasoconstrictive effect is principally a result of enhanced NO generation [50]. However, specific inhibition of the vasoconstrictor systems indicate that, at least in the early stages of cirrhosis, they contribute to the maintenance of basal vascular tone [68,69]. At present, the sustained systemic vasodilatation in spite of all vasoconstrictor systems being highly activated is most likely related to a combination of changes in receptor affinity, down-regulation of receptors and several post-receptor defects; however, future research should further disclose the pathophysiology.

Hepatosplanchnic Circulation

In portal hypertensive patients, the clinical picture is dominated by severe complications such as bleeding from oesophageal varices. From a haemodynamic point of view, hepatic vascular resistance and portal in-flow determine the level of portal pressure. Factors that determine the former include both structural and dynamic components [70]. Histological characteristics such as steatosis, fibrosis and regeneration nodules are among the structural components. Dynamic structures include cells with contractile properties such as hepatic stellate cells, myofibroblasts and smooth muscle cells [70]. Portal venous in-flow is mainly determined by the degree of splanchnic vasodilatation. Patients with portal hypertension have a substantial portosystemic collateral circulation and an increased mesenteric in-flow of up to several litres per minute (Table 1) [70]. Thus, a large part of the increased cardiac output is returned through portosystemic collaterals. The azygos blood flow is especially important, as it drains oesophageal varices, and an increase in azygos flow is associated with an increased risk of variceal bleeding [28]. Beta-blockers, nitrates, octreotide, terlipressin, etc., can reduce the increased hepatosplanchnic blood flow pharmacologically, and infusion of these drugs may in part reverse the hyperkinetic mesenteric circulation [70]. As outlined above, there seems to be a defective sinusoidal ecNOS-derived production of NO [36]. In addition, recent investigations of endogenous vasoactive substances have focused on ET-1, angiotensin II, catecholamines and leukotrienes in increased hepatic-sinusoidal resistance [19,71,72]. The haemodynamic imbalance with a predominant sinusoidal constriction may also be an important target for treatment.

Table 3. Characterization of cirrhotic cardiomyopathy

Definition
A cardiac dysfunction in patients with cirrhosis characterised by impaired contractile responsiveness to stress, and/or altered diastolic relaxation with electrophysiological abnormalities in the absence of over known cardiac disease
Diagnostic criteria
Systolic dysfunction
Blunted increase in cardiac output with exercise, volume challenge or pharmacological stimuli
Resting EF <55%
Diastolic dysfunction
E/A ratio <1.0 (age corrected)
Prolonged deceleration time (>200 msec)
Prolonged isovolumetric relaxation time (>80 msec)
Supportive criteria
Electrophysiological abnormalities
Abnormal chronotropic response
Electromechanical uncoupling/dyssynchrony
Prolonged Q-T interval
Enlarged left atrium
Increased myocardial mass
Increased BNP and pro-BNP
Increased troponin I

BNP: brain natriuretic peptide; E/A: early diastolic/atrial filling ratio; EF: left ventricular ejection fraction.

The Heart in Cirrhosis

Deterioration in liver function was first associated with dysfunction of the cardiovascular system via a hyperdynamic circulation described in cirrhosis more than 50 years ago [73]. Later, results of pathophysiological studies directed focus upon the complex relations between cardiac output, plasma volume expansion, an inappropriate central blood volume and cardiac loading conditions [26]. Thus, redistribution of the circulating blood volume results in a reduced central and arterial blood volume with 'effective' hypovolaemia [19]. The combination of low effective blood volume and arterial hypotension leads to activation of potent vasoconstricting systems, including the SNS [74]. This further aggravates hyperdynamic circulation and cardiac strain. Results of experimental and clinical studies have shown impaired myocardial contractility as well as electrophysiological abnormalities in cirrhosis, which have crystallized the clinical entity 'cirrhotic cardiomyopathy' [11,75]. This term denotes chronic cardiac dysfunction, characterized by blunted contractile responsiveness to stress and altered diastolic relaxation with electrophysiological abnormalities, such as prolongation of the Q–T interval, all occurring in the absence of any other cardiac disease (Table 3) [2,76]. This cardiac dysfunction may affect patient prognosis and aggravate the course during invasive procedures such as surgery, insertion of transjugular intrahepatic portosystemic shunts (TIPS) and liver transplantation [77,78]. The pathophysiological mechanisms include changes in the cardiomyocyte plasma membrane, attenuated function of the β-adrenergic pathway and greater activity of inhibitory systems [79]. Other studies have focused on negative inotropic effects of NO, nitration of cardiac proteins, carbon monoxide, endogenous cannabinoids, bile acids and endotoxins [75,80].

Systolic Dysfunction

In patients with cirrhotic cardiomyopathy, cardiac failure may become manifest only under conditions of haemodynamic stress. Thus, left ventricular end-diastolic pressure increases after exercise, but the expected increases in cardiac stroke index and left ventricular ejection fraction (LVEF) are absent or subnormal, which indicates an inadequate response in the ventricular reserve to a rise in filling pressure [81]. A 30% vasoconstrictor-induced increase in the left ventricular afterload results in a doubling in pulmonary capillary wedge pressure, with no change in cardiac output [29]. This response may be useful in diagnosing cirrhotic cardiomyopathy. A similar pattern is seen after insertion of TIPS, but the raised cardiac pressures tend to normalize with time [82,83]. Some patients (12%) may develop manifest cardiac failure in association with the TIPS insertion [84]. A failure to increase cardiac output, despite increased ventricular filling pressure, indicates that normalization of the afterload impairs cardiac performance and unmasks left ventricular dysfunction [29].

LVEF reflects systolic function, even though it is very much influenced by preload and afterload. It has been reported to be normal at rest in some studies, but reduced in one study of a subgroup of patients with ascites [29,81,85]. After exercise, LVEF increases less in cirrhotic patients than in controls [75,81,86]. The reduced functional capacity may be attributed to a combination of blunted heart rate response to exercise, reduced myocardial reserve, and profound skeletal muscle wasting with impaired oxygen extraction [87,88].

Diastolic Dysfunction

The clinical significance of diastolic dysfunction and its importance in cirrhotic cardiomyopathy has been questioned, as overt cardiac failure is not a prominent feature of cirrhosis. However, there are several reports of unexpected death from heart failure following liver transplantation, surgical portocaval shunts and TIPS [84,89]. These procedures involve a rapid increase in cardiac preload. In a less compliant heart, the diastolic dysfunction could be enough to cause pulmonary oedema and heart failure. This is consistent with the findings of an increase in pulmonary artery pressure, preload and diastolic dysfunction after TIPS [82]. Diastolic dysfunction affecting left ventricular filling may progress to systolic dysfunction [29,90]. The pathological basis of the increased stiffness of the left ventricle seems to be cardiac hypertrophy, patchy fibrosis and subendothelial oedema [29,86,91]. Determinants of diastolic dysfunction on a Doppler echocardiogram are a decreased ratio of early to late diastolic filling (E/A) and delayed early diastolic transmitral filling with prolonged deceleration and isovolumetric relaxation times [29,85,92]. Liver transplantation has recently been shown to reverse cardiac changes, including diastolic dysfunction [86].

Electrophysiological Abnormalities

There is a large body of evidence for electrophysiological abnormalities in cirrhosis, primarily comprising prolonged repolarization time and increased dispersion of the electromechanical time interval [76,93]. In cirrhotic patients, the Q–T interval is prolonged and significantly related to the severity of the liver disease, portal hypertension, portosystemic shunts, elevated brain type natriuretic peptide (BNP) and pro-BNP, elevated plasma noradrenaline, decreased heart rate variability and reduced survival [76,77,94–96]. The prolongation of the Q–T interval is partly reversible after liver transplantation and beta-blocker treatment [94,97]. The prolonged Q–T interval in cirrhosis should be considered an element in cirrhotic cardiomyopathy and may be of potential use in identifying patients at risk.

Peripheral Circulation

Cutaneous and muscular circulations may be increased in patients with cirrhosis [19]. Palmar erythema, spider naevi and potatory face were recognized early on as clinical signs of cutaneous hyperperfusion. These types of circulatory abnormalities illustrate capillary hyperperfusion and the presence of arteriovenous fistulae. Muscular circulation is reported to be increased, normal or reduced in patients with cirrhosis [98,99]. Evaluation of brachial and femoral artery blood flow by Doppler techniques has failed to disclose a clear hyperdynamic perfusion of the limbs [98–100]. Recently, however, it has been shown that blockade of NOS causes peripheral vasoconstriction in the forearm in cirrhosis and that this system contributes to the regulation of peripheral vascular tone and to the hyperdynamic state [101]. Measurement of skin blood flow by nuclear medicine techniques have shown normal capillary skin blood flow in cirrhotic patients [102]. At present it can be concluded that the increased cardiac output in patients with cirrhosis covers systemic vascular beds with various degrees of perfusion, owing to an imbalanced state of vasoconstriction and vasodilatation. The exact distribution of the increased cardiac output to the different organs, tissues and types of vessels remains to be clarified.

Vascular Hyporeactivity

The hyporeactivity of the vascular system in chronic liver disease is a result of a differential balance between vasoconstricting and vasodilating forces in different vascular areas (Figure 4). Generally, however, the vascular system in cirrhosis is very yielding, as reflected by an overall increase in vascular and arterial compliance [13,103,104]. Systemic arterial compliance, defined as an increase in intra-arterial volume relative to an increase in transmural arterial blood pressure, is especially increased in patients with decompensated cirrhosis [55]. This is because of structural as well as dynamic changes in the arterial wall that are also closely associated with the circulatory and homoeostatic derangement [13,56]. Therefore, the changes in arterial mechanics are partly reversible. The arteriolar tone adjusts the level of blood pressure and may therefore also affect large artery compliance. The increased arterial compliance is directly related to the severity of liver disease and to the circulating vasodilator CGRP, but it is inversely related to circulating adrenaline [56,105]. Arterial compliance is not affected by β-adrenergic blockade, but terlipressin almost normalizes it [106]. It is an important determinant of the coupling between the heart and the arterial system, and of the dynamics of intravascular volume relocation [107]. An element in the elevated arterial compliance in advanced cirrhosis is reduced arterial blood volume and blood pressure [56].

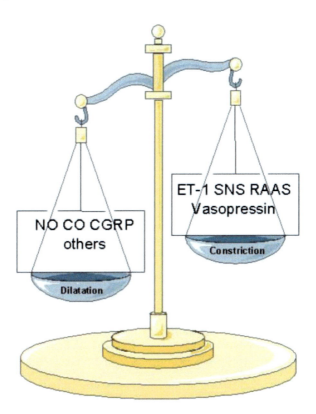

Figure 4. Imbalance between major vasoconstricting and vasodilating forces in end-stage liver disease. CGRP: calcitonin gene related peptide; CO: carbon monoxide; ET-1: endothelin-1; NO: nitric oxide; RAAS: renin-angiotensin-aldosterone system; SNS: sympathetic nervous system.

Arterial compliance is an integral variable for vascular responsiveness, together with systemic vascular resistance. Changed dynamic and static function of the arterial tree may contribute to the abnormal reactions of volume and baroreceptors and may have implications for the abnormal circulatory regulation and potentially for therapy with vasoactive drugs. These aspects are, however, a topic for further research. In conclusion, arterial compliance is elevated in advanced cirrhosis.

Besides a relationship with age, body size, gender and the level of arterial blood pressure, arterial compliance is directly related to the severity of cirrhosis and the hyperdynamic circulatory derangement.

Autonomic Dysfunction

Cirrhosis is often associated with autonomic dysfunction, as has become evident from studies on haemodynamic responses to standard cardiovascular reflex tests such as heart rate variability and isometric exercise [21,108–111]. Most studies on these issues have found a high prevalence of autonomic dysfunction in cirrhosis, with associations with liver dysfunction and survival [110,112,113]. The autonomic dysfunction may be temporary and seems reversible after liver transplantation [97]. Most studies have focused on enhanced activity and defects in the SNS, but the importance of a vagal impairment for sodium and fluid retention has also been shown [19,108,109,112,114]. Sympathetic responses to dynamic exercise appear to be normal in patients with cirrhosis, whereas those to isometric exercise are clearly impaired [115]. Similarly, blood pressure responses to orthostasis are impaired, probably because of a blunted baroreflex function [21,74,116]. Abnormal cardiovascular responses to pharmacological stimulation with angiotensin II, noradrenaline and vasopressin in terms of impaired responses in blood flow and blood pressure have been reported in patients with cirrhosis [19,117]. In addition, it has been shown experimentally that haeme oxygenase mediates hyporeactivity to phenylephrine in the mesenteric vessels of cirrhotic rats with ascites [118]. Administration of captopril partly corrects autonomic dysfunction in cirrhosis, which indicates that the vagal component is to a certain extent caused by neuromodulation by angiotensin II [112]. Involvement of the RAAS is also supported by data that show normalization of cardiac responses to postural changes after administration of canrenone, an aldosterone antagonist, to compensated cirrhotic patients [116]. Interestingly, the hyporeactivity to vasoconstrictors seems to be reversible by antioxidants such as vitamin C, which indicates that oxidative stress plays a role in vascular hyporeactivity and that antioxidant therapy could thus play a role in these complications in cirrhosis [119].

Potential pathophysiological explanations of autonomic dysfunction are summarized in Figure 5. However, the relationship between the severity of liver disease, mortality and reversibility after liver transplantation point to hepatic metabolism and increased NO production and reduced vasoconstrictor sensitivity as a post-receptor defect.

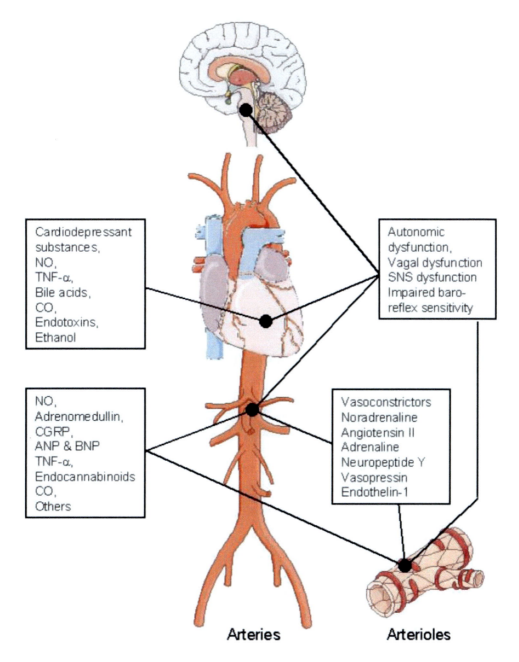

Figure 5. Vascular hyporeactivity in cirrhosis originates in the central nervous system, the autonomic nervous system, from local mediators, or within the smooth muscle cell/heart muscle cell. Autonomic dysfunction acts at cardiac, arterial and arteriolar levels. Vasodilators and vasoconstrictors may act variably at cardiac, arterial and arteriolar levels. At the smooth cellular (arteriolar) level, hyporeactivity may be caused by increased concentrations of vasodilators [atrial natriuretic peptide (ANP), brain natriuretic peptide (BNP), calcitonin gene related peptide (CGRP), carbon monoxide (CO), endocannabinoids, nitric oxide (NO), tumour necrosis factor-alpha (TNF-α)] and decreased sensitivity to vasoconstrictors (endothelin-1).

Arterial Blood Pressure Regulation

The level of arterial blood pressure depends on cardiac output and systemic vascular resistance. The latter is determined by the tone of the smooth muscle cells in the small arteries and arterioles, which are governed by complex local and central neurohumoral regulation [13]. In cirrhosis, arterial blood pressure is kept low normal or low, depending on the state of the disease, as a circulatory compromise between the vasodilating and counter-regulatory vasoconstricting forces that affect both vascular resistance and compliance. Previous studies have shown a relationship between the degree of arterial hypotension in cirrhosis and the severity of hepatic dysfunction, signs of decompensation and survival [19,28]. SNS, RAAS and vasopressin are all highly activated, and recent clinical studies suggest that the ET system also contributes to the maintenance of arterial blood pressure in cirrhosis [19,120]. Arterial blood pressure has a circadian variation. Twenty-four-hour determinations in cirrhotic patients show that during the day, systolic, diastolic and mean arterial blood pressures are substantially reduced, whereas at night the values are normal [121]. The combination of normal blood pressure and increased heart rate at night suggests abnormal regulation of the circulation in cirrhosis. The upright position further aggravates central hypovolaemia, and normal arterial blood pressure cannot be maintained, even when the heart rate and cardiac output are increased [20,21,23].

A resetting of the baroreceptors is still discussed in relation to wall tension of the fibroelastic tissues in the vessels and stretch-induced activation of sodium-potassium channels [25].

As mentioned above, autonomic dysfunction is well established in cirrhosis, and impaired baroreceptor reflex sensitivity has been shown to occur in cirrhosis as part of a general cardiovascular autonomic dysfunction [21,114,122–126]. In a study of 105 patients with cirrhosis, a reduced baroreflex –sensitivity was found that was significantly related to central haemodynamics and biochemical characteristics [74]. These results suggest that a reduced baroreflex sensitivity owing to the severity of the liver disease is associated with cardiac dysfunction in cirrhosis. Since regulation of the arterial blood pressure plays an important role in the development of fluid retention and renal function, reduced baroreflex sensitivity will further impair renal sodium and water excretion in these patients. Low arterial blood pressure, abnormal distribution of the circulating medium and diurnal variation in arterial blood pressure, and marked activation of neurohumoral systems are all features of the abnormal homoeostatic regulation in patients with cirrhosis. There are only a few reports on arterial hypertension in cirrhosis. However, the prevalence of arterial hypertension in cirrhotic patients seems substantially reduced, especially in advanced cirrhosis [127].

Renal Circulation

Although cardiac output in cirrhosis is increased, reflecting a substantial overall vasodilatation, it covers hyperperfused, normoperfused and hypoperfused vascular areas. In the kidney, vasoconstriction prevails and plays a pivotal role in the development of hepatic nephropathy with a decreased renal blood flow and glomerular filtration rate and increased sodium and water reabsorption (Table 1)[128]. Liver dysfunction, central hypovolaemia, arterial hypotension and neurohumoral activation with renal vasoconstriction are of major importance. Recent results suggest that a decrease in cardiac output in the face of severe splanchnic vasodilatation and activation of the SNS and RAAS is an important determinant of the HRS [128,129]. The vasoconstricting and vasodilating forces are illustrated in Figure 4. Angiotensin II mainly acts on the efferent arteriole, and a low dose of an ACE inhibitor may induce a significant reduction in glomerular filtration and a further reduction in sodium excretion, even in the absence of a change in arterial blood pressure. This suggests that the integrity of the RAAS is important for maintenance of renal function in cirrhotic patients, and that RAAS overactivity does not solely contribute to the adverse renal vasoconstriction. The renal perfusion pressure is low and critically dependent on counter-regulatory systems. For these reasons, blockers of these systems by ACE inhibitors (captopril), angiotensin II antagonists (losartan), β-adrenergic blockers and V1 vasopressin antagonist may further decrease renal blood flow [130]. The HRS denotes a functional and reversible impairment of renal function with a poor prognosis in patients with severe cirrhosis [128]. Treatment is directed towards improving liver function, arterial hypotension and central hypovolaemia, and reducing renal vasoconstriction, for instance with the combined use of splanchnic vasoconstrictors such as terlipressin and plasma expanders such as human albumin [128,131]. Recently, it has been suggested that low cardiac output as part of a cardiorenal syndrome adversely affects renal function and outcome in patients with refractory ascites and HRS [132]. In patients with advanced cirrhosis and severe vasodilatation, activation of the SNS and RAAS, impaired renal function and a reduced systolic function (a decrease in cardiac output) appear to be major determinants for the development of the HRS [129]. Spontaneous bacterial peritonitis is a well-known risk factor for the HRS and after resolution of the infection, suppression of systolic function appears to be more pronounced in patients who develop renal failure, and thus maintenance of cardiac contractility appears to be an important factor in the prevention of renal failure [133]. These observations have stimulated speculations on the presence of a cardiorenal syndrome in cirrhosis [132,133].

Pulmonary Circulation

In cirrhosis, pulmonary vascular resistance is most often decreased [134]. Analysis of the pulmonary circulation in relation to lung function may be obscured by the presence of cardiac dysfunction or the fact that many patients with alcoholic cirrhosis are heavy smokers [135]. Thus, substantial chronic obstructive lung disease may exist in addition to hepatic dysfunction. However, independent of smoking status, these patients have compromised lung function with reduced diffusing lung capacity (DLCO) and ventilation/perfusion abnormalities [54,135–137]. It has now been documented that areas with a high perfusion rate in relation to alveolar ventilation exist in a substantial number of patients (Table 4) [54,135,138]. Besides the abnormal ventilation:perfusion ratio and the presence of regular pulmonary arteriovenous shunts, portopulmonary shunts have also been described [134,135,137,139].

Hepatopulmonary Syndrome

A syndrome with reduced DLCO, abnormal ventilation:perfusion ratio or shunts, low arterial oxygen saturation and pulmonary hyperdynamics has been termed the 'hepatopulmonary syndrome' [137,140,141]. Fallon et al. reported increased pulmonary vascular endothelial NOS and ET-receptor expression and NO-dependent pulmonary vasodilatation in experimental studies [142,143], and this is supported by clinical studies showing increased NO in exhaled air from cirrhotic patients [144,145]. The hepatopulmonary syndrome has been successfully reversed by orthotopic liver transplantation in some patients [137,146,147], and surprisingly by TIPS [148,149]. The frequency of hepatopulmonary syndrome among patients with cirrhosis is not settled at present. Different reports have given varying frequencies of reduced arterial oxygen saturation in cirrhotic patients, from about 10% to as high as 70% [17,150–152].

The reduced DLCO has been related to an increased amount of blood in the lung capillaries [135,153]. However, this seems to be a misconception as there is a direct relationship between the number of the red blood cells in the lung capillaries and DLCO in normal physiology and in other pathological conditions [154].

Table 4. Diagnostic discrimination between hepatopulmonary syndrome and portopulmonary syndrome

Hepatopulmonary syndrome	Portopulmonary hypertension
Presence of liver disease, intrapulmonary shunts, and moderate hypoxaemia	Presence of liver disease and portal hypertension, with no or mild hypoxaemia
Normal or low pulmonary arterial pressure	Mean pulmonary arterial pressure >25 mmHg
Normal or low pulmonary vascular resistance	Pulmonary vascular resistance >240 dyn·s·cm^{-5}
P_{A-a},O_2 >15 mmHg (>2 kPa)	Left atrial pressure <15 mmHg
Positive contrast-enhanced echocardiography	Negative contrast echocardiography
Extrapulmonary shunt fraction >6%	Extrapulmonary shunt fraction <6%

P_{A-a},O_2: alveolar-arterial oxygen gradient.

Moreover, it has been shown that a direct relationship exists between the central and arterial blood volume on the one hand and DLCO on the other in patients with cirrhosis [54]. In addition, a direct relationship between low pulmonary blood volume and reduced DLCO has been described [155]. These observations have been further confirmed by Degano et al., who described associations between low DLCO, high alveolar-arterial oxygen gradient ($P_{A-a}O_2$) and decreased lung capillary blood volume in cirrhotic patients [156].

Thus, it may be concluded that in cirrhotic patients without chronic obstructive lung disease a hyperkinetic condition with reduced pulmonary vascular resistance exists, but when these patients develop chronic obstructive lung disease, pulmonary hypertension with increased pulmonary vascular resistance may follow as in other patients with chronic pulmonary dysfunction.

Portopulmonary Syndrome

The association between portal hypertension and pulmonary arterial hypertension is termed 'portopulmonary hypertension' and is defined as specified in Table 4. It is seen infrequently in cirrhosis, with a prevalence of 1–4% [157]. Symptoms are typically progressive and include fatigue, dyspnoea and oedema [137]. Systemic vascular resistance and cardiac output are similar to those in cirrhotic patients without portopulmonary hypertension, whereas arterial oxygenation is impaired in this group [158]. The histological appearance of pulmonary vessels is similar to that seen in primary pulmonary arterial hypertension, and includes smooth muscle proliferation and hypertrophy [159]. Local vasoconstrictor systems, such as the ET system, may play a role; recently, administration of a mixed ET antagonist has produced beneficial effects in portopulmonary hypertension [160,161].

Cerebral Circulation

Although a considerable increase in our understanding of cerebral perfusion has appeared within the last decade, most studies have been directed towards patients with cerebral ischaemia, hypertension, stroke and related conditions. Only a few and conflicting studies have been performed in cirrhosis. In patients without encephalopathy, cerebral perfusion seems to be normal [162,163]. Patients with early encephalopathy may have reduced cerebral perfusion, but reduced as well as increased perfusion with cerebral oedema have been reported in comatose patients [164]. In patients with fulminant hepatic failure, autoregulation is absent and cerebral blood flow changes parallel with alterations in arterial blood pressure [165]. Generally, the autoregulation of the cerebral blood flow is preserved in patients with cirrhosis, but the lower limit may be changed in some patients with advanced disease [163,165]. In other patients, however, regional cerebral blood flow may be impaired and the abnormalities may reverse after liver transplantation [166,167]. In addition, acute changes in cerebral blood flow have been reported in relation to TIPS insertion [168]. Recently, Mani et al. described decreased heart rate variability in cirrhosis relating to the presence and degree of hepatic encephalopathy and to the level of inflammatory cytokines, suggesting common pathogenetic mechanisms [111]. However, regulation of cerebral circulation in patients with cirrhosis is complex and should be the topic of much future research.

Conclusion

Complications of cirrhosis relating to hyperdynamic circulation and the liver are part of multi-organ failure and may significantly affect a patient's prognosis. The function of the central circulation in cirrhosis is disturbed, with increased cardiac output and heart rate and decreased central and arterial blood volume. Cardiac pressures and performance, and the systolic and diastolic functions are clearly impaired and vary according to the degree of liver dysfunction. The cirrhotic heart is overloaded with a high-output failure and is at the same time hyperdynamic and dysfunctional, and strain may unmask latent heart failure. Cirrhotic cardiomyopathy implies systolic and diastolic dysfunction and electrophysiological abnormalities, and can be unmasked by procedures that stress the heart. Lung function is disturbed in the majority of patients with cirrhosis and in particular in those with hepatopulmonary syndrome. Caution should be exercised with respect to stressful procedures, such as large volume paracentesis with adequate plasma volume expansion, TIPS insertion, peritoneovenous shunting and surgery. In general, cardiopulmonary complications should be treated non-specifically and supportively (Table 5).

Table 5. Principles in prevention and therapy of cardiovascular complications in cirrhosis

Sodium and water restriction
Adequate plasma volume expansion after paracentesis
Treatment with albumin and vasoconstrictors
Treatment with diuretics, including aldosterone antagonists
Treatment with beta-adrenergic blockers
Avoid angiotensin converting enzyme inhibitors
Liver transplantation

Major questions still remain to be resolved, but there is no doubt that circulatory and neuroendocrine derangements play important roles in the clinical aggravation of circulatory, cardiac, renal and pulmonary vascular reactivity. Future studies should be directed towards a demarcation of the clinical importance of these organ-specific haemodynamic complications. Until we have achieved more knowledge on these aspects it is difficult to say how patients, in particular those with cardiovascular complications, should be treated and whether they should be treated specifically.

References

[1] Iwakiri Y, Groszmann RJ. The hyperdynamic circulation of chronic liver diseases: from the patient to the molecule. *Hepatology* 2006;43(2 Suppl 1):S121–31.
[2] Møller S, Henriksen JH. Cardiovascular complications of cirrhosis. *Gut* 2008;57(2):268–78.
[3] Schrier RW, Arroyo V, Bernardi M, Epstein M, Henriksen JH, Rodés J. Peripheral artery vasodilatation hypothesis: a proposal for the initiation of renal sodium and water retention in cirrhosis. *Hepatology* 1988;5:1151–7.
[4] Schrier RW. Renin-angiotensin in preascitic cirrhosis: evidence for primary peripheral arterial vasodilatation. *Gastroenterology* 1998;115(2):489–91.
[5] Møller S, Bendtsen F, Henriksen JH. Vasoactive substances in the circulatory dysfunction of cirrhosis. *Scand. J. Clin. Lab. Invest* .2001;61(6):421–9.

[6] Iwakiri Y. The molecules: mechanisms of arterial vasodilatation observed in the splanchnic and systemic circulation in portal hypertension. *J. Clin. Gastroenterol.* 2007;41(Suppl 3):S288–94.

[7] Arroyo V, Fernandez J, Ginès P. Pathogenesis and treatment of hepatorenal syndrome. *Semin. Liver Dis* .2008;28(1):81–95.

[8] Gerbes AL. The patient with refractory ascites. *Best Pract. Res. Clin. Gastroenterol.* 2007;21(3):551–60.

[9] Ginès P, Schrier RW. Renal failure in cirrhosis. *N. Engl. J. Med* .2009;361(13):1279–90.

[10] Witte CL, Witte MH. The portocardiorenal axis and refractory ascites: the underfilled cup runneth over. *Hepatology* 1989;10(1):114–16.

[11] Alqahtani SA, Fouad TR, Lee SS. Cirrhotic cardiomyopathy. *Semin. Liver. Dis.* 2008;28(1):59–69.

[12] Møller S, Krag A, Henriksen JH, Bendtsen F. Pathophysiological aspects of pulmonary complications of cirrhosis. *Scand. J. Gastroenterol.* 2007;42(4):419–27.

[13] Henriksen JH, Fuglsang S, Bendtsen F, Christensen E, Møller S. Arterial compliance in patients with cirrhosis. High stroke volume/pulse pressure ratio as an index of elevated arterial compliance. *Am. J. Physiol* .2001;280:G584–94.

[14] Llach J, Ginés P, Arroyo V, Rimola A, Titó L, Badalamenti S, et al. Prognostic value of arterial pressure, endogenous vasoactive systems, and renal function in cirrhotic patients admitted to the hospital for the treatment of ascites. *Gastroenterology* 1988;94:482–7.

[15] Braillon A, Cales P, Valla D, Gaudy D, Geoffroy P, Lebrec D. Influence of the degree of liver failure on systemic and splanchnic haemodynamics and on response to propranolol in patients with cirrhosis. *Gut* 1986;27:1204–9.

[16] Møller S. Systemic haemodynamics in cirrhosis and portal hypertension with focus on vasoactive substances and prognosis. *Dan. Med. Bull.* 1998;45(1):1–14.

[17] Møller S, Hillingsø J, Christensen E, Henriksen JH. Arterial hypoxaemia in cirrhosis: fact or fiction? *Gut* 1998;42(6):868–74.

[18] Hobolth L, Dümcke CW, Bendtsen F, Møller S. Determinants of the hyperdynamic circulation and central hypovolaemia in cirrhosis and portal hypertension. *J. Hepatol.* 2009;50:S80.

[19] Møller S, Henriksen JH. The systemic circulation in cirrhosis. In: Ginès P, Arroyo V, Rodés J, Schrier RW, editors. *Ascites and renal dysfunction in liver disease.* 2nd edn. Malden: Blackwell; 2005; pp. 139–55.

[20] Bernardi M, Fornalè L, Di Marco C, Trevisani F, Baraldini M, Gasbarrini A, et al. Hyperdynamic circulation of advanced cirrhosis: A re-appraisal based on posture-induced changes in hemodynamics. *J. Hepatol* .1995;22:309–18.

[21] Laffi G, Barletta G, Lavilla G, Delbene R, Riccardi D, Ticali P, et al. Altered cardiovascular responsiveness to active tilting in nonalcoholic cirrhosis. *Gastroenterology* 1997;113:891–8.

[22] Gentilini P, Romanelli RG, Laffi G, Barletta G, Del Bene R, Messeri G, et al. Cardiovascular and renal function in normotensive and hypertensive patients with compensated cirrhosis: effects of posture. *J. Hepatol.* 1999;30(4):632–8.

[23] Møller S, Nørgaard A, Henriksen JH, Frandsen E, Bendtsen F. Effects of tilting on central hemodynamics and homeostatic mechanisms in cirrhosis. *Hepatology* 2004;40(4):811–19.

[24] Brinch K, Møller S, Bendtsen F, Becker U, Henriksen JH. Plasma volume expansion by albumin in cirrhosis. Relation to blood volume distribution, arterial compliance and severity of disease. *J. Hepatol.* 2003;39(1):24–31.

[25] Schrier RW. Water and sodium retention in edematous disorders: role of vasopressin and aldosterone. *Am. J. Med* .2006;119(7 Suppl 1):S47–53.

[26] Møller S, Bendtsen F, Henriksen JH. Effect of volume expansion on systemic hemodynamics and central and arterial blood volume in cirrhosis. *Gastroenterology* 1995;109:1917–25.

[27] Kiszka-Kanowitz M, Henriksen JH, Møller S, Bendtsen F. Blood volume distribution in patients with cirrhosis: aspects of the dual-head gamma-camera technique. *J. Hepatol.* 2001;35(5):605–12.

[28] Møller S, Bendtsen F, Christensen E, Henriksen JH. Prognostic variables in patients with cirrhosis and oesophageal varices without prior bleeding. *J. Hepatol.* 1994;21:940–6.

[29] Møller S, Henriksen JH. Cardiovascular dysfunction in cirrhosis. Pathophysiological evidence of a cirrhotic cardiomyopathy. *Scand. J. Gastroenterol.* 2001;36(8):785–94.

[30] Bendtsen F, Henriksen JH, Sørensen TIA. Long-term effects of oral propranolol on splanchnic and systemic haemodynamics in patients with cirrhosis and oesophageal varices. *Scand. J. Gastroenterol* .1991;26:933–9.

[31] Groszmann RJ. Vasodilatation and hyperdynamic circulatory state in chronic liver disease. In: Bosch J, Groszmann RJ, editors. *Portal hypertension. Pathophysiology and treatment.* 1st edn. Oxford: Blackwell; 1994; pp. 17–26.

[32] Arroyo V, Colmenero J. Ascites and hepatorenal syndrome in cirrhosis: pathophysiological basis of therapy and current management. *J. Hepatol.* 2003;38 (Suppl 1):S69–89.

[33] Møller S, Henriksen JH. Circulatory abnormalities in cirrhosis with focus on neurohumoral aspects. *Semin. Nephrol.* 1997;17(6):505–19.

[34] Schrier RW, Ecder T. Unifying hypothesis of body fluid volume regulation: implications for cardiac failure and cirrhosis. *Mt. Sinai J. Med.* 2001;68(6):350–61.

[35] Martin PY, Ginès P, Schrier RW. Mechanisms of disease: nitric oxide as a mediator of hemodynamic abnormalities and sodium and water retention in cirrhosis. *N. Engl. J. Med* .1998;339(8):533–41.

[36] Wiest R, Groszmann RJ. The paradox of nitric oxide in cirrhosis and portal hypertension: too much, not enough. *Hepatology* 2002;35(2):478–91.

[37] Møller S, Bendtsen F, Schifter S, Henriksen JH. Relation of calcitonin gene-related peptide to systemic vasodilatation and central hypovolaemia in cirrhosis. *Scand. J. Gastroenterol* .1996;31:928–33.

[38] Hori N, Okanoue T, Sawa Y, Kashima K. Role of calcitonin gene-related peptide in the vascular system on the development of the hyperdynamic circulation in conscious cirrhotic rats. *J. Hepatol.* 1997;26:1111–19.

[39] Guevara M, Ginès P, Jiménez W, Sort P, Fernández-Esparrach G, Escorsell A, et al. Increased adrenomedullin levels in cirrhosis: relationship with hemodynamic abnormalities and vasoconstrictor systems. *Gastroenterology* 1998;114:336–43.

[40] Batkai S, Jarai Z, Wagner JA, Goparaju SK, Varga K, Liu J, et al. Endocannabinoids acting at vascular CB1 receptors mediate the vasodilated state in advanced liver cirrhosis. *Nat. Med.* 2001;7(7):827–32.

[41] Moezi L, Gaskari SA, Lee SS. Endocannabinoids and liver disease. V. endocannabinoids as mediators of vascular and cardiac abnormalities in cirrhosis. *Am. J. Physiol. Gastrointest. Liver Physiol.* 2008;295(4):G649–53.

[42] Ros J, Claria J, To-Figueras J, Planaguma A, Cejudo-Martin P, Fernandez-Varo G, et al. Endogenous cannabinoids: a new system involved in the homeostasis of arterial pressure in experimental cirrhosis in the rat. *Gastroenterology* 2002;122(1):85–93.

[43] Farzaneh-Far R, Moore K. Nitric oxide and the liver. *Liver* 2001;21(3):161–74.

[44] Rockey DC, Chung JJ. Reduced nitric oxide production by endothelial cells in cirrhotic rat liver: endothelial dysfunction in portal hypertension. *Gastroenterology* 1998;114:344–51.

[45] McNaughton L, Puttagunta L, Martinez-Cuesta MA, Kneteman N, Mayers I, Moqbel R, et al. Distribution of nitric oxide synthase in normal and cirrhotic human liver. *Proc. Natl. Acad. Sci. U S A* 2002;99(26):17161–6.

[46] Tazi KA, Barriere E, Moreau R, Heller J, Sogni P, Pateron D, et al. Role of shear stress in aortic eNOS up-regulation in rats with biliary cirrhosis. *Gastroenterology* 2002;122(7):1869–77.

[47] Lee F-Y, Colombato LA, Albillos A, Groszmann RJ. N omega-nitro-L-arginine administration corrects peripheral vasodilatation and systemic capillary hypotension and ameliorates plasma volume expansion and sodium retention in portal hypertensive rats. *Hepatology* 1993;17:84–90.

[48] Niederberger M, Martin P-Y, Ginès P, Morris K, Tsai P, Xu D-L, et al. Normalization of nitric oxide production corrects arterial vasodilation and hyperdynamic circulation in cirrhotic rats. *Gastroenterology* 1995;109:1624–30.

[49] La Villa G, Barletta G, Pantaleo P, Del Bene R, Vizzutti F, Vecchiarino S, et al. Hemodynamic, renal, and endocrine effects of acute inhibition of nitric oxide synthase in compensated cirrhosis. *Hepatology* 2001;34(1):19–27.

[50] Helmy A, Newby DE, Jalan R, Johnston NR, Hayes PC, Webb DJ. Nitric oxide mediates the reduced vasoconstrictor response to angiotensin II in patients with preascitic cirrhosis. *J. Hepatol*.2003;38(1):44–50.

[51] Fernandez M, Mejias M, Angermayr B, Garcia-Pagan JC, Rodés J, Bosch J. Inhibition of VEGF receptor-2 decreases the development of hyperdynamic splanchnic circulation and portal-systemic collateral vessels in portal hypertensive rats. *J. Hepatol.* 2005;43(1):98–103.

[52] Gupta S, Morgan TR, Gordan GS. Calcitonin gene-related peptide in hepatorenal syndrome. *J. Clin. Gastroenterol*.1992;14:122–6.

[53] Bendtsen F, Schifter S, Henriksen JH. Increased circulating calcitonin gene-related peptide (CGRP) in cirrhosis. *J. Hepatol*.1991;12:118–23.

[54] Møller S, Becker U, Schifter S, Abrahamsen J, Henriksen JH. Effect of oxygen inhalation on systemic, central, and splanchnic haemodynamics in cirrhosis. *J. Hepatol*.1996;25:316–28.

[55] Henriksen JH, Møller S, Schifter S, Bendtsen F. Increased arterial compliance in decompensated cirrhosis. *J. Hepatol.* 1999;31(4):712–18.

[56] Henriksen JH, Møller S, Schifter S, Abrahamsen J, Becker U. High arterial compliance in cirrhosis is related to elevated circulating calcitonin gene-related peptide (CGRP) and low adrenaline, but not to activated vasoconstrictor systems. *Gut* 2001;49:112–18.

[57] Richards AM, Nicholls MG, Lewis L, Lainchbury JG. Adrenomedullin. *Clin. Sci.* 1996;91:3–16.

[58] Fábrega E, Casafont F, Crespo J, de la Peña J, San Miguel G, de las Heras G, et al. Plasma adrenomedullin levels in patients with hepatic cirrhosis. *Am. J. Gastroenterol* .1997;92(10):1901–4.

[59] Genesca J, Gonzalez A, Catalan R, Segura R, Martinez M, Esteban R, et al. Adrenomedullin, a vasodilator peptide implicated in hemodynamic alterations of liver cirrhosis: relationship to nitric oxide. *Digest Dis. Sci* .1999;44(2):372–6.

[60] Heinemann A, Wachter CH, Fickert P, Trauner M, Stauber RE. Vasopressin reverses mesenteric hyperemia and vasoconstrictor hyporesponsiveness in anesthetized portal hypertensive rats. *Hepatology* 1998;28(3):646–54.

[61] Newby DE, Jalan R, Masumori S, Hayes PC, Boon NA, Webb DJ. Peripheral vascular tone in patients with cirrhosis: role of the renin-angiotensin and sympathetic nervous systems. *Cardiovasc. Res.* 1998;38(1):221–8.

[62] Bandi JC, Fernández M, Bernadich C, De Lacy AM, García-Pagán JC, Bosch J, et al. Hyperkinetic circulation and decreased sensitivity to vasoconstrictors following portacaval shunt in the rat. Effects of chronic nitric oxide inhibition. *J. Hepatol.* 1999;31(4):719–24.

[63] Jaue DN, Ma ZH, Lee SS. Cardiac muscarinic receptor function in rats with cirrhotic cardiomyopathy. *Hepatology* 1997;25:1361–5.

[64] Moreau R, Komaichi H, Kirstetter P, Ohsuga M, Cailmail S, Lebrec D. Altered control of vascular tone by adenosine triphosphate-sensitive potassium channels in rats with cirrhosis. *Gastroenterology* 1994;106:1016–23.

[65] Heinemann A, Wachter CH, Holzer P, Fickert P, Stauber RE. Nitric oxide-dependent and -independent vascular hyporeactivity in mesenteric arteries of portal hypertensive rats. *Br. J. Pharmacol* .1997;121(5):1031–7.

[66] Gerbes AL, Remien J, Jüngst D, Sauerbruch T, Paumgartner G. Evidence for down-regulation of beta-2-adrenoceptors in cirrhotic patients with severe ascites. *Lancet* 1986;1:1409–11.

[67] Lee SS, Pak JM, Medlicott SM, Bomzon A. Vasodilatory responses of isolated arteries of cirrhotic rats. *Clin. Sci* .1995;89:227–32.

[68] Helmy A, Jalan R, Newby DE, Hayes PC, Webb DJ. Role of angiotensin II in regulation of basal and sympathetically stimulated vascular tone in early and advanced cirrhosis. *Gastroenterology* 2000; 118(3):565–72.

[69] Helmy A, Jalan R, Newby DE, Johnston NR, Hayes PC, Webb DJ. Altered peripheral vascular responses to exogenous and endogenous endothelin-1 in patients with well-compensated cirrhosis. *Hepatology* 2001;33(4):826–31.

[70] Bosch J, Abraldes JG, Groszmann R. Current management of portal hypertension. *J. Hepatol* .2003;38:S54–68.

[71] Rockey DC. Hepatic blood flow regulation by stellate cells in normal and injured liver. *Semin. Liver Dis.* 2001;21(3):337–49.

[72] Schepke M, Werner E, Biecker E, Schiedermaier P, Heller J, Neef M, et al. Hemodynamic effects of the angiotensin II receptor antagonist irbesartan in patients with cirrhosis and portal hypertension. *Gastroenterology* 2001;121(2):389–95.

[73] Kowalski HJ, Abelmann WH. The cardiac output at rest in Laennec's cirrhosis. *J. Clin. Invest*.1953;32:1025–33.

[74] Møller S, Iversen JS, Henriksen JH, Bendtsen F. Reduced baroreflex sensitivity in alcoholic cirrhosis: relations to hemodynamics and humoral systems. *Am J Physiol Heart Circ. Physiol.*2007;292(6):H2966–72.

[75] Møller S, Henriksen JH. Cirrhotic cardiomyopathy: a pathophysiological review of circulatory dysfunction in liver disease. *Heart* 2002;87(1):9–15.

[76] Zambruni A, Trevisani F, Caraceni P, Bernardi M. Cardiac electrophysiological abnormalities in patients with cirrhosis. *J. Hepatol.* 2006;44:994–1002.

[77] Bernardi M, Calandra S, Colantoni A, Trevisani F, Raimondo ML, Sica G, et al. Q-T interval prolongation in cirrhosis: prevalence, relationship with severity, and etiology of the disease and possible pathogenetic factors. *Hepatology* 1998;27:28–34.

[78] Rabie RN, Cazzaniga M, Salerno F, Wong F. The use of E/A ratio as a predictor of outcome in cirrhotic patients treated with transjugular intrahepatic portosystemic shunt. *Am. J. Gastroenterol.* 2009;104(8):2458–66

[79] Liu H, Gaskari SA, Lee SS. Cardiac and vascular changes in cirrhosis: pathogenic mechanisms. *World J. Gastroentero.* 2006;12:837–42.

[80] Mani AR, Ippolito S, Ollosson R, Moore KP. Nitration of cardiac proteins is associated with abnormal cardiac chronotropic responses in rats with biliary cirrhosis. *Hepatology* 2006;43:847–56.

[81] Wong F, Girgrah N, Graba J, Allidina Y, Liu P, Blendis L. The cardiac response to exercise in cirrhosis. *Gut* 2001;49(2):268–75.

[82] Huonker M, Schumacher YO, Ochs A, Sorichter S, Keul J, Rössle M. Cardiac function and haemodynamics in alcoholic cirrhosis and effects of the transjugular intrahepatic portosystemic stent shunt. *Gut* 1999;44(5):743–8.

[83] Merli M, Valeriano V, Funaro S, Attili AF, Masini A, Efrati C, et al. Modifications of cardiac function in cirrhotic patients treated with transjugular intrahepatic portosystemic shunt (TIPS). *Am. J. Gastroenterol.* 2002;97(1):142–8.

[84] Ginès P, Uriz J, Calahorra B, Garcia-Tsao G, Kamath PS, Del Arbol LR, et al. Transjugular intrahepatic portosystemic shunting versus paracentesis plus albumin for refractory ascites in cirrhosis. *Gastroenterology* 2002;123(6):1839–47.

[85] Pozzi M, Carugo S, Boari G, Pecci V, de Ceglia S, Maggiolini S, et al. Evidence of functional and structural cardiac abnormalities in cirrhotic patients with and without ascites. *Hepatology* 1997;26(5):1131–7.

[86] Torregrosa M, Aguade S, Dos L, Segura R, Gonzalez A, Evangelista A, et al. Cardiac alterations in cirrhosis: reversibility after liver transplantation. *J. Hepatol.* 2005;42(1):68–74.

[87] Grose RD, Nolan J, Dillon JF, Errington M, Hannan WJ, Bouchier IAD, et al. Exercise-induced left ventricular dysfunction in alcoholic and non-alcoholic cirrhosis. *J. Hepatol* .1995;22:326–32.

[88] Epstein SK, Ciubotaru RL, Zilberberg MD, Kaplan LM, Jacoby C, Freeman R, et al. Analysis of impaired exercise capacity in patients with cirrhosis. *Dig. Dis. Sci.* 1998;43(8):1701–7.

[89] Myers RP, Lee SS. Cirrhotic cardiomyopathy and liver transplantation. *Liver Transpl.* 2000;6(4 Suppl 1):S44–52.

[90] Pozzi M, Redaelli E, Ratti L, Poli G, Guidi C, Milanese M, et al. Time-course of diastolic dysfunction in different stages of chronic HCV related liver diseases. *Minerva Gastroenterol. Dietol.* 2005;51(2):179–86.

[91] Gaskari SA, Honar H, Lee SS. Therapy insight: cirrhotic cardiomyopathy. *Nat Clin Pract. Gastroenterol. Hepatol.* 2006;3(6):329–37.

[92] Finucci G, Desideri A, Sacerdoti D, Bolognesi M, Merkel C, Angeli P, et al. Left ventricular diastolic function in liver cirrhosis. *Scand J Gastroenterol* 1996;31:279–84.

[93] Henriksen JH, Fuglsang S, Bendtsen F, Christensen E, Møller S. Dyssynchronous electrical and mechanical systole in patients with cirrhosis. *J Hepatol* 2002;36(4):513–20.

[94] Henriksen JH, Bendtsen F, Hansen EF, Møller S. Acute non-selective beta-adrenergic blockade reduces prolonged frequency-adjusted Q-T interval (QTc) in patients with cirrhosis. *J. Hepatol* .2004;40(2):239–46.

[95] Henriksen JH, Gøetze JP, Fuglsang S, Christensen E, Bendtsen F, Møller S. Increased circulating pro-brain natriuretic peptide (proBNP) and brain natriuretic peptide (BNP) in patients with cirrhosis: relation to cardiovascular dysfunction and severity of disease. *Gut* 2003;52(10):1511–17.

[96] Genovesi S, Prata Pizzala DM, Pozzi M, Ratti L, Milanese M, Pieruzzi F, et al. QT interval prolongation and decreased heart rate variability in cirrhotic patients: relevance of hepatic venous pressure gradient and serum calcium. *Clin. Sci. (Lond)* 2009;116(12):851–9.

[97] Mohamed R, Forsey PR, Davies MK, Neuberger JM. Effect of liver transplantation on QT interval prolongation and autonomic dysfunction in end-stage liver disease. *Hepatology* 1996;23:1128–34.

[98] Maroto A, Ginès P, Arroyo V, Ginès A, Saló J, Clària J, et al. Brachial and femoral artery blood flow in cirrhosis : relationship to kidney dysfunction. *Hepatology* 1993;17:788–93.

[99] Luca A, García-Pagán JC, Feu F, Lopez-Talavera JC, Fernández M, Bru C, et al. Noninvasive measurement of femoral blood flow and portal pressure response to propranolol in patients with cirrhosis. *Hepatology* 1995;21:83–8.

[100] Campillo B, Chabrier PE, Pelle G, Sediame S, Atlan G, Fouet P, et al. Inhibition of nitric oxide synthesis in the forearm arterial bed of patients with advanced cirrhosis. *Hepatology* 1995;22:1423–9.

[101] Ferguson JW, Dover A, Chia S, Cruden N, Hayes PC, Newby D. Inducible nitric oxide synthase activity contributes to the regulation of peripheral vascular tone in patients with cirrhosis and ascites. *Gut* 2005;55(4):542–6.

[102] Carella M, Hunter JO, Fazio S, Del Piano C, Bartoli GC. Capillary blood flow to the skin of forearm in cirrhosis. *Angiology* 1992;43:969–74.

[103] Hadengue A, Moreau R, Gaudin C, Bacq Y, Champigneulle B, Lebrec D. Total effective vascular compliance in patients with cirrhosis: a study of the response to acute blood volume expansion. *Hepatology* 1992;15:809–15.

[104] Andreu V, Perello A, Moitinho E, Escorsell A, García-Pagán JC, Bosch J, et al. Total effective vascular compliance in patients with cirrhosis. Effects of propranolol. *J. Hepatol.* 2002;36(3):356–61.

[105] Møller S, Gulberg V, Becker U, Gerbes AL, Henriksen JH. Elevated arterial compliance in patients with cirrhosis is not related to arterial endothelin-1. *Scand J. Gastroenterol.* 2002;37(9):1064–9.

[106] Møller S, Hansen EF, Becker U, Brinch K, Henriksen JH, Bendtsen F. Central and systemic haemodynamic effects of terlipressin in portal hypertensive patients. *Liver* 2000;20(1):51–9.

[107] Rowell LB. *Human cardiovascular control.* Oxford: Oxford University Press; 1993.

[108] Hendrickse MT, Triger DR. Vagal dysfunction and impaired urinary sodium and water excretion in cirrhosis. *Am. J. Gastroenterol.* 1994;89(5):750–7.

[109] Trevisani F, Sica G, Mainquà P, Santese G, De Notariis S, Caraceni P, et al. Autonomic dysfunction and hyperdynamic circulation in cirrhosis with ascites. *Hepatology* 1999;30(6):1387–92.

[110] Rangari M, Sinha S, Kapoor D, Mohan JC, Sarin SK. Prevalence of autonomic dysfunction in cirrhotic and noncirrhotic portal hypertension. *Am. J. Gastroenterol.* 2002;97(3):707–13.

[111] Mani AR, Montagnese S, Jackson CD, Jenkins CW, Head IM, Stephens RC, et al. Decreased heart rate variability in patients with cirrhosis relates to the presence and severity of hepatic encephalopathy. *Am. J. Physiol. Gastrointest Liver Physiol.* 2009;296(2):G330–8.

[112] Dillon JF, Nolan J, Thomas H, Williams BC, Neilson JMM, Bouchier IAD, et al. The correction of autonomic dysfunction in cirrhosis by captopril. *J. Hepatol*.1997;26:331–5.

[113] Ates F, Topal E, Kosar F, Karincaoglu M, Yildirim B, Aksoy Y, et al. The relationship of heart rate variability with severity and prognosis of cirrhosis. *Dig. Dis. Sci* .2006;51(9):1614–8.

[114] Barron HV, Alam I, Lesh MD, Strunk A, Bass NM. Autonomic nervous system tone measured by baroreflex sensitivity is depressed in patients with end-stage liver disease. *Am. J. Gastroenterol.* 1999;94(4):986–9.

[115] Bernardi M, Rubboli A, Trevisani F, Cancellieri C, Ligabue A, Baradini M, et al. Reduced cardiovascular responsiveness to exercise-induced sympathoadrenergic stimulation in patients with cirrhosis. *J. Hepatol* .1991;12:207–16.

[116] Villa GL, Barletta G, Romanelli RG, Laffi G, Del Bene R, Vizzutti F, et al. Cardiovascular effects of canrenone in patients with preascitic cirrhosis. *Hepatology* 2002;35(6):1441–8.

[117] MacGilchrist AJ, Sumner D, Reid JL. Impaired pressor reactivity in cirrhosis: evidence for a peripheral vascular defect. *Hepatology* 1991;13:689–94.

[118] Bolognesi M, Sacerdoti D, Di Pascoli M, Angeli P, Quarta S, Sticca A, et al. Haeme oxygenase mediates hyporeactivity to phenylephrine in the mesenteric vessels of cirrhotic rats with ascites. *Gut* 2005;54(11):1630–6.

[119] Ferlitsch A, Pleiner J, Mittermayer F, Schaller G, Homoncik M, Peck-Radosavljevic M, et al. Vasoconstrictor hyporeactivity can be reversed by antioxidants in patients with advanced alcoholic cirrhosis of the liver and ascites. *Crit. Care Med.* 2005;33(9):2028–33.

[120] Tripathi D, Therapondos G, Ferguson JW, Newby DE, Webb DJ, Hayes PC. Endothelin-1 contributes to maintenance of systemic but not portal haemodynamics in patients with early cirrhosis: a randomised controlled trial. *Gut* 2006;55(9):1290–5.

[121] Møller S, Wiinberg N, Henriksen JH. Noninvasive 24-hour ambulatory arterial blood pressure monitoring in cirrhosis. *Hepatology* 1995;22:88–95.
[122] Veglio F, Melchio R, Calva S, Rabbia F, Gallo V, Melino P, et al. Noninvasive assessment of spontaneous baroreflex sensitivity in patients with liver cirrhosis. *Liver* 1998;18(6):420–6.
[123] Laffi G, Lagi A, Cipriani M, Barletta G, Bernardi L, Fattorini L, et al. Impaired cardiovascular autonomic response to passive tilting in cirrhosis with ascites. *Hepatology* 1996;24:1063–7.
[124] Lazzeri C, Lavilla G, Laffi G, Vecchiarino S, Gambilonghi F, Gentilini P, et al. Autonomic regulation of heart rate and QT interval in nonalcoholic cirrhosis with ascites. *Digestion* 1997;58:580–6.
[125] Hansen S, Møller S, Bendtsen F, Jensen G, Henriksen JH. Diurnal variation and dispersion in QT interval in cirrhosis: relation to haemodynamic changes. *J. Hepatol.* 2007;47(3):373–80.
[126] Dumcke CW, Møller S. Autonomic dysfunction in cirrhosis and portal hypertension. *Scand. J. Clin. Lab. Invest* .2008;25:1–11.
[127] Henriksen JH, Møller S. Hypertension and liver disease. *Curr. Hypertens. Rep.* 2004;6(6):453–61.
[128] Arroyo V, Terra C, Ginès P. New treatments of hepatorenal syndrome. *Semin. Liver Dis.* 2006;26(3):254–64.
[129] Ruiz-del-Arbol L, Monescillo A, Arocena C, Valer P, Ginès P, Moreira V, et al. Circulatory function and hepatorenal syndrome in cirrhosis. *Hepatology* 2005;42:439–47.
[130] Gonzàlez-Abraldes J, Albillos A, Bañares R, del Arbol LR, Moitinho E, Rodríguez C, et al. Randomized comparison of long-term losartan versus propranolol in lowering portal pressure in cirrhosis. *Gastroenterology* 2001;121(2):382–8.
[131] Salerno F, Gerbes A, Ginès P, Wong F, Arroyo V. Diagnosis, prevention and treatment of the hepatorenal syndrome in cirrhosis. *Gut* 2007;56:1310–8.
[132] Krag A, Bendtsen F, Henriksen JH, Møller S. Low cardiac output predicts development of hepatorenal syndrome and survival in patients with cirrhosis and ascites. *Gut* 2010;59(1):105–10.
[133] Ruiz-del-Arbol L, Urman J, Fernandez J, Gonzalez M, Navasa M, Monescillo A, et al. Systemic, renal, and hepatic hemodynamic derangement in cirrhotic patients with spontaneous bacterial peritonitis. *Hepatology* 2003;38(5):1210–18.
[134] Hervé P, Lebrec D, Brenot F, Simonneau G, Humbert M, Sitbon O, et al. Pulmonary vascular disorders in portal hypertension. *Eur. Resp. J.*1998;11(5):1153–66.
[135] Agusti AGN, Roca J, Rodriguez-Roisin R. Mechanisms of gas exchange impairment in patients with liver cirrhosis. *Clin. Chest Med.* 1996;17(1):49–66.
[136] Krowka MJ. Hepatopulmonary syndromes. *Gut* 2000;46(1):1–4.
[137] Fallon MB, Abrams GA. Pulmonary dysfunction in chronic liver disease. *Hepatology* 2000;32(4 Pt 1):859–65.
[138] Söderman C, Juhlin-Dannfelt A, Lagerstrand L, Eriksson LS. Ventilation-perfusion relationships and central haemodynamics in patients with cirrhosis. Effects of a somatostatin analogue. *J. Hepatol.* 1994;21:52–7.

[139] Abrams GA, Nanda NC, Dubovsky EV, Krowka MJ, Fallon MB. Use of macroaggregated albumin lung perfusion scan to diagnose hepatopulmonary syndrome: a new approach. *Gastroenterology* 1998;114:305–10.

[140] Rodríguez-Roisin R, Agustí A, Roca J. The hepatopulmonary syndrome: new name, old complexities. *Thorax.* 1992;47:897–902.

[141] Krowka MJ, Cortese DA. Hepatopulmonary syndrome: current concepts in diagnostic and therapeutic considerations. *Chest* 1994;105:1528–37.

[142] Fallon MB, Abrams GA, Luo B, Hou ZY, Dai J, Ku DD. The role of endothelial nitric oxide synthase in the pathogenesis of a rat model of hepatopulmonary syndrome. *Gastroenterology* 1997;113:606–14.

[143] Luo B, Liu L, Tang L, Zhang J, Stockard CR, Grizzle WE, et al. Increased pulmonary vascular endothelin B receptor expression and responsiveness to endothelin-1 in cirrhotic and portal hypertensive rats: a potential mechanism in experimental hepatopulmonary syndrome. *J. Hepatol.* 2003;38(5):556–63.

[144] Söderman C, Leone A, Furst V, Persson MG. Endogenous nitric oxide in exhaled air from patients with liver cirrhosis. *Scand. J. Gastroenterol* .1997;32:591–7.

[145] Rolla G, Brussino L, Colagrande P, Dutto L, Polizzi S, Scappaticci E, et al. Exhaled nitric oxide and oxygenation abnormalities in hepatic cirrhosis. *Hepatology* 1997;26:842–7.

[146] Meyers C, Low L, Kaufman L, Druger G, Wong LL. Trendelenburg positioning and continuous lateral rotation improve oxygenation in hepatopulmonary syndrome after liver transplantation. *Liver Transpl. Surg.*.1998;4(6):510–12.

[147] Martínez GP, Barberà JA, Visa J, Rimola A, Paré JC, Roca J, et al. Hepatopulmonary syndrome in candidates for liver transplantation. *J. Hepatol.* 2001;34(5):651–7.

[148] Allgaier HP, Haag K, Ochs A, Hauenstein KH, Jeserich M, Krause T, et al. Hepatopulmonary syndrome: successful treatment by transjugular intrahepatic portosystemic stent-shunt (TIPS). *J Hepatol* 1995;23:102.

[149] Riegler JL, Lang KA, Johnson SP, Westerman JH. Transjugular intrahepatic portosystemic shunt improves oxygenation in hepatopulmonary syndrome. *Gastroenterology* 1995;109:978–83.

[150] Thorens JB, Junod AF. Hypoxaemia and liver cirrhosis: a new argument in favour of a "diffusion-perfusion defect". *Eur Resp J* 1992;5(16):754–6.

[151] Rodríguez-Roisin R, Krowka MJ. Is severe arterial hypoxaemia due to hepatic disease an indication for liver transplantation? A new therapeutic approach. *Eur. Resp. J.* 1994;7:839–42.

[152] Schenk P, Fuhrmann V, Madl C, Funk G, Lehr S, Kandel O, et al. Hepatopulmonary syndrome: prevalence and predictive value of various cut offs for arterial oxygenation and their clinical consequences. *Gut* 2002;51(6):853–9.

[153] Krowka MJ. Hepatopulmonary syndrome versus portopulmonary hypertension: distinctions and dilemmas. *Hepatology* 1997;25:1282–4.

[154] Cotes JE. Lung function. Assessment and application in medicine. 5th edn. Oxford: Blackwell; 1993.

[155] Møller S, Burchardt H, Ogard CG, Schiodt FV, Lund JO. Pulmonary blood volume and transit time in cirrhosis: relation to lung function. *Liver Int.* 2006;26(9):1072–8.

[156] Degano B, Mittaine M, Guénard H, Rami J, Garcia G, Kamar N, et al. Nitric oxide and carbon monoxide lung transfer in patients with advanced liver cirrhosis. *J. Appl. Physiol.* 2009;107(1):139–43.

[157] Hadengue A, Kamal KB, Lebrec D, Benhamou JP. Pulmonary hypertension complicating portal hypertension: prevalence and relation to splanchnic hemodynamics. *Gastroenterology* 1991;100:520–8.

[158] Katsuta Y, Zhang XJ, Kato Y, Shimizu S, Komeichi K, Ohsuga M, et al. Hemodynamic features and impaired arterial oxygenation in patients with portopulmonary hypertension. *Hepatol. Res.* 2005;32:79–88.

[159] Rodríguez-Roisin R, Krowka MJ, Hervé P, Fallon MB. Pulmonary-hepatic vascular disorders (PHD). *Eur Respir J* 2004;24(5):861–80.

[160] Kuntzen C, Gülberg V, Gerbes AL. Use of a mixed endothelin receptor antagonist in portopulmonary hypertension: a safe and effective therapy? *Gastroenterology* 2005;128(1):164–8.

[161] Hoeper MM, Halank M, Marx C, Hoeffken G, Seyfarth HJ, Schauer J, et al. Bosentan therapy for portopulmonary hypertension. *Eur. Respir. J.* 2005;25(3):502–8.

[162] Almdal T, Schroeder T, Ranek L. Cerebral blood flow and liver function in patients with encephalopathy due to acute and chronic liver diseases. *Scand. J. Gastroenterol.* 1989;24:299–303.

[163] Larsen FS, Olsen KS, Ejlersen E, Hansen BA, Paulson OB, Knudsen GM. Cerebral blood flow autoregulation and transcranial Doppler sonography in patients with cirrhosis. *Hepatology* 1995;22:730–6.

[164] Ede RJ, Gimson AES, Bihari D, Williams R. Controlled hyperventilation in the prevention of cerebral oedema in fulminant hepatic failure. *J Hepatol* 1986;2:43–51.

[165] Larsen FS, Knudsen GM, Hansen BA. Pathophysiological changes in cerebral circulation, oxidative metabolism and blood–brain barrier in patients with acute liver failure. Tailored cerebral oxygen utilization. *J. Hepatol*.1997;27(1):231–8.

[166] Lagi A, La Villa G, Barletta G, Cencetti S, Bacalli S, Cipriani M, et al. Cerebral autoregulation in patients with cirrhosis and ascites . A transcranial Doppler study. *J. Hepatol.* 1997;27:114–20.

[167] Dam M, Burra P, Tedeschi U, Cagnin A, Chierichetti F, Ermani M, et al. Regional cerebral blood flow changes in patients with cirrhosis assessed with Tc-99m-HM-PAO single-photon emission computed tomography: effect of liver transplantation. *J. Hepatol*.1998;29(1):78–84.

[168] Jalan R, Newby DE, Damink SW, Redhead DN, Hayes PC, Lee A. Acute changes in cerebral blood flow and metabolism during portasystemic shunting. *Liver Transpl* 2001;7(3):274–8.

[169] Ring-Larsen H. Renal blood. *Scand. J. Clin. Lab. Invest.* 1977;37:635–42

In: Cardiovascular Diseases and Liver Transplantation
Editor: Zoka Milan, pp. 31-48
ISBN: 978-1-61122-910-3
© 2011 Nova Science Publishers, Inc.

Chapter II

Coronary Artery Disease and Liver Transplantation

James Y. Findlay[*]

Department of Anesthesiology and Critical Care Medicine
Mayo Clinic, Rochester MN 55905, USA

Abstract

Coronary artery disease (CAD) is common in patients undergoing evaluation for liver transplantation and its prevalence in this population will likely increase as liver transplantation is offered to a wider range of candidates, particularly older patients. A significant percentage of this CAD is previously undiagnosed. Cardiovascular events are one of the leading causes of mortality and morbidity after liver transplantation and patients with CAD who undergo liver transplantation have a higher morbidity and mortality than controls. Identification of CAD in the transplant candidate is problematic as the symptoms of liver disease confound clinical suspicion and conventional non-invasive screening tests are reported as having poor diagnostic accuracy in this population when used as part of typical screening algorithms. The optimum management of the patient with CAD prior to liver transplantation is currently unknown, current practice suggests correcting identifiable significant lesions percutaneously where possible and providing optimum medical management as per current guidelines. Acceleration of known CAD and the development of CAD are significant issues in the post-transplant population. Modifiable cardiovascular risk factor identification and risk reduction management should be actively undertaken.

Introduction

Cardiovascular disease is one of the leading causes of post-transplant mortality after liver transplantation [1-3]. In 1996 Plotkin reported high morbidity and mortality in 32 patients

---

[*] Correspondence: James Y. Findlay, Consultant, Department of Anesthesiology and Critical Care Medicine, Mayo Clinic, First St S.W., Rochester MN 55905, USA, E-mail: Findlay.James@mayo.edu.

with known coronary artery disease (CAD) undergoing liver transplantation [4]. He found a 50% three year mortality (30% at 3 months) and 81% morbidity. This concerning finding led to recommendations for the screening of liver transplant candidates for CAD [5] with many programs incorporating CAD screening into their pre-operative evaluation. More recently Diedrich re-examined the outcomes for CAD patients undergoing liver transplantation and found that patients with known CAD had significantly worse three year cardiovascular morbidity (38%) and mortality (26%) at three years than matched controls without CAD [6]. Three month mortality was 2% in both cases and controls [6]. Whilst not as striking as Plotkin's original report it appears that, despite advances in both the screening of liver transplant candidates and the management of CAD [7-9], patients with CAD continue to have worse outcomes than those without. Hence the continued interest in identifying CAD in liver transplant candidates and in assessing strategies for the optimum management of these patients.

Prevalence of CAD in Liver Disease

There has for many years been a debate over whether there is a protective effect of cirrhosis on the cardiovascular system and the coronary arteries in particular. Older studies suggested a low prevalence of CAD in cirrhotic patients [10] and more recent pathological studies have suggested a lower plaque burden in individuals with chronic liver disease [11]. This position is, however, controversial [12] and a recent comparison of cirrhotic patients to matched controls found CAD to be significantly more prevalent in the cirrhotic group (20% versus 12%) [13]. That CAD occurs in the cirrhotic population is not in doubt - in 1995 Carey undertook coronary angiography in OLT candidates over 50 years of age [14] and reported an overall prevalence of moderate to severe CAD of 27%. This is consistent with a recent study where coronary angiography was used to identify CAD in patients over 45 years being evaluated for OLT where a 20% prevalence was found [15]. Also notable is the prevalence of previously unsuspected CAD in the pre-transplant population: in the Carey study this was 13% of the total [14], more recently Aydinalp found that 15% of transplant candidates had previously undiagnosed CAD, again by coronary angiography in a cohort of patients [16]. Various other prevalence estimates, mostly lower, are quoted in the literature, a number of factors may account for the variability. Few investigators have performed coronary angiography on every member of a study cohort, most frequently this is only done in selected subgroups thus the true prevalence of coronary lesions is unknown. The definitions used to identify CAD are variable; even within the studies in which coronary angiography is undertaken the degree (percentage of vessel occluded), extent and anatomic position of the lesions used to define CAD (and its various sub-categorizations) differ. Furthermore those patients presenting for transplantation are a selected subgroup of the overall population of patients with end stage liver disease. To reach transplantation they must be identified, referred to a transplant center and be considered worthy of further evaluation with the possibility of selection bias at every stage in the procedure – for example a patient with end stage liver disease but known CAD may never be referred for transplant evaluation due to a belief on the part of his physician that he would not be a suitable candidate. This possibility of a referral bias in current practice should be borne in mind since as the outcomes from liver transplantation improve there is a resultant widening of the range of patients considered suitable candidates. As more patients are referred the prevalence of CAD in liver transplant candidates seen in transplant centers will probably rise.

CAD Risk Factors and Liver Disease

Advancing age is one of the major risk factors for CAD. The incidence of CAD and CAD related events increases markedly with age [17]. At all ages males have more disease than females, however in post-menopausal women the incidence and severity of CAD increases rapidly resulting in a narrowing of the sex ratio at older ages [18]. Thus as liver transplantation is offered as a therapeutic option to older patients the prevalence of CAD in those presenting for transplant will increase. Additionally patients presenting for transplantation are predominantly male, reflecting the predominance of males in those with alcoholic cirrhosis [19, 20] and hepatitis C [21].

Conventional cardiac risk factors for CAD are common in liver transplant candidates. Table 1 gives representative percentages, with similar findings in a number of series [13, 15, 22, 26]. In comparing a cohort of cirrhotic patients with matched controls from the general population a significantly higher prevalence of diabetes mellitus and arterial hypertension were noted in the cirrhotic patients [13].

The etiology of the underlying liver disease influences the prevalence of CAD. Non-alcoholic fatty liver disease has been found to be an independent predictor of CAD [27] even in the absence of metabolic syndrome [28]. The "J-curve" in mortality associated with alcohol consumption is worthy of mention - whilst alcohol consumption at moderate doses seems to have a protective effect on the cardiovascular system [29] at higher doses concordant with those resulting in end stage liver disease the effect may be towards an increase in disease [30] and an increased morbidity and mortality.

Identifying CAD in Liver Transplant Candidates

Given that patients with CAD have poorer outcomes after liver transplantation than those without there is a desire by clinicians to identify such individuals during the pre-transplant evaluation. This allows the identification of CAD, the institution of appropriate management and, if necessary, the re-addressing of candidacy for liver transplantation. As the prevalence of undiagnosed CAD in the population presenting for liver transplantation is in the order of 15% [14,16] this involves the screening of patients. When evaluating the literature on screening for CAD in the liver transplant population there are a number of issues that should be kept in mind.

Table 1. Approximate prevalence of cardiovascular risk factor in patients presenting for liver transplantation

Risk factor	Prevalence (%)
Hypertension	25
Diabetes mellitus	30
Smoker (current or previous)	35
Hyperlipidemia	15
Family history CAD	10
Risk factor per patient	
1	14
2	33
≥ 3	14

CAD-coronary artery disease.
Adapted from Safadi [24], Tiukinhoy [15] and Findlay [23].

Firstly, the utility of any screening test is dependent on the prevalence of the disease sought. Whilst at around 15% the prevalence of undiagnosed CAD of seems quite frequent a cursory review of the studies suggest a much lower value, frequently around 1-3%. Whilst the true value is likely higher than this since not every subject had a definitive assessment for CAD it would seem unlikely to be low by a factor of 5-10. This suggests that the populations appearing in these studies are selected from the general population of patients with end-stage liver disease, potentially for reasons mentioned earlier. It also means that any screening test will be of less utility as the ratio of false positives to true positives rises with diminishing prevalence.

Secondly, what is the outcome of interest? Is it demonstrating CAD, or is it predicting transplant related cardiovascular morbidity and mortality? Whilst these were once regarded as synonymous [31] cirrhotic cardiomyopathy has been identified recently as both prevalent in end-stage liver disease [32] and as a potential cause of cardiovascular complications in these patients [33]. Thus, depending on the outcome measure, the utility of a screening test may be to a greater or lesser extent independent of its ability to detect CAD. Also, in terms of outcomes, what is the time period of interest – short term perioperative or long term? In relation to perioperative outcomes there are intraoperative factors during liver transplantation that may influence cardiovascular morbidity and mortality which may be unrelated to CAD. Hypotension and hypoperfusion secondary to blood loss, myocardial dysrhythmias and dysfunction at the time of reperfusion are well recognized intraoperative events. Studies have identified adverse intraoperative hemodynamic events as associated with perioperative myocardial injury [23], 6 month cardiovascular mortality and morbidity [3] and overall post-transplant outcome [34]. Finally, there is no consistent classification of cardiovascular outcomes in the published studies. Cardiovascular events considered range from troponin elevation through to death, some studies consider the identification of pre-operative CAD an adverse perioperative outcome. This variability makes comparison between studies difficult.

Thirdly, which patients were screened, and what was the screening algorithm? The studied population varies from all candidates through "intermediate risk" candidates to "high risk" candidates", with differing definitions and with differing algorithms for who actually undergoes the test under investigation. Again, the selection criteria can be expected to influence the utility of the test – it is not the test alone that is being evaluated but the test in the setting of the screening algorithm used. Additionally some studies exclude "high risk" candidates, often those with several major clinical risk factors who would be the group of patients in which a useful test would be expected to have the best positive predictive value.

Fourthly, what is the confidence in the results from the available literature? The majority of studies have small patient numbers and hence have low power. Even in those with larger total patient numbers, the number of outcomes is small. To take one example Tsutsui report a 50% mortality in patients with an abnormal DSE myocardial perfusion scan who underwent liver transplant [25], however this was 2 deaths in 4 patients. One or two less events (or a few more uneventful cases) and the result could be much less impressive.

These caveats should be borne in mind when considering the published literature and in evaluating future studies in this area.

Risk Factors

Cardiovascular risk factors are an established method for the stratification of perioperative cardiovascular risk in non-cardiac surgery, with the presumption that perioperative cardiovascular morbidity occurs in those with underlying CAD. The most commonly used approach is based the revised cardiac risk index described by Lee [35]. This scores the type of surgery along with the presence of clinical predictors (ischemic heart disease, compensated or prior heart failure, diabetes mellitus, renal insufficiency and cerebrovascular disease, Table 2). Higher scores predict more perioperative cardiovascular complications. The use of stratification by these "major" risk factors is the basis of current guidelines for perioperative cardiovascular assessment for non-cardiac surgeries [36, 37] specifically relating to liver transplantation the relationship between cardiovascular risk factors and 30 day cardiovascular outcomes (death and myocardial infarction) was recently investigated by Safadi and colleagues [24]. They found that on multivariate analysis the independent predictors were a history of CAD (odds ratio 4), prior stroke (odds ratio 6.6), as well as post-operative sepsis. When only perioperative myocardial infarction (MI) was considered as the outcome of interest history of stroke remained a predictor. The utility of using a risk-factor based assessment for CAD in liver transplant patients remains to be established.

Non-Invasive Testing

The use of non-invasive testing to identify CAD is well established in cardiology practice and has formed part of the standard guidelines for the cardiovascular evaluation of patients for non-cardiac surgery for many years [38,39]. Commonly used modalities are exercise testing and pharmacological stress testing.

Table 2. Major risk factors for perioperative cardiovascular complications

History of ischemic heart disease
Compensated or prior heart failure
Diabetes mellitus
Renal insufficiency
Cerebrovascular disease

Adapted from Lee [35], Fleisher [36] and Poldermans [37].

It should be noted that the recommended approach in most guidelines is to proceed to non-invasive testing in patients who have a number (usually 3 or greater) of major risk factors [36,37] whilst in the published studies in the pre-liver transplant population the indications are in general much broader. This approach will result in the performance of the non-invasive test under scrutiny in a population which most likely has a lower prevalence of CAD, affecting the utility of the non-invasive test in the manner alluded to already - the false positive rate will be higher than in a more restricted population.

Exercise Testing

Exercise testing is not frequently performed in the liver transplant population. Patients with end-stage liver disease frequently have fatigue and limited exercise tolerance; the frequency of severe exercise limitation in this group has been assessed at almost 50% [40,41]. Thus obtaining satisfactory workloads to make theses tests valid is often not possible. Additionally it has been reported that ST segment changes with exercise in the cirrhotic population may not reflect CAD [42]. For more details about exercise testing see chapter 6.

Pharmacologic Testing

Dobutamine stress echocardiography (DSE) and stress (dipyridamole or adenosine) thallium isotope perfusion imaging with single proton emission computed tomography (SPECT) are the most established pharmacologic methods of non-invasive cardiac testing. There have been many studies of the utility of these modalities in assessment for non-cardiac surgery; a recent meta-analysis suggests that DSE has better negative predictive characteristics (negative study predicting low chance of perioperative complications) with positive predictive characteristics similar [43]. With regards to liver transplantation it has been suggested that the physiologic changes induced by dobutamine are similar to those occurring during liver transplantation [5], thus potentially increasing the utility of DSE in this population. Over the years a number of studies have used DSE in the preoperative evaluation of liver transplant candidates [22-26,31,44,45], these are summarized in Table 3. Unfortunately the results have been generally disappointing: reported negative predictive values have been generally acceptable (75-100%) but the positive predictive values poor (0-33%).

Table 3. Studies evaluating dobutamine stress echocardiography in liver transplant candidates

Study	DSE criteria	N (total assessed/DSE)	DSE positive	Cor Angio/CAD present	Transplanted	Transplant Events
Donovan [22], 1996	Clinical suspicion Age >45, HTN, DM, history	190/165	11	9/3	71 CAD excluded	1 MI, 4 LV failure – all neg DSE
Plotkin [31], 1998	Age>50 + 2 risk factors, Age>60, DM, clinical suspicion	220/80	6	6/2	31 None DSE pos	0 complications
Williams [45], 2000	Age>60, HTN, DM, smoking history. Known CAD excluded	?/121	2 67 non-diagnostic	-	61 (25/34/2 neg/non-diag/pos DSE	CV events 5/3/0
Findlay [23], 2005	Age>50, clinical suspicion, FH, CAD, HTN, DM, obesity	117/73	8	7/1	117	Elevated troponin 2/8 pos DSE 8/65 neg DSE
Tsutsui [25], 2006	Exclusion: age<18, unstable, recent MI, unstable angina	?/230 DSE with myocardial perfusion imaging	18 (abnormal perfusion) 5 (RWMA)	17/7	85	Hospital death 2/4 abnormal perfusion 2/81 normal perfusion
Umphrey [26], 2007	Age>45, DM, PVD, 2 risk factors	284/157	0 58 non-diagnostic	9/0	284	CV events at 4mo 9/58 non-diagnostic 7/226 negative
Harinstein [44], 2007	? (All had DSE + cor angio)	?/105	9 of 78 27 non-diagnostic 14 known CAD*	9/4 (pos DSE)† 55/20 (neg DSE)	21	1 CV event at 1yr CAD excluded
Safadi [24], 2009	"routine"	403/356	22	-	403	48 MI or death in 30d Pos DSE not predictive

CAD - coronary artery disease, cor angio -coronary angiography, CV- cardiovascular, DSE-doutamine stress echocardiography, DM - diabetes mellitus, FH - family history, HTN -hypertension, MI - myocardial infarction, PVD - peripheral vascular disease, RWMA - regional wall motion
* patients with known CAD excluded from further analysis.
† using >50% stenosis as definition.

Some reasons for this have been touched on above, in addition the proportion of non-diagnostic tests (did not reach the target heart rate) is generally high, which may affect the utility of the test – although Umphrey does reports that a non-diagnostic test was a risk factor for adverse outcome [26]. The high proportion of inadequate heart rate responses may be related to the frequent use of beta-blockade to control portal hypertension in this group and also possibly to the chronotropic incompetence seen with cirrhotic cardiomyopathy [46]. The results with isotope perfusion imaging have been similar, again generally good negative predictive values are reported, but poor positive prediction [16,47-49]. Whilst disappointing for the clinician searching for a test to identify CAD the results in liver transplant candidates are not dissimilar to those reported for stress testing in the general population of non-cardiac surgery patients. Reviewing 32 studies of perfusion imaging and 16 of DSE in non-cardiac surgery candidates Fleisher reports positive predictive values ranging from 2-20% for perfusion imaging and 0-33% for DSE with negative predictive values of around 99% and 93-100% respectively [36]. Part of the issue may be the too frequent use of stress testing (that is using it in a group with a low disease prevalence), several investigators have noted that if only those patients with more risk factors go forward to stress testing the positive utility of the results is improved without affecting the negative prediction value [40,50,51].

Considering the current body of evidence it seems that pharmacologic stress testing as it currently stands may be of value in identifying those at low risk of perioperative cardiac events (using the seemingly good negative predictive value), but is inadequate alone to identify high risk patients. False positives are common hence a non-invasive result suggesting CAD needs confirmation. Future refinements in non-invasive testing may hold promise for improved utility: Tsustsui has reported the use of DSE and real-time myocardial imaging using echo-contrast [25] and dobutamine stress magnetic resonance imaging is also being investigated [52]. In the meantime clinicians developing screening guidelines for liver transplant patients within their own program should consider the available evidence, particularly that related to the false positive rate associated with the use of non-invasive screening tests and the consequent rate of coronary angiography, and select a strategy that best suits their goals.

Coronary Angiography

Coronary angiography definitively identifies coronary artery disease. Given the limitations of risk factor and non-invasive testing based risk stratification a proportion of liver transplant candidates will undergo this to define their CAD status. Whilst there have been recommendations that some sub-groups of the liver transplant population go directly to angiography without non-invasive testing [47] this approach is currently not recommended in the most recent ACC/AHA or ESC/ESA guidelines [36,37]. Concern has been raised about the frequency of cardiac catheterization associated complications in liver transplant candidates. Sharma recently reported a case-control study [53] finding that the end-stage liver disease patients required more blood and blood products and had a higher incidence of post-procedure pseudoaneurysm than the control group: however the overall conclusion was that cardiac catheterization can be safely accomplished in these patients with appropriate attention to per-procedural coagulation. An additional concern is that of contrast-induced nephropathy given the frequency of renal insufficiency seen in liver transplant candidates. A recent series examining coronary angiography performed in patients with advanced kidney disease was reassuring, reporting that there was no acceleration in renal decline post-angiography [54]. Thus, whilst not without risk, it seems that coronary angiography is a reasonable procedure to perform in liver transplant candidates, particularly when the results may potentially influence transplant candidacy and pre-operative management.

Currently interest is increasing in the use of multislice-CT coronary angiography as a non-invasive means of directly evaluating coronary artery lesions [55]. This modality has shown promise in the evaluation of patients for CAD and its role in perioperative evaluation has begun to be assessed [56].

Other Tests

Coronary artery calcification is associated with CAD and adverse cardiac outcomes [57]. Coronary artery calcification score in end-stage liver disease patients has been associated with CAD risk factors [58], how this relates to outcome predication is as yet unknown.

Biomarkers have shown some promise in cardiovascular risk prediction. In renal transplant candidates and recipients elevated pre-transplant troponin was recently demonstrated to be a powerful independent predictor of cardiovascular outcome irrespective of other cardiovascular risk factors [59,60]. No similar information is available for liver transplant patients however this finding does suggest a route for further research.

CAD and Transplant Candidacy

Before leaving the topic of assessment of liver transplant candidates for CAD there is one further issue that should be discussed: what is the purpose of the evaluation? Whilst this may seem self-evident initially - the purpose is to identify candidates with CAD - the subsequent issue is how the information gained is used. Currently there is no good evidence to determine which, if any, patients with CAD have a severity of disease such that they are unlikely to benefit from liver transplantation. There are also no published guidelines suggesting risk stratification to assist clinicians and programs in making decisions about the appropriateness of transplantation in either individuals or groups of patient with CAD, indeed the current evidence is such that the basis of any such guidelines would be questionable. However, the presence and severity of CAD undoubtedly figures into decisions about whether to proceed with or deny transplantation to individual patients.

A corollary may be drawn with renal transplantation. Here transplantation confers a survival benefit for patients with and without CAD. Outcomes are, however, worse for patients with CAD than for those without (although still improved over no transplant) [61]. Studies have documented that a diagnosis of CAD reduces access to transplantation [62] and the identification of CAD may not only lead to a denial of transplantation but may not result in appropriate referral for management of CAD [63]. Thus the screening may confer no benefit on the individual patient although the population outcome for those transplanted may be improved. Whilst adequate reliable data for liver transplantation is not available it is likely to be similar – the limited evidence is that CAD confers a worse outcome after transplant than no CAD and it is likely that transplanted patients with end-stage liver disease and CAD have better survival than those not transplanted. The moral and ethical issues raised by this, given the limited supply of organs, are beyond the scope of this chapter but should be considered by the individual clinician when faced with a liver transplant candidate with CAD and also by liver transplant programs when planning their policies for such patients. Until better data is available the best approach that can be suggested is that the presence of CAD, particularly severe CAD, is one of the factors considered in deciding on the candidacy, however for each individual patient this is considered along with all relevant factors.

Management of the Patient with CAD

Revascularization

The liver transplant candidate with identified CAD requires the clinician to make decisions regarding the appropriateness of proceeding to liver transplantation and, if proceeding to transplantation, how to manage the CAD. The liver transplant specific literature on this topic is scant. In Plotkin's original series of 32 CAD patients undergoing liver transplantation with a 50% mortality [4] the majority (20) had undergone coronary artery bypass grafting (CABG) surgery with 9 medically managed and one percutaneous transluminal coronary angioplasty (PTCA) there was no difference in outcome in the CABG patients versus those medically managed. A more recent series [6] has, as would be expected, a greater proportion of patients with percutaneous interventions (PCI) (40% of the CAD patients) and reported lower overall mortality (26%) but did not differentiate between the treatment groups. In the surgical population in general the appropriate approach to patients with CAD undergoing non-cardiac surgery has been controversial. When compared to medical management prior revascularization was shown to decrease mortality and myocardial infarction after high risk non-cardiac surgery (including abdominal and vascular procedures) [64] and percutaneous interventions have been found to be as efficacious as CABG in this regard [65]. However no outcome benefit to pre-operative revascularization (either surgical or percutaneous) has been demonstrated in randomized studies of at risk patients undergoing vascular surgery [66,67]. The extensive literature on this topic is recently reviewed in the latest ACC/AHA guidelines for preoperative cardiac evaluation for non-cardiac surgery [36] The current recommendations from this group are for revascularization for patients with stable angina and left main disease, 3-vessel disease, 2-vesel disease with proximal LAD stenosis, unstable angina or non-ST-elevation MI. Additionally PCI is recommended in symptomatic patients. For the group of patients most often identified during liver transplantation assessment – those with abnormal non-interventional testing the guidelines state that the usefulness of revascularization is 'not well established' and prophylactic revascularization for stable CAD is not recommended.

Where does this leave the clinician faced with a liver transplant candidate with CAD? Clearly, in need of better quality evidence. However, until that becomes available a suggested approach follows.

For the patient with a non-invasive test result suggesting CAD coronary angiography should be undertaken to define the coronary anatomy. If significant coronary artery lesions are found and these are amenable to PCI then this should be undertaken. Once this has been undertaken then the patient should be considered for transplantation. CABG prior to liver transplantation may not a realistic option given the poor outcomes in advanced liver disease [68] but a combined procedure may be considered [69].

For the patient with known CAD a non-invasive study should be performed. If this is consistent with inducible ischemia or reduced flow reserve, then proceed to coronary angiography and intervention, if advisable and feasible, as above. If the non-invasive test is not concerning, proceed to transplant.

PCI and Coronary Artery Stents

When PCI is performed often coronary artery stents are deployed in the vessel post angioplasty. Two general types are currently used – bare-metal and drug-eluting stents (DES). For both a period of dual antiplatelet therapy (aspirin plus a thienopyridine) is recommended to prevent re-thrombosis, currently for 1 month after bare-metal and for ideally 12 months after DES [70]. Premature discontinuation of dual anti-platelet therapy has been reported to result in a 29% re-thrombosis rate [71]. Patients with coronary artery stents undergoing non-cardiac surgery are at risk of post-procedure cardiac events related to stent thrombosis, the frequency of these events depends on the type of stent and time from placement – for bare-metal stents this falls from 10% at less than 30 days to 3% at 90 days [72]; with DES this is 6.4% at less that 30 days and 3% at over 1 year [73]. Given these findings the recommendation is to place bare-metal stents in patients anticipated to undergo surgery within 12 months [70], with the provision of at least one month of dual anti-platelet therapy; this would apply to liver transplant candidates anticipate to have a one-month or more wait for an organ. An alternative approach of performing only balloon angioplasty has been proposed; this avoids the issues associated with stents in the peri-operative period. However, re-angioplasty may be required. More definitive management can be addressed post-surgery. This approach may be more appropriate for a liver transplant candidate anticipated to proceed to transplant within one month of PCI.

Intraoperative Management

Patients with CAD undergoing liver transplantation should have the same routine invasive monitoring as other liver transplant patients. Anesthesia management should be with the usual care and diligence of a specialized team. Aside from the exhortation to "avoid hypoxia, hypotension and tachycardia" one specific perioperative strategy that has potential benefit in the CAD patient during liver transplantation is beta blockade. Safadi found that the use of beta-blockers in the perioperative period was an independent predictor of favorable cardiac outcome [24]. In non-cardiac surgery in general the use of perioperative beta-blockade had been recently heavily scrutinized after the results of the POISE trial [74]. This found that whilst perioperative beta-blockade decreased post-operative myocardial infarction there was an excess of deaths in the beta-blockade group, potentially due to detrimental effects in low cardiac risk patients versus beneficial effects in higher cardiac risk patients [75]. Current recommendations would support the use of perioperative blockade in intermediate and high cardiac risk liver transplantation patients, with these patients defined by the presence of one or more major cardiac risk factor [76]. Patients beta-blocked prior to transplantation should have this continued through the peri-operative period.

Post-Transplant Management

The prominence of cardiovascular related morbidity and mortality in the longer term post-transplantation [1,2] implies that management of CAD should be aggressively pursued in this population. Along with the pre-existing risk factors for CAD that patients may bring to transplantation the immunosuppressive medications employed post-transplantation can themselves cause or exacerbate risk factors for CAD and have been implicated directly in CAD development [77]. Currently there are no specific recommendations for liver transplant patients, however patients with known CAD should continue to be followed up post-transplantation and managed as suggested by the most recent guidelines [78]. In patients transplanted without known CAD clinicians should have a high index of suspicion for the development of CAD in the post-transplant years and risk factors should be sought and appropriately managed with the hope that such interventions will decrease and/or delay the development of significant CAD and its attendant complications and mortality [79].

Conclusion

CAD is prevalent in end-stage liver disease and is a significant contributor to post-liver transplant morbidity and mortality. Currently the optimum approach to identifying CAD in liver transplant candidates is unclear with controversy regarding the best approach and whether this should differ from the approach to other non-cardiac surgeries. Also unclear are the optimum management strategies for patients identified as having CAD both in the perioperative and in the longer term post liver transplantation. These important areas merit further thoughtful clinical investigations. Whilst awaiting clearer evidence clinicians should carefully consider the available evidence when deciding how to approach individual patients and in setting up protocols for their transplant programs.

References

[1] Johnston SD, Morris JK, Cramb R, Gunson BK, Neuberger J. Cardiovascular morbidity and mortality after orthotopic liver transplantation. *Transplantation* 2002; 73: 901-6.
[2] Pruthi J, Medkiff KA, Esrason KT, Donovan JA, Yoshida EM, Erb SR et al. Analysis of causes of death in liver transplant recipients who survived more than 3 years. *Liver Transpl* 2001; 7: 811-5.

[3] Fouad TR, Abdel-Razek WM, Burak KW, Bain VG, Lee SS. Prediction of cardiac complications after liver transplantation. *Transplantation* 2009; 87: 763-770.

[4] Plotkin JS, Scott VL, Pinna A, Dobsch BP, De Wolf AM, Kang Y. Morbidity and mortality in patients with coronary artery disease undergoing orthotopic liver transplantation. *Liver Transpl Surg* 1996; 2: 426-30.

[5] Plevak DJ. Stress echocardiography identifies coronary artery disease in liver transplant candidates. *Liver Transpl. Surg* 1998; 4: 337-9.

[6] Diedrich DA, Findlay JY, Harrison BA, Rosen CB. Influence of coronary artery disease on outcomes after liver transplantation. *Transplant. Proc* 2008; 40: 3554-7.

[7] Fraker TD, Jr., Fihn SD, Gibbons RJ, Abrams J, Chatterjee K, Daley J et al. 2007 chronic angina focused update of the ACC/AHA 2002 guidelines for the management of patients with chronic stable angina: a report of the American College of Cardiology/American Heart Association Task Force on Practice Guidelines Writing Group to develop the focused update of the 2002 guidelines for the management of patients with chronic stable angina. *J Am Coll Cardio.* 2007; 50: 2264-74.

[8] Hansson GK. Inflammation, atherosclerosis, and coronary artery disease. *N Engl J Med* 2005;352: 1685-95.

[9] Smith EJ, Jain AK, Rothman MT. New developments in coronary stent technology. *J Interv Cardiol* 2006;19: 493-9.

[10] Howell WL, Manion WC. The low incidence of myocardial infarction in patients with portal cirrhosis of the liver: A review of 639 cases of cirrhosis of the liver from 17,731 autopsies. *Am Heart J* 1960; 60: 341-4.

[11] Otsubo R, Higuchi Mde L, Gutierrez PS, Benvenuti LA, Massarollo PC, Costa AL, Ramires JA. Influence of chronic liver disease on coronary atherosclerosis vulnerability features. *Int J Cardiol* 2006; 109: 387-391.

[12] Parrish HM, Eberly AL, Jr. Negative association of coronary atherosclerosis with liver cirrhosis and chronic alcoholism--a statistical fallacy. JJ *Indiana State Med Assoc* 1961; 54: 341-7.

[13] Kalaitzakis E, Rosengren A, Skommevik T, Bjornsson E. Coronary artery disease in patients with liver cirrhosis. *Dig Dis Sci* 2010; 55: 467-75.

[14] Carey WD, Dumot JA, Pimentel RR, Barnes DS, Hobbs RE, Henderson JM et al. The prevalence of coronary artery disease in liver transplant candidates over age 50. *Transplantation* 1995; 59: 859-64.

[15] Tiukinhoy-Laing SD, Rossi JS, Bayram M, De Luca L, Gafoor S, Blei A et al. Cardiac hemodynamic and coronary angiographic characteristics of patients being evaluated for liver transplantation. *Am J Cardio* 2006; 98: 178-81.

[16] Aydinalp A, Bal U, Atar I, Ertan C, Aktas A, Yildirir A et al. Value of stress myocardial perfusion scanning in diagnosis of severe coronary artery disease in liver transplantation candidates. *Transplant Proc* 2009; 41: 3757-60.

[17] Lerner DJ, Kannel WB. Patterns of coronary heart disease morbidity and mortality in the sexes: a 26-year follow-up of the Framingham population. *Patterns of coronary heart disease morbidity and mortality in the sexes: a 26-year follow-up of the Framingham population* 1986;111: 383-90.

[18] Gordon T, Kannel WB, Hjortland MC, McNamara PM. Menopause and coronary heart disease. The Framingham Study. *Ann Intern Med* 1978; 89: 157-61.

[19] Reuben A. Alcohol and the liver. *Curr Opin Gastroenterol* 2006; 22: 263-71.

[20] Sofair AN, Barry V, Manos MM, Thomas A, Zaman A, Terrault NA et al. The Epidemiology and Clinical Characteristics of Patients With Newly Diagnosed Alcohol-related Liver Disease: Results From Population-based Surveillance. *J Clin Gastroenterol* 2010; 44: 301-7

[21] Te HS, Jensen DM. Epidemiology of hepatitis B and C viruses: a global overview. *Clin Liver Dis* 2010; 14: 1-21

[22] Donovan CL, Marcovitz PA, Punch JD, Bach DS, Brown KA, Lucey MR, Armstrong WF. Two-dimensional and dobutamine stress echocardiography in the preoperative assessment of patients with end-stage liver disease prior to orthotopic liver transplantation. *Transplantation* 1996; 61: 1180-8.

[23] Findlay JY, Keegan MT, Pellikka PP, Rosen CB, Plevak DJ. Preoperative dobutamine stress echocardiography, intraoperative events, and intraoperative myocardial injury in liver transplantation. *Transplant Proc* 2005; 37: 2209-13.

[24] Safadi A, Homsi M, Maskoun W, Lane KA, Singh I, Sawada SG, Mahenthiran J. Perioperative risk predictors of cardiac outcomes in patients undergoing liver transplantation surgery. *Circulation* 2009;120: 1189-94.

[25] Tsutsui JM, Mukherjee S, Elhendy A, Xie F, Lyden ER, O'Leary E et al. Value of dobutamine stress myocardial contrast perfusion echocardiography in patients with advanced liver disease. *Liver Transpl* 2006;12: 592-9.

[26] Umphrey LG, Hurst RT, Eleid MF, Lee KS, Reuss CS, Hentz JG et al. Preoperative dobutamine stress echocardiographic findings and subsequent short-term adverse cardiac events after orthotopic liver transplantation. *Liver Transpl* 2008;14: 886-92.

[27] Arslan U, Turkoglu S, Balcioglu S, Tavil Y, Karakan T, Cengel A. Association between nonalcoholic fatty liver disease and coronary artery disease. *Coron Artery Dis* 2007;18: 433-6.

[28] Assy N, Djibre A, Farah R, Grosovski M, Marmor A. Presence of coronary plaques in patients with nonalcoholic fatty liver disease. *Radiology 2010;* 254: 393-400.

[29] Gronbaek M. Epidemiologic evidence for the cardioprotective effects associated with consumption of alcoholic beverages. *Pathophysiology* 2004;10: 83-92.

[30] Corrao G, Rubbiati L, Bagnardi V, Zambon A, Poikolainen K. Alcohol and coronary heart disease: a meta-analysis. *Addiction* 2000; 95: 1505-23.

[31] Plotkin JS, Benitez RM, Kuo PC, Njoku MJ, Ridge LA, Lim JW et al. Dobutamine stress echocardiography for preoperative cardiac risk stratification in patients undergoing orthotopic liver transplantation. *Liver Transpl Surg* 1998;4(4):253-7.

[32] Henriksen JH, Moller S. Cardiac and systemic haemodynamic complications of liver cirrhosis. *Scand Cardiovasc J* 2009; 43: 218-25.

[33] Rabie RN, Cazzaniga M, Salerno F, Wong F. The use of E/A ratio as a predictor of outcome in cirrhotic patients treated with transjugular intrahepatic portosystemic shunt. *Am J Gastroenterol* 2009;104: 2458-66.

[34] Reich DL, Wood RK, Jr., Emre S, Bodian CA, Hossain S, Krol M, Feierman D. Association of intraoperative hypotension and pulmonary hypertension with adverse outcomes after orthotopic liver transplantation. *J Cardiothorac Vasc Anesth* 2003;17: 699-702.

[35] Lee TH, Marcantonio ER, Mangione CM, Thomas EJ, Polanczyk CA, Cook EF et al. Derivation and prospective validation of a simple index for prediction of cardiac risk of major noncardiac surgery. *Circulation* 1999;100: 1043-49.

[36] Fleisher LA, Beckman JA, Brown KA, Calkins H, Chaikof EL, Fleischmann KE et al. ACC/AHA 2007 guidelines on perioperative cardiovascular evaluation and care for noncardiac surgery: a report of the American College of Cardiology/American Heart Association Task Force on Practice Guidelines (Writing Committee to Revise the 2002 Guidelines on Perioperative Cardiovascular Evaluation for Noncardiac Surgery) developed in collaboration with the American Society of Echocardiography, American Society of Nuclear Cardiology, Heart Rhythm Society, Society of Cardiovascular Anesthesiologists, Society for Cardiovascular Angiography and Interventions, Society for Vascular Medicine and Biology, and Society for Vascular Surgery. *J Am Col. Cardiol* 2007; 50): e159-241.

[37] Poldermans D, Bax JJ, Boersma E, De Hert S, Eeckhout E, Fowkes G et al. Guidelines for pre-operative cardiac risk assessment and perioperative cardiac management in non-cardiac surgery: the Task Force for Preoperative Cardiac Risk Assessment and Perioperative Cardiac Management in Non-cardiac Surgery of the European Society of Cardiology (ESC) and endorsed by the European Society of Anaesthesiology (ESA). *Eur. Heart J* 2009;30: 2769-2812.

[38] Eagle KA, Berger PB, Calkins H, Chaitman BR, Ewy GA, Fleischmann KE et al. ACC/AHA guideline update for perioperative cardiovascular evaluation for noncardiac surgery--executive summary: a report of the American College of Cardiology/American Heart Association Task Force on Practice Guidelines (Committee to Update the 1996 Guidelines on Perioperative Cardiovascular Evaluation for Noncardiac Surgery). *J Am Coll Cardiol* 2002; 39: 542-53.

[39] Fleisher LA, Beckman JA, Brown KA, Calkins H, Chaikof EL, Fleischmann KE et al. ACC/AHA 2007 Guidelines on Perioperative Cardiovascular Evaluation and Care for Noncardiac Surgery: Executive Summary: A Report of the American College of Cardiology/American Heart Association Task Force on Practice Guidelines (Writing Committee to Revise the 2002 Guidelines on Perioperative Cardiovascular Evaluation for Noncardiac Surgery) Developed in Collaboration With the American Society of Echocardiography, American Society of Nuclear Cardiology, Heart Rhythm Society, Society of Cardiovascular Anesthesiologists, Society for Cardiovascular Angiography and Interventions, Society for Vascular Medicine and Biology, and Society for Vascular Surgery. *J Am Coll Cardio.* 2007; 50: 1707-32.

[40] Dharancy S, Lemyze M, Boleslawski E, Neviere R, Declerck N, Canva V et al. Impact of impaired aerobic capacity on liver transplant candidates. *Transplantation* 2008; 86: 1077-83.

[41] Iscar M, Montoliu MA, Ortega T, Rodriguez B, Rodriguez M, Glez-Pinto I, Alonso P. Functional capacity before and after liver transplantation. *Transplant Proc* 2009; 41: 1014-5.

[42] Mori T, Nomura M, Hori A, Kondo N, Bando S, Ito S. Mechanism of ST segment depression during exercise tests in patients with liver cirrhosis. *J Med Invest* 2007; 54: 109-115.

[43] Beattie WS, Abdelnaem E, Wijeysundera DN, Buckley DN. A meta-analytic comparison of preoperative stress echocardiography and nuclear scintigraphy imaging. *Anesth. Analg.* 2006;102: 8-16.

[44] Harinstein ME, Flaherty JD, Ansari AH, Robin J, Davidson CJ, Rossi JS et al. Predictive value of dobutamine stress echocardiography for coronary artery disease detection in liver transplant candidates. *Am J Transplant* 2008;8: 1523-28.

[45] Williams K, Lewis JF, Davis G, Geiser EA. Dobutamine stress echocardiography in patients undergoing liver transplantation evaluation. *Transplantation* 2000;69: 2354-6.

[46] Wong F, Girgrah N, Graba J, Allidina Y, Liu P, Blendis L. The cardiac response to exercise in cirrhosis. *Gut* 2001;49: 268-75.

[47] Davidson CJ, Gheorghiade M, Flaherty JD, Elliot MD, Reddy SP, Wang NC et al. Predictive value of stress myocardial perfusion imaging in liver transplant candidates. *Am J Cardiol.*2002;89: 359-60.

[48] Zoghbi GJ, Patel AD, Ershadi RE, Heo J, Bynon JS, Iskandrian AE. Usefulness of preoperative stress perfusion imaging in predicting prognosis after liver transplantation. *Am J Cardiol* 2003;92: 1066-71.

[49] Kryzhanovski VA, Beller GA. Usefulness of preoperative noninvasive radionuclide testing for detecting coronary artery disease in candidates for liver transplantation. *Am J Cardiol* 1997;79: 986-8.

[50] Das MK, Pellikka PA, Mahoney DW, Roger VL, Oh JK, McCully RB, Seward JB. Assessment of cardiac risk before nonvascular surgery: dobutamine stress echocardiography in 530 patients. *J Am Coll Cardiol* 2000;35: 1647-53.

[51] Morgan PB, Panomitros GE, Nelson AC, Smith DF, Solanki DR, Zornow MH. Low utility of dobutamine stress echocardiograms in the preoperative evaluation of patients scheduled for noncardiac surgery. *Anesth. Analg.* 2002; 95: 512-16.

[52] Nagel E, Lehmkuhl HB, Bocksch W, Klein C, Vogel U, Frantz E et al. Noninvasive diagnosis of ischemia-induced wall motion abnormalities with the use of high-dose dobutamine stress MRI: comparison with dobutamine stress echocardiography. *Circulation* 1999; 99: 763-70.

[53] Sharma M, Yong C, Majure D, Zellner C, Roberts JP, Bass NM et al. Safety of cardiac catheterization in patients with end-stage liver disease awaiting liver transplantation. *Am J Cardiol* 2009;103: 742-6.

[54] Kumar N, Dahri L, Brown W, Duncan N, Singh S, Baker C et al. Effect of elective coronary angiography on glomerular filtration rate in patients with advanced chronic kidney disease. *Clin J Am Soc Nephrol* 2009; 4: 1907-13.

[55] Schuijf JD, Pundziute G, Jukema JW, Lamb HJ, van der Hoeven BL, de Roos A et al. Diagnostic accuracy of 64-slice multislice computed tomography in the noninvasive evaluation of significant coronary artery disease. *Am J Cardiol* 2006; 98: 145-8.

[56] Buffa V, De Cecco CN, Cossu L, Fedeli S, Vallone A, Ruopoli R et al. Preoperative coronary risk assessment with dual-source CT in patients undergoing noncoronary cardiac surgery. *Radiol. Med 2010; 115: 1028-37*

[57] Pletcher MJ, Tice JA, Pignone M, Browner WS. Using the coronary artery calcium score to predict coronary heart disease events: a systematic review and meta-analysis. *Arch Intern Med* 2004; 164: 1285-92.

[58] McAvoy NC, Kochar N, McKillop G, Newby DE, Hayes PC. Prevalence of coronary artery calcification in patients undergoing assessment for orthotopic liver transplantation. *Liver Transpl* 2008;14: 1725-31.

[59] Hickson LJ, Cosio FG, El-Zoghby ZM, Gloor JM, Kremers WK, Stegall MD et al. Survival of patients on the kidney transplant wait list: relationship to cardiac troponin T. *Am J Transplant* 2008; 8: 2352-9.

[60] Hickson LT, El-Zoghby ZM, Lorenz EC, Stegall MD, Jaffe AS, Cosio FG. Patient survival after kidney transplantation: relationship to pretransplant cardiac troponin T levels. *Am J Transplant* 2009; 9: 1354-61.

[61] Bittar J, Arenas P, Chiurchiu C, de la Fuente J, de Arteaga J, Douthat W, Massari PU. Renal transplantation in high cardiovascular risk patients. *Transplant. Rev. (Orlando).* 2009; 23: 224-34.

[62] Stel VS, van Dijk PC, van Manen JG, Dekker FW, Ansell D, Conte F et al. Prevalence of co-morbidity in different European RRT populations and its effect on access to renal transplantation. *Nephrol Dial Transplant* 2005; 20: 2803-11.

[63] Patel RK, Mark PB, Johnston N, McGeoch R, Lindsay M, Kingsmore DB et al. Prognostic value of cardiovascular screening in potential renal transplant recipients: a single-center prospective observational study. *Am. J Transplant* 2008; 8: 1673-83.

[64] Eagle KA, Rihal CS, Mickel MC, Holmes DR, Foster ED, Gersh BJ. Cardiac risk of noncardiac surgery: influence of coronary disease and type of surgery in 3368 operations. CASS Investigators and University of Michigan Heart Care Program. Coronary Artery Surgery Study. *Circulation* 1997; 96(6): 1882-7.

[65] Hassan SA, Hlatky MA, Boothroyd DB, Winston C, Mark DB, Brooks MM, Eagle KA. Outcomes of noncardiac surgery after coronary bypass surgery or coronary angioplasty in the Bypass Angioplasty Revascularization Investigation (BARI). *Am. J Med.* 2001;110: 260-6.

[66] McFalls EO, Ward HB, Moritz TE, Goldman S, Krupski WC, Littooy F et al. Coronary-artery revascularization before elective major vascular surgery. *N Engl J Med* 2004;351: 2795-2804.

[67] Poldermans D, Schouten O, Vidakovic R, Bax JJ, Thomson IR, Hoeks SE et al. A clinical randomized trial to evaluate the safety of a noninvasive approach in high-risk patients undergoing major vascular surgery: the DECREASE-V Pilot Study. *J Am. Coll Cardiol* 2007;49: 1763-9.

[68] Filsoufi F, Salzberg SP, Rahmanian PB, Schiano TD, Elsiesy H, Squire A, Adams DH. Early and late outcome of cardiac surgery in patients with liver cirrhosis. *Liver Transpl* 2007;13: 990-5.

[69] Axelrod D, Koffron A, Dewolf A, Baker A, Fryer J, Baker T et al. Safety and efficacy of combined orthotopic liver transplantation and coronary artery bypass grafting. *Liver Transp.* 2004;10: 1386-90.

[70] Grines CL, Bonow RO, Casey DE, Jr., Gardner TJ, Lockhart PB, Moliterno DJ et al. Prevention of premature discontinuation of dual antiplatelet therapy in patients with coronary artery stents: a science advisory from the American Heart Association, American College of Cardiology, Society for Cardiovascular Angiography and Interventions, American College of Surgeons, and American Dental Association, with representation from the American College of Physicians. *J Am Coll Cardiol* 2007;49: 734-39.

[71] Iakovou I, Schmidt T, Bonizzoni E, Ge L, Sangiorgi GM, Stankovic G et al. Incidence, predictors, and outcome of thrombosis after successful implantation of drug-eluting stents. *JAMA* 2005;293: 2126-30.

[72] Nuttall GA, Brown MJ, Stombaugh JW, Michon PB, Hathaway MF, Lindeen KC et al. Time and cardiac risk of surgery after bare-metal stent percutaneous coronary intervention. *Anesthesiology* 2008;109: 588-95.

[73] Rabbitts JA, Nuttall GA, Brown MJ, Hanson AC, Oliver WC, Holmes DR, Rihal CS. Cardiac risk of noncardiac surgery after percutaneous coronary intervention with drug-eluting stents. *Anesthesiology* 2008;109: 596-604.

[74] Devereaux PJ, Yang H, Yusuf S, Guyatt G, Leslie K, Villar JC et al. Effects of extended-release metoprolol succinate in patients undergoing non-cardiac surgery (POISE trial): a randomised controlled trial. *Lancet* 2008;371: 1839-47.

[75] Lindenauer PK, Pekow P, Wang K, Mamidi DK, Gutierrez B, Benjamin EM. Perioperative beta-blocker therapy and mortality after major noncardiac surgery. *N Engl J Med.* 2005; 353: 349-61.

[76] Fleischmann KE, Beckman JA, Buller CE, Calkins H, Fleisher LA, Freeman WK et al. 2009 ACCF/AHA focused update on perioperative beta blockade: a report of the American college of cardiology foundation/American heart association task force on practice guidelines. *Circulation* 2009;120: 2123-51.

[77] Miller LW. Cardiovascular toxicities of immunosuppressive agents. *Am. J Transplant* 2002;2: 807-18.

[78] Smith SC, Jr., Allen J, Blair SN, Bonow RO, Brass LM, Fonarow GC et al. AHA/ACC guidelines for secondary prevention for patients with coronary and other atherosclerotic vascular disease: 2006 update endorsed by the National Heart, Lung, and Blood Institute. *J Am Coll Cardiol* 2006;47: 2130-9.

[79] Mells G, Neuberger J. Reducing the risks of cardiovascular disease in liver allograft recipients. *Transplantation* 2007;83: 1141-50.

In: Cardiovascular Diseases and Liver Transplantation
Editor: Zoka Milan, pp. 49-65
ISBN: 978-1-61122-910-3
© 2011 Nova Science Publishers, Inc.

Chapter III

Cardiac Arrhythmias and Liver Transplantation

Andrea Vannucci and Ivan Kangrga[*]
Department of Anesthesiology, Washington University School of Medicine
St. Louis, MO 63110, USA

Abstract

Cardiovascular events are a leading cause of morbidity and mortality in OLT. Pre-existing or perioperative arrhythmias are common in OLT but their incidence and impact on outcomes have not been systematically addressed.

Prolonged QT interval is a manifestation of cirrhotic cardiomyopathy but there is no consensus on its prognostic value or best management.

Reperfusion arrhythmias are common intraoperative complications of possible prognostic value for long-term outcomes. Preventative and best treatment strategies have not been defined.

Other serious arrhythmias, such as atrial fibrillation or ventricular arrhythmias, are not specifically related to ESLD or OLT but are prevalent in general population, particularly perioperatively.

The aim of this Chapter is to summarize reports of arrhythmias in OLT literature and to provide suggestions for perioperative management based on current knowledge of arrhythmias and clinical challenges of OLT.

Introduction

Patients with end-stage liver disease (ESLD) presenting for orthotopic liver transplantation (OLT) have multiple risk factors predisposing them to serious arrhythmias.

---

[*] Correspondence: Dr Ivan Kangrga, MD, PhD, Chief, Vascular, Hepatobiliary, Liver Transplant Anesthesia, Washington University School of Medicine, 660 S. Euclid Ave, Box 8054, St. Louis, MO 63110, Tel: +1 314-747-2858, Fax: +1 314-362-1185, E-mail: kangrgai@anest.wustl.edu.

First, cirrhotic cardiomyopathy, a cardiomyopathy of ESLD irrespective of etiology, is associated with myocardial repolarization abnormalities, such as the prolonged QT interval [1, 2, 3]. These abnormalities constitute a predisposition toward life-threatening ventricular arrhythmias and sudden cardiac death in general patient population. Second, there has recently been a trend of transplanting older and sicker recipients, with higher cardiovascular burden [4]. One implication of this trend is that perioperative physicians are more likely to encounter recipients with coronary artery disease and other cardiovascular comorbidities predisposing them for arrhythmias. An example of an arrhythmia which dramatically increases in incidence with age is atrial fibrillation. Finally, OLT itself creates a number of conditions favoring serious arrhythmias, such as hypothermia and electrolyte and metabolic derangements associated with graft reperfusion, embolic events or myocardial ischemia.

Despite the above, and the fact that cardiac complications are a leading cause of mortality after OLT, evidence for arrhythmia in liver transplant literature remains surprisingly sparse. In two case series [5,6] arrhythmias were frequent (6-15 %) intra- and post-operative complications in patients undergoing OLT. In one of these reports serious intraoperative arrhythmias appeared to be associated with increased perioperative mortality [5]. In addition, several case reports of arrhythmias complicating OLT underscored their possible etiology; unrecognized prolonged QT for torsade de pointes [7, 8], air-embolism for ventricular fibrillation [9], or hypomagnesemia for atrial fibrillation [10]. Finally, bradyarrhythmia, leading to cardiac arrest, has been a recognized component of the reperfusion syndrome since its first description [11] and may be related to long term survival after OLT [12, 13, 14].

The available evidence pertains to arrhythmias only as complications of OLT, but not as preexisting arrhythmias. Whereas other advanced cardiopulmonary conditions, such as severe coronary artery or structural heart disease, and severe pulmonary hypertension, are widely accepted contraindications to OLT [15, 16], the impact of arrhythmias on preoperative evaluation, risk stratification, management and outcomes, of OLT has not been systematically reported and remains largely unknown.

As the general topic of arrhythmias is broad, we will focus on common and clinically relevant arrhythmias for cirrhotic patients presenting for OLT, such as the reperfusion arrhythmias and prolonged QT interval, and on those that have not been described in literature but that we have encountered in our practice and found difficult to manage. An example of the latter is atrial fibrillation. We will attempt to address important clinical questions pertaining to the preoperative evaluation and perioperative management of an OLT candidate with arrhythmia, the impact of some common arrhythmias on outcomes, and whether arrhythmias constitute a contraindication to OLT.

General Approach to Patient with Arrhythmia

The two main goals of the preoperative evaluation of an OLT candidate with arrhythmia are assessment of eligibility for transplant, by ruling out severe underlying heart disease (i.e., coronary artery or severe valvular or structural disease, CHF), and medical optimization. Ideally, OLT candidates with significant arrhythmias should have completed cardiology diagnostics, addressing the underlying etiology, anatomic and physiologic abnormalitis and the degree of functional disability according to New York Heart Association. In patients that have not been evaluated, symptoms concerning for arrhythmias, such as pre-syncope or syncope, palpitations, or chest pains should always warrant a complete cardiology work up.

A thorough history and ECG are pivotal in diagnosing arrhythmias. Physical examination and further testing inform of possible underlying cardiopulmonary disease. The aggressiveness of the evaluation and treatment are typically commensurate with the severity of symptoms. Most common tests, in addition to a 12-lead ECG, include exercise test monitoring, long-term electrocardiographic recordings (i.e. Holter monitoring, event recording, etc.), echocardiography, and in select cases, invasive electrophysiological studies. Heart rate and QT variability, and signal averaged electrocardiography (i.e., late potentials and T wave alternans) have prognostic value for an increased risk of ventricular arrhythmia [17].

Frequent premature ventricular beats (PVCs) and supraventricular tachycardia (SVT) are commonly encountered on the preoperative assessment. PVCs do not carry high prognostic value when not associated with structural heart disease. However, PVCs associated with underlying structural heart disease and present with runs of ventricular tachycardia, have prognostic significance for sudden cardiac death and warrant full evaluation [18] Supraventricular tachycardias are usually not associated with structural heart disease, although there are exceptions (e.g., the presence of accessory pathways associated with hypertrophic cardiomyopathy or Ebstein's anomaly). Pharmacological management (usually beta or calcium channel blockers) is effective in most patients. Patients with recurrent symptomatic episodes, heart rates over 200 beats per minute, or with rapid antegrade conduction over an accessory pathway, should be considered for catheter ablation.

In conclusion, prevalence of clinically significant arrhythmias in OLT candidates is not known. Life-threatening intraoperative arrhythmias in OLT have been reported in up to 3% [5, 19, 20]. There is no evidence-based approach to the assessment and management of liver transplant candidates with arrhythmia. The effect of ESLD on pharmacokinetics of antiarrhythmic agents should be considered [21, 22]. Based on general knowledge, our opinion is that arrhythmias may be considered a contraindication for OLT if they are associated with severe uncompensated structural or ischemic heart disease, or if they cause recurring hemodynamic instability poorly controlled by medical or interventional treatment.

Prolonged QT Interval

Prolonged QT interval (LQT) is a common electrophysiological abnormality in ESLD. LQT reflects prolonged ventricular electrical systole. The main underlying mechanism is a decrease in the delayed rectifier (I_{Kr}), an outward potassium current responsible for rapid repolarization of myocyte action potentials [23]. In other clinical settings, LQT is of great significance because of its association with polymorphic ventricular arrhythmias, torsades de pointes (TdP), and sudden cardiac death [24]. The impact of LQT on outcomes and perioperative management of liver transplant recipients is not fully understood.

QT interval is measured from the beginning of QRS complex to the end of T wave, or in case of a prominent U wave, to the nadir between T and U waves. QT duration varies in standard ECG leads, and the longest measured in leads II and V5 or V6 is typically reported [25, 26, 27]. Commonly used is standardized, heart *rate-corrected QT* interval (QTc), based on the Bazett formula (QTc=QT/√(R-R interval). Clinically relevant ranges of QTc values are presented in Table 1. QTc is longer in women and QTc > 500 ms is considered highly abnormal in both sexes and identifies patients at high risk of ventricular arrhythmia.

The difference between the longest and the shortest QT interval in a 12-lead ECG is *QT dispersion* (QTd). QTd reflects spatial heterogeneity of myocardial repolarization. Elevated QTd (> 50-70 ms) may be a better predictor of TdP than LQT [28, 29]. Other parameters that correlate with dispersion of myocardial repolarization, are T wave peak-to-end interval and T-wave alternans may be better predictors of TdP [29], but have not been described in ESLD.

LQT is common in cirrhosis of all etiologies. Its prevalence correlates with the severity of liver disease [30, 31]. LQT was reported in 20-25% of Child-Pugh class A and in up to 60-80% of class C patients, compared to only 5% in control [32, 33]. Furthermore, LQT is significantly related to elevated plasma levels of brain-type natriuretic peptide (BNP), pro-BNP, and noradrenaline [34-37], and is considered a manifestation of cirrhotic cardiomyopathy.

LQT is associated with increased mortality in patients with ESLD [32, 34] but the relation to survival in OLT is largely unknown. A single study found no relation between QTc and postoperative mortality in pediatric recipients [38]. Normalization of LQT was reported in more than 50% of patients following OLT [33, 38]. Evidence for QT dispersion in cirrhosis is controversial. A 24-hour Holter monitor study of 23 cirrhotic patients found prolonged QTc but normal QT dispersion [39]. In contrast, a small study demonstrated a high prevalence (45%, n=33 patients) of increased corrected QT dispersion, and found it to be an independent predictor of mortality [40].

There are very few reports of LQT-related life-threatening arrhythmias in the OLT literature [7, 8]. It has been suggested that this is possibly due to normal QTd observed in some studies [39, 33, 37].

Clinical assessment. Although cirrhosis is the likely cause of LQT in a transplant candidate, other etiologies should be considered. Congenital LQT, particularly in children and adolescents, or myocardial ischemia and dilated cardiomyopathy in adults, should be ruled out. History of palpitations and syncope, or sudden death of a family member, should be queried. Medications (Table 2) and electrolyte disturbances (hypokalemia, hypocalcemia, and hypomagnesemia) implicated in LQT should be reviewed.

ECG should be analyzed for QT/QTc. Review of serial ECGs may show trends in QTc that can be reconciled with electrolyte abnormalities or medications. QTc > 500 ms and female gender constitute higher risk for development of life-threatening arrhythmias in non-cirrhotic patients [25]. QT dispersion is not a part of a routine automated ECG report and can be assessed manually.

Intraoperative management. The principal goal is to avoid further prolongation of QT interval and protect against development of ventricular arrhythmias.

Table 1. Normal and pro;onged QTc values (ms)

	Male	Female
Normal	<440	<450
Borderline	440-460	450-470
Prolonged	>460	>470
Highly Abnormal	>500	>500

QTc - Heart rate-corrected QT interval.

Table 2. Drugs associated with QT prolongation or TdP

Inhalational anesthetics	**Narcotics**
Sevoflurane	Methadone
Halothane	**Antimicrobials**
Desflurane	Clarythromycin
Antiarrhytmics	Erythromycin
Quinidine (IA)	Pentamidine
Procainamide (IA)	Halofantrine
Disopyramide (IA)	Sparfloxacine
Dofetilide (III)	Fluconazole
Ibutilide (III)	Ketoconazole
Sotalol (III)	**Antiemetics**
Amiodarone (III)	Domperidone
Bepridil (IV)	Droperidol
Nonsedating antihistamines	Ondansetron
Terfenadine	Dolasetron
Astemizole	**Immunosuppressants**
Psychotropics	Tacrolimus
Phenothiazines	**Antihypertensives**
Butyrophenones	Dihydralazine
Pimozide	Diltiazem
Miscellaneous	Nicardipine
Vasopressin	Verapamil
Cisapride	Mibefradil
Vitamins, supplements, herbals	
Cesium	
Licorice	

TdP - Torsade de pointes
Adapted from [41] and [48].
A comprehensive list is available at www.qtdrugs.org

No special intraoperative monitoring of LQT has been proposed during OLT. It should be noted that some newer monitors allow continuous real-time display of QTc and of QTc trends (Figure 1). Accuracy and usefulness of such monitoring have not been validated, but one could speculate that continuous QTc monitoring could possibly allow early detection of unfavorable trends and help guide therapeutic interventions.

Multiple anesthetic and adjunct drugs known to prolong QT interval or to be associated with TdP should be avoided or used judiciously. Sevoflurane, desflurane, and barbiturates prolong QTc whereas propofol, etomidate and isoflurane seem to be better choices [41, 42].

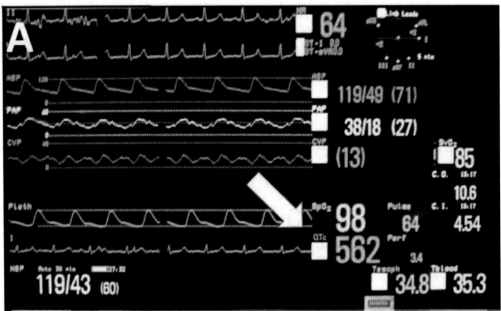

QTc - Heart rate-corrected QT interval, QTc - Heart rate-corrected QT interval.

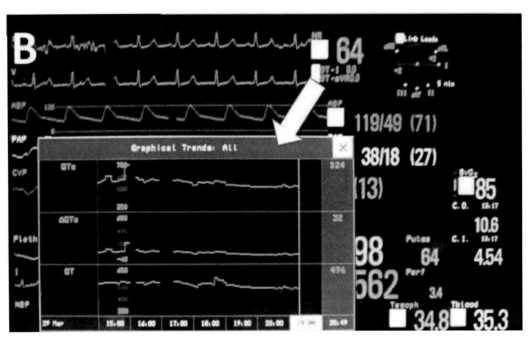

Figure 1. Intraoperative screen shots of a Philips Intelliveiw MP70 monitor taken during an liver transplantation (LT). A: continuous QTc monitoring on a dedicated ECG lead showing an instantaneous QTc value of 562 ms (arrow). B: a window displaying five-hour trending of QT, QTc, and ΔQTc (arrow) during the same case.

Succinylcholine, by inducing bradycardia, prolongs QT while vecuronium or atracurim have no appreciable effects. QTc and QTd may increase with induction and endotracheal intubation in coronary artery disease patients and this increase can be attenuated with beta blockers and fentanyl [43-45]. Such data do not exist for OLT.

Electrolytes (Ca, K, Mg) should be kept in normal range. Significant changes of plasma electrolytes occur particularly with transfusion and graft reperfusion [46, 47]. Routine administration of 2 g of MgSO$_4$ is benign, and although it does not shorten the QT interval, it is thought to be protective. High normal range of potassium is considered protective for TdP [48], but reperfusion- hyperkalemia may render this intervention risky.

Hypothermia can prolong QT interval [49] and this should be a consideration in the reperfusion period. All efforts should be made to maintain normal body temperature and minimize postreperfusion hypothermic insult.

Use of β-blockers in patients with LQT during OLT has not been studied. In congenital LQT and in healthy and coronary artery disease patients undergoing induction of general anesthesia, β-blockade shortens QTc and QTd, and is presumably antiarrhythmogenic effect [25, 44, 45, 50]. Similarly, in cirrhotic patients with LQT, β-blockers tend to normalize QTc [51, 52] but whether this intervention is protective is not known. Conversely, in a rare well documented OLT case, a patient with LQT and increased QTd who developed TdP was successfully treated by positive chronotropy induced by glycopyrrolate and isoproterenol [7].

Torsade de pointes are treated with intravenous magnesium sulfate (30 mg/kg) regardless of the magnesium serum level. Sustained or hemodynamically unstable TdP, or ensuing ventricular fibrillation, requires immediate nonsynchronized defibrillation. Overdrive transvenous pacing (90-110 bpm) is effective in preventing TdP recurrence in refractory congenital LQT. Preoperative placement of pads for transcutaneous pacing and cardioversion-defibrillation should be considered in patients assessed to be at high risk for developing TdP or ventricular fibrillation.

Postoperative considerations. Information regarding the LQT should be transferred to the ICU. Intraoperative principles are continued postoperatively. As the risk of TdP increases significantly with concurrent use of more than one QT prolonging drug [27, 29, 48], attention should be paid at multiple medications routinely used in the postoperative care of liver transplant patients that have been implicated in prolongation of QT interval or associated with torsades. Continuous telemetry may be considered after discharge from the ICU.

In conclusion, LQT is a common complication of cirrhosis whose underlying cellular mechanisms are largely understood. Only few long QT-related arrhythmias have been reported in OLT literature. However, perioperative physicians should recognize this common condition and be aware of multiple medications and factors that may prolong QT interval and precipitate life-threatening arrhythmias. Intraoperative monitoring of QT interval is possible with new monitors but not widely reported.

Atrial Fibrillation

Atrial fibrillation (AF) is a supraventricular arrhythmia characterized by uncoordinated atrial activation and consequent deterioration of mechanical function [53]. AF is the most common arrhythmia in North America and Europe, with estimated prevalence of 0.4% in patients younger than 70 years, and 2% to 4% in older patients [54]. Risk factors include age, hypertension, coronary or valvular heart disease, pericardial disease, congestive heart failure, diabetes mellitus, hyperthyroidism, and COPD [55]. The most feared consequence of AF is stroke, increasing in incidence with age. Other complications include hypotension, congestive heart failure, and myocardial ischemia.

Diagnosis is typically made based on the irregular heart rate on physical examination, and uneven RR interval with occasional *f* waves on the ECG. Further evaluation includes echocardiogram and stress test to rule out structural or ischemic myocardial disease. Common risk factors, hypertension, coronary artery and valvular disease, diabetes, kidney disease and hyperthyroidism, should be sought.

AF is clinically classified based on the temporal pattern of occurrence [53, 56]. *Newly-discovered* AF is the first presentation of AF for which the actual onset is not known. *Paroxysmal* and *persistent* AF are both recurrent, but the former is self-terminating within 7 days, while the latter requires cardioversion to restore sinus rhythm. When attempts to convert to sinus rhythm are unsuccessful or abandoned, the AF is classified as *permanent*. The classification has prognostic and therapeutic implications. Although the specific management depends upon the type, etiology, clinical manifestations and risk of complications from AF or from the treatment, the principles of management are common for all AF. Cornerstones of management are conversion to sinus rhythm or ventricular rate control, prevention of recurrence, and prevention of stroke and other thromboembolic events.

Clinical Challenges in the Peritransplant Management of Patients with AF

Is atrial fibrillation a contraindication to OLT? Postoperative atrial fibrillation ranges in incidence from up to 8% in non cardiac surgery, to up to 33% in cardiac surgery [57]. There is not much evidence in literature regarding the incidence of AF in OLT, or the impact of AF on OLT outcomes. Fouad recently reported on cardiac complications in 197 patients older than 40 years undergoing OLT [5]. Preoperative AF was not reported. A presumed new-onset AF was detected in 1 patient intraoperatively, and in 5 patients postoperatively. The patient who developed intraoperative AF died of cardiac death within one week. Autopsy indicated alcoholic cardiomyopathy.

A review of 600 patients transplanted at Washington University over last 7 years identified 8 patients with pre-existing AF. Four were men and four women, ranging in age from 48 to 69. The observed 1.3% incidence of AF is similar to the incidence in the general population for the same age category. Two patients had a ventricular pacemaker placed to prevent bradycardia induced by treatment. In all cases OLT was performed using piggy-back technique without major intraoperative complications. Post-operative course was complicated in 3 patients. One patient died of heart failure approximately two months after surgery. The autopsy showed a severe mitral stenosis, erroneously estimated only as mild on the preoperative echocardiographic assessment. One developed pulmonary edema requiring mechanical ventilation for more than 24 hours post-operatively. The third patient had an unremarkable early recovery and was discharged six days post surgery. She was readmitted several days later, and treated successfully for a new episode of AF with rapid ventricular response. Our limited experience suggests that safe OLT is possible in patients who are medically well optimized and in whom AF is not associated with severe underlying heart disease.

Antiarrhythmic therapy: rate vs. rhythm control. Decision regarding rate vs. rhythm control strategy in an OLT candidate with AF should be made by a cardiology consultant, according to ACC/AHA/ESC or NICE guidelines, and irrespective of the transplant. The antiarrhythmic regimen should be continued throughout the perioperative period. Sinus rhythm is clearly more desirable because it offers better hemodynamic stability, but conversion to sinus rhythm, i.e., *rhythm control*, is indicated only in specific subsets of patients with AF. Rhythm control is the preferred strategy in symptomatic patients, younger patients, those presenting for the first time with lone atrial fibrillation, and those in whom the precipitating factor has been corrected. In contrast, *rate control* is typically the preferred initial strategy in patients with permanent AF, and in elderly patients with persistent AF (over 65 years) in whom cardioversion is unsuitable. The ideal ventricular rate control is controversial, but AF is generally considered reasonably well controlled if heart rates are 60-80 bpm at rest and 90-115 bpm after exercise [53]. Specific antiarrhythmic drug selection is usually based on the 2006 Guidelines, although the Guidelines are not entirely evidence-based in this respect. For rhythm control fewer patients are on Class I and more on Class III antiarrhythmics (amiodarone, sotalol) largely due to toxicity profile. Both Class III drugs should be used with caution in patients with LQT. For rate control, beta blockers and calcium channel blockers are commonly used.

In general patient population, maintenance of sinus rhythm had no added benefit over rate control strategy in decreasing mortality or rate of stroke in the AFFIRM trial [58]. In fact, prolongation of QT interval and TdP, and pulmonary and gastrointestinal complications, were less frequent in the rate controlled patients.

Antithrombotic therapy in an OLT candidate with AF. The decision to use antithrombotic therapy and the choice of therapy is based on an estimated risks and benefits of the therapy, and the risk of stroke. ACC/AHA/ESC guidelines for general patient population recommend thromboembolic prophylaxis with aspirin or vitamin K antagonists (VKA) in all patients except in those with lone AF or those with contraindications to thromboprophylaxis. Target INR is between 2 and 3, or higher, in patients at high risk of thromboembolization (prosthetic valves, prior thromboembolism, persistent left atrial thrombus) [53]. An OLT candidate with AF presents several challenges with respect to thromboembolic prophylaxis. First, a common perioperative strategy, to replace VKA with low molecular weight heparin several days before the surgery, is clearly not applicable because of the unpredictable timing of the transplant. Second, in patients with varices, thrombocytopenia, and abnormal clotting, benefits of antithrombotic therapy should be carefully weighed against the higher risk of bleeding. And finally, a common notion that the patient with ESLD and prolonged INR is coagulopathic may be misleading. Prolonged INR in liver disease is a better index of reduced synthetic function (thus a part of MELD score) than a predictor of bleeding, because it does not reflect the true balance between pro and anticoagulant factors [59]. Thus, to assume that prolonged INR in liver disease confers additional protective anticoagulant effect may be erroneous.

In eight patients with moderate risk of stroke transplanted at our institution, thromboprophylaxis with aspirin only, was not associated with any clinically evident thromboembolic events. In another single case report, low molecular weight heparin was successfully used off-label for thromboprophylaxis in a post-OLT patient with AF sensitized to coumarins [60]. In absence of evidence-based guidelines for management of anticoagulation in patients with AF and ESLD, individual patient approach that includes stroke risk stratification and assessment of bleeding risk, is essential.

A new oral direct thrombin inhibitor, Dabigatran etexilate, is currently undergoing initial clinical evaluation in patients with AF. This is a promising agent because of its short half-life and predominant kidney elimination [61]. Additionally, new percutaneous interventional treatments are under development, such as left atrial appendage transcatheter occlusion for patients unable to take warfarin [62]. These new modalities may become relevant in the treatment of AF in patients with ESLD.

Intraoperative considerations. Our practice is to place external defibrillator pads in all patients with a diagnosis of major arrhythmias undergoing OLT. In patients with paroxysmal or persistent AF who develop acute rapid ventricular response and hemodynamic instability, the goal is immediate cardioversion . In hemodynamically stable patients, a more conservative approach is reasonable: assess and correct possible triggers, such as electrolyte abnormalities or atrial distention assessed by TEE, ensure adequate oxygenation and ventilation, and adequate depth of anesthesia. If unsuccessful, or in patients with borderline hemodynamics and ventricular rates continuously at or above 100, pharmacological rate control or conversion to sinus rhythm is indicated (Table 3). We favor amiodarone as the first line pharmacological treatment of AF in conditions of low systemic vascular resistance (SVR). Amiodarone should be used cautiously in patients with LQT because it may precipitate TdP [63]. Beta blockers are an alternative, particularly esmolol because of its short half-life [64, 65]. Calcium channel blockers are less desirable in OLT because of their depressant effects on SVR and contractility. Digoxin is less effective in controlling excessive heart rates, particularly during high adrenergic states such as the surgical stress [56].

In permanent AF, intraoperative conversion to sinus rhythm is not desirable because of the risk of thromobembolic complications. We still advocate placement of external pads because we consider these patients at higher risk for developing ventricular arrhythmias or requiring pacing. Acute rapid ventricular rate should be managed pharmacologically, as described above.

In patients that develop new-onset AF intraoperatively, immediate cardioversion is indicated only in case of rapid ventricular response and hemodynamic instability, according to Advance Cardiac Life Support (ACLS) guidelines. In more stable hemodynamics, the priority is pharmacological conversion to sinus rhythm within a few hours. The reason is that a new-onset AF lasting more than 48 hours or managed by cardioversion, ideally requires prolonged (several weeks) anticoagulation which would increase the risk of bleeding in the postoperative period.

It seems prudent to monitor intraoperatively all AF patients with TEE. TEE can detect spontaneous ECHO contrast indicative of a low-flow state in the atrial appendage, or frank atrial or pericatheter intracardiac thrombi. Other advantages are detection of regional wall motion abnormalities and guiding volume management.

Intraoperative use of antifibrinoytics in OLT patients with AF poses another challenge. As thromboembolic potential is increased in AF, we do not advocate routine prophylactic antifibrinolytics. We would consider judicious use of antifibrinolytics in the presence of laboratory and clinical signs suggestive of fibrinolysis. Rapid turnover of clotting test results by point-of-care testing is extremely useful for early detection of fibrinolysis. Thromboelastogram (TEG) or thromboelastometry (ROTEM) are uniquely helpful in detecting hypercoagulable states.

Table 3. Pharmacological management of an acute intraoperative AF

	Dosage (IV)	Efficacy	Side Effects	Comments
Diltiazem	Bolus 20 mg or 25 mcg/kg over 2 min, then 5-15 mg/hr	Good	Heart block, ↓HR, ↓BP	95% hepatic elimination Inhibits metabolism and potentiates toxicity of calcineurin inhibitors Hepatic dosing not defined, caution advised
Metoprolol	1-5 mg bolus every 15 min up to 15 mg	Good	Heart block, ↓HR, ↓BP Bronchospasm	Primarily metabolized in the liver Potential decreased therapeutic effect due to β-receptor downregulation in cirrhosis
Esmolol	Bolus 0.5 mg/kg, then 0.05 mg/kg/min	Good	Heart block, ↓HR, ↓BP Bronchospasm	Metabolised by red blood cell cytosol esterases, unchanged dosing in hepatic disease
Amiodarone	5-7 mg/kg or 150 mg over 10 min, then 0.5-1.0 mg/kg/min up to 1500 mg/24 hrs	Good	↓HR, ↓BP Thrombophlebitis Hepatic and pulmonary injury with long term use	Hepatic metabolism and elimination Inhibits metabolism and potentiates toxicity of calcineurin inhibitors Useful in hypotension Torsades described in cirrhosis and long QT Consider decreased hepatic dosing for longer adminstration
Digoxin	0.25 mg every 2 hrs, up to 1.5 mg/24 hrs	Low to Moderate	Delayed-onset AV slowing	Small amount metabolized by the liver, 30-50% eliminated unchanged in urine. Hepatic dosing unchanged; caution in hepatorenal syndrome. Electrolyte imbalance potentiates toxicity

AF-atrial fibrillation, HR-heart rate, BP-blood pressure.

In cardiac surgery, where AF prevalence is high, beta-blockers, amiodarone, ACE-inhibitors, sartans, statins, and steroids seem to have a protective effect [66-69]. The efficacy of steroids is of potential interest in OLT as most immunosuppressive regimens include intraoperative steroid administration. It is not known if patients receiving steroid-free protocols have higher incidence of perioperative AF [70, 71].

An OLT candidate with AF merits a consideration with respect to the surgical technique. In our experience, piggy-back technique offers relatively stable hemodynamic conditions throughout the procedure. Changes in preload associated with portocaval shunt are manageable. A surgical approach that involves total IVC cross-clamping without veno-venous bypass may not be well tolerated by a patient in AF because of a reduced capacity for maintaining cardiac output under the conditions of decreased preload and possibly rapid ventricular rate.

In conclusion, evidence regarding the incidence of AF in OLT candidates and its impact on outcomes is lacking. Our experience suggests that good outcomes are possible in patients in whom AF is not associated with a severe underlying structural or ischemic cardiomyopathy. Intraoperative and postoperative complications, including mortality, are possibly increased. Perioperative management of AF warrants additional considerations and cardiology consultation. In absence of OLT specific guidelines, individual patient management strategy is essential. It must consider type of AF, stroke risk stratification, response to antiarrhythmic drugs and extent of comorbidities.

Post-Reperfusion and other Intraoperative Arrhythmias

Post-reperfusion syndrome (PRS) occurring in 25-55% of OLTs, is associated with adverse outcomes, including increased blood loss and blood product requirements, higher incidence of postoperative allograft loss, kidney failure, and early mortality [11-14].

The most common reperfusion arrhythmia is bradycardia, often resistant to chronotropic agents, and occasionally progressing to asystole [5, 11, 72, 73]. The mechanisms behind bradycardia and reperfusion syndrome are not yet fully understood. Various factors have been implicated, such vasoactive substances from the graft or the recipient gut (potassium, acids, prostanoids, bradykinin, interleukins), hypovolemia, hypothermia, or small air or thromboemboli.

No universally accepted preventative strategies have been developed. Common interventions include pretreatment with chronotropic and vasoconstrictor agents and optimization of temperature, pH and electrolytes, including magnesium. Acosta reported successful prevention of postreperfusion bradycardia by pretreatment with atropine (0.2 mg/kg) immediately before reperfusion. Their immediate mean prereperfusion heart rates were 115-120 bpm [74]. Our common practice is to administer glycopyrrolate (0.2 – 0.4 mg) targeting heart rates of at least 80 – 90 bpm. Glycopyrrolate in this dose is usually effective in preventing vagal reflexes without causing excessive increase in heart rate that could be detrimental in many older OLT recipients.

In three other reports (462 patients) incidence of major intraoperative arrhythmias, including asystolic cardiac arrest, ventricular tachycardia, atrial fibrillation and ventricular fibrillation, ranged from 2.5 to 6.6% [5, 19, 75]. Although majority of these arrhythmias were successfully treated, almost 17% of the patients who developed serious intraoperative arrhythmia died within the first 24 hours.

A prospective study of 105 OLT patients [76] reported high incidence of ventricular ectopy, including two episodes of sustained ventricular tachycardia and fibrillation, upon insertion and removal of the pulmonary artery catheter. The arrhythmias were not associated with mortality.

In conclusion, serious intraoperative arrhythmias during liver transplantation seem to be associated with increased morbidity and mortality. The incidence is significant, but predicting arrhythmia in an individual patient remains elusive. General preventative measures are careful maintenance of oxygenation and ventilation, temperature, electrolyte and acid-base balance, and hemodynamics. Available drugs and equipment for resuscitation, and anesthesia team proficient in ACLS are essential.

Conclusion

Arrhythmias are common in patients undergoing OLT. Symptomatic arrhythmias require focused diagnostic workup to guide medical optimization and exclude an underlying heart disease that may constitute a contraindication for OLT. LQT is a marker of cirrhotic cardiomyopathy but its impact on OLT outcomes is not fully understood. Serious intraoperative arrhythmias, particularly reperfusion arrhtythmias, are associated with worse outcomes but there is no consensus regarding the value or modality of preventive strategies. Patients with pre-existing AF can successfully undergo OLT but require multidisciplinary approach and individualized management, balancing the risk and benefits of antithrombotic therapy against the risk of bleeding.

There is an overall lack of evidence-based knowledge regarding arrhythmias in OLT. Large database reviews and future prospective studies are needed to provide important information pertaining to incidence, risk factors, prevention and best treatment of arrhythmias in this high-risk patient population.

References

[1] Henriksen JH, Fuglsang S, Bendtsen F, Christensen E, Møller S. Dyssynchronous electrical and mechanical systole in patients with cirrhosis. *J. Hepatol.* 2002; 36 (4): 513-20

[2] Moller S, Henricksen JH. Cardiovascular complications of cirrhosis. *Gut* 2008;58:268-78

[3] Wong, F. Cirrhotic cardiomyopathy. Hepatol Int. 2009, 3, 294-304.3. Xia VW, Taniguchi M, Steadman RH. The changing face of patients presenting for liver transplantation. *Curr. Opin. Organ. Transplant* .2008;13 (3): 280-4

[4] Xia, VW, Taniguchi M; Steadman, RH. The changing face of patients presenting for liver transplantation. *Curr. Opin. Organ. Trasplant.* 2008, 13(3), 280-4.

[5] Fouad TR, Abdel-Razek WM, Burak KW, Bain VG, Lee SS. Prediction of cardiac complications after liver transplantation. *Transplantation* 2009; 87(5):763-70

[6] Johnston SD, Morris JK, Cramb R, Gunson BK, Neuberger J. Cardiovascular morbidity *Transplantation* 2002;73(6):901-6

[7] Lustik SJ, Eichelberger JP, Chhibber AK, Bronsther, O. Torsade de pointes during orthotopic liver transplantation. *Anesth. Analg.* 1998;87:300-3

[8] Biancofiore G, Valentini C, Cellai F, Filipponi F, Mosca F, Vagelli A. Report of a life-threatening arrhythmia after hospital discharge in a liver transplant recipient with previously unknown congenital long QT syndrome. *Digest Liver Dis* 2001;33:432-4

[9] Yeh,PA; Chen,HP; Tsai,YC; Lin,YJ; Liu,YC. Successful management of air embolism-induced ventricular fibrillation in orthotopic liver transplantation. *Acta Anaesthesiol Taiwan* 2005, 43, 243-68.

[10] Ranasinghe DN and Mallet SV. Hypomagnesaemia, cardiac arrhythmias and orthotopic liver transplantation. *Anaesthesia* 1994;49:403-5
[11] Aggarwal S, Kang Y, Freeman JA, Fortunato FL, Pinsky MR. Postreperfusion syndrome: cardiovascular collapse following hepatic reperfusion during liver transplantation. *Transplant. Proc.* 1987; 19(4 Suppl 3):54-5
[12] Hilmi, I, Horton CN, Planinsic RM, Sakai T; Nicolau-Raducu, R, Damian D et al. The impact of postreperfusion syndrome *Liver Transpl.* 2008, 14, 504-8.
[13] Nanashima A, Pillay P, Crawford M, Nakasuji M, Verran DJ, Painter D. Analysis of postrevascularization syndrome *J. Hepatobiliary Pancreat. Surg.* 2001;8(6):557-63
[14] Paugam-Burtz C, Kavafyan J, Merckx P, Dahmani S, Sommacale D, Ramsay M et al. Postreperfusion syndrome *Liver Transp.* 2009;15(5):522-9
[15] Gallegos-Orozco JF, Vargas HE. Liver transplantation: from Child to MELD. *Med Clin North Am* 2009;93(4):931-50
[16] Murray KF and Carithers, RL Jr., AASLD practice guidelines: Evaluation of the patient for liver transplantation. *Hepatolog* .2005;41(6):1407-32
[17] Stein KM. Non invasive risk stratification for sudden death: signal-averaged electrocardiography, non sustained ventricular tachycardia, Heart rate variability, baroreflex sensitivity, and QRS duration. *Progress in Cardiovasc Dis.* 2008;51(2):106-17
[18] Zipes DP, Camm AJ, Borggrefe M, Buxton AE, Chaitman B, Fromer M et al. ACC/AHA/ESC 2006 Guidelines for management of patients with ventricular arrhythmias and prevention of sudden cardiac death. *Circulation* 2006;114:1088-1132.
[19] Therapondos, G; Flapan, AD; Plevris, JN; Hayes, PC. Cardiac morbidity and mortality related to orhtotopic liver transplantation. *Liver Transpl.* 2004, 1441-1453.
[20] Humphrey LG, Hurst TR, Eleid MF, Lee KS, Reuss CS, Hentz JG et al. Preoperative dobutamine stress echocardiographic findings and subsequent short-term adverse cardiac events after orthotopic liver transplantation. *Liver Transpl.*2008;14:886-92
[21] Verbeeck, RK. Pharmacokinetics and dosage adjustment in patients with hepatic dysfunction. *Eur. J. Clin. Pharmacol* .2008;64:1147-61
[22] Shu, J, Zhou, J, Patel C, Yan GX. Pharmacotherapy of cardiac arrhythmias – basic science for clinicians. *PACE* 2009;32:1454-65
[23] Ward CA, Ma Z, Lee SS, Giles WR. Potassium currents in atrial and ventricular myocytes from a rat model of cirrhosis. *Am. J. Physiol* .1997;273:G537-G544
[24] Day CP, McComb JM, Campbell RWF. QT dispersion: an indication of arrhythmia risk in patients with long QT intervals. *Br. Heart J* .1990;63:342-4
[25] Goldenberg I, Moss AJ, Zareba W. QT interval: how to measure it and what is "normal". *J Cardiovasc Electrophysiol* 2006;102(17):333-668 Goodman S, Weiss Y, Weissman C. Update on cardiac arrhythmias in the ICU. *Curr. Opin. Crit. Care* 2008;14:549-554
[26] Goodman, S; Weiss, Y; Weissman, C. Update on cardiac arrhythmias in the ICU. *Curr Opin. Crit. Care* 2008, 14:549-554
[27] Drew BJ, Ackerman MJ, Funk M, Gibler BW, Kligfield P, Menon V et al. Prevention of Torsade de Pointes in Hopsital Settings. A Scientific Statement from the American Heart Association and the American College of Cardiology Foundation. *J. Am. Col. Cardiol.* 2010;55(9):934-47

[28] Darbar D, Luck J, Davidson N, Pringle T, Main G, McNeill et al. Sensitivity and specificity of QTC dispersion for identification of risk of cardiac death in patients with peripheral vascular disease. *Brit. Med. J.* 1996;312:874-8

[29] Kannankeril PJ, Roden DM. Drug-induced long QT and torsades de pointes: recent advances. *Curr. Opin. Cardiol.* 2007;22:39-43

[30] Henricksen JH, Gulberg V, Fuglsang S, Schifter S, Bendtsen F, Gerbes AL et al. Q-T interval (QTc) in patients with cirrhosis: relation to vasoactive peptides and heart rate. *Scand J. Clin Lab. Invest.* 2007; 67:643-53

[31] Genovesi S, Prata Pizzala DM, Pozzi M, Ratti L, Milanese, Pieruzzi F et al. QT interval prolongation and decreased heart rate variability in cirrhotic patients: relevance of hepatic venous pressure gradient and serum calcium. *Clincal Science* 2009;116:851-859

[32] Bernardi M, Calandra S, Trevisan F, Raimondo ML, Sica G, Schepis F et al. Q-T interval prolongation in cirrhosis: prevalence, relationship with severity and etiology of the disease and possible pathogenetic factors. *Hepatology* 1998;23:28-34

[33] Mohamed, R, Forsey PR, Davies MK, Neuberger JM. Effect of liver transplantation on QT interval prolongation and autonomic dysfunction in end-stage liver disease. *Hepatolog* .1996;23:1128-34.

[34] Bal J-S, Thuluvath PJ. Prolongation of QTc interval: relationship with etiology and severity of liver disease, mortality and liver transplantation. *Liver International* 2003;23:243-8

[35] Henricksen JH, Goetze JP, Fuglsang S, Christensen E, Bendtsen F, Moller S. Increased circulating pro-brain natriuretic peptide (pro-BNP) and brain natriuretic peptide (BNP) in patients with cirrhosis: a relation to cardiovascular disfunction and severity of disease. *Gut* 2003;52:1511-7

[36] Yitting H, Henricksen JH, Fuglsang S, Bendtsen F, Moller S, Prolonged Q-Tc interval in mild portal hypertensive cirrhosis. *J. Hepatol.* 2005;43:637-43.

[37] Zambruni, A, Trevisani, F, Caraceni, P, Bernardi M. Cardiac electrophysiological abnormalities in patients with cirrhosis. *J. Hepatol.* 2006;44:994-1002.

[38] Arikan C, Kilic M, Tumgor G, Levent E, Yuksekkaya HA, Yagci RV et al. Impact of liver transplantation on rate-corrected QT interval in children with chronic liver disease. *Pediatric Transplantation* 2009;13:300-6

[39] Hansen S, Moler S, Bendtsen F, Jesen G, Henricksen JH. Diurnal variation and dispersion in QT interval in cirrhosis: relation to haemodynamic changes. *J. Hepatol.* 2007;47:373-80

[40] Kosar F, Fehmi A, Sahin I, Karincaoglu M, Yildrim B. QT interval analysis in patients with chronic liver disease: a prospective study. *Angiology* 2007;58:218-24

[41] Kies S, Pabelick CM, Hurley HA, White RD, Ackerman MJ. Anesthesia for patients with congenital long QT syndrome. *Anesthesiology* 2005;102: 204-10

[42] Nakao S, Hatano K, Sumi C, Masuzawa M, Sakamoto S, Ikeda S, Shingu K. Sevoflurane causes greater QTc interval prolongation in elderly patients than in young patients. *Anesth. Analg* .2010;110:775-9

[43] Ay B, Fak AS, Toprak A, Gogus YF, Oktay A. QT dispersion increases during intubation in patients with coronary artery disease. *J. Electrocardiol.* 2004;37:81-90

[44] Erdil S, Demirbilek S, Begec E, Ozturk A, But A, Ozcan Ersoy M. The effect of esmolol on the QTc interval during induction of anesthesia in patients with coronary artery disease. *Anaesthesia* 2009;64:246-50

[45] Kaneko M, Hamaguchi S, Egawa H, Fujii K, Ishikawa K, Kitajima T et al. Effects of landiolol on QT interval and QT dispersion during induction of anesthesia using computerized measurement. *J. Clin. Anesth.* 2009;21:555-61

[46] Scott VI, De Wolf AM, Kang Y, Altura BT, Virji MA, Cook DR et al. Ionized hypomagnesemia in patients undergoing orhtotopic liver transplantation: a complication of citrate intoxication. *Liver Transpl. Surg* 1996;2:343-47.

[47] Acosta F, Sansano T, Contreras RF, Reche M, Beltran R, Roques V et al. Changes in serum *Transplant Proc.* 1999:31(6);2382-3

[48] Gupta A, Lawrence AT, Krishnan K, Kavinsky C, Throman RG. Current concepts in the mechanism and management of drug-induced QT prolongation and torsade de pointes. *Am. Heart J* .2007;153:891-9

[49] Khan JN, Prasad N, Glancy JM. QTc prolongation during therapeutic hypothermia: are we giving it attention it deserves? *Europac* 2010;12:266-70

[50] Kaufman E. Mechanisms and clinical management of inherited channelopathies: Long QT syndrome, Brugada syndrome, catecholaminergic polymorphic ventricular tachycardia, and short QT syndrome. *Heart Rhythm.* 2009; S51-S55

[51] Henricksen JH, Bnedtsen F, Hanse EF, Moller S. Acute non-selective beta-adrenergic blockade reduces prolonged frequency-adjusted QT interval (QTc) in patients with cirrhosis. *J. Hepatol.* 2008;48:415-21

[52] Micoli AD, Zambruni A, Bracci E, Benazzi B, Zappoli P, Berzigotti A et al. "Torsade de pointes" during amiodarone infusion in a cirrhotic woman with a prolonged QT interval. *Digestive and Liver Disease* 2009;41:535-8

[53] Fuster V, Rydén LE, Cannom DS, Crijns HJ, Curtis AB, Ellenbogen KA et al. ACC/AHA/ESC Guidelines for Management of Patients with Atrial Fibrillation. *Circulation* 2006;114:257-354

[54] Jongnarangasin K, Oral H. Postoperative atrial fibrillation. *Med. Clin. N. Am.* 2008;92:87-99

[55] Indik JH, Alpert JS. The patient with atrial fibrillation. *The American Journal of Medicine* 2009;122: 415-8

[56] Lip GYH, Tse, HF. Management of Atrial fibrillation. *The Lancet* 2007;370:604-18.

[57] Mayson, SE; Greenspon, AJ; Adams, S; Decaro, MV; Sheth, M; Weitz, HH; Whellan, DJ. The changing face of postoperative atrial fibrillation prevention: a review of current medical therapy. *Cardiol. Rev.* 2007, 15, 231-41.

[58] Wyse DG, Waldo AL, DiMarco JP, Domanski MJ, Rosenberg Y, Schron, EB et al. The Atrial Fibrillation Follow-up Investigation of Rhythm Management (AFFIRM) Investigators. A comparison of rate control and rhythm control in patients with atrial fibrillation. *N. Engl. J. Med.* 2002; 347(23):1825-33

[59] Tripodi A, Mannucci PM. Abnormalities of hemostasis in chronic liver disease: reappraisal of their clinical significance and need for clinical and laboratory research. *J Hepatol* .2007;46:727-33

[60] Bertsche T, Fritz R, Sauer P. Encke J, Haefeli WE, Walter-Sack I. Off-label use in long-term anticoagulation after liver transplantation due to phenprocoumom-induced hepatic failure. *Med. Monatsschr. Pahrm.* 2006;29:257-62

[61] Van Ryn J, Stangier J, Haertter S, Liesenfeld KH, Wienen W, Feuring M et al. Dabigatran etexilate - a novel, reversible, oral direct thrombin inhibitor: Interpretation

of coagulation assays and reversal of anticoagulant activity. *Thromb Haemost.* 2010;103(6) : 1116-27

[62] Block PC, Burstein S, Casale PN, Kramer PH, Teirstein P, Williams DO et al. Percutaneous left atrial appendage occlusion for patients in atrial fibrillation suboptimal for warfarin therapy: 5-year results of the PLAATO (Percutaneous Left Atrial Appendage Transcatheter Occlusion) Study. *JACC Cardiovasc. Interv.* 2009;7:594-600

[63] Di Micoli A, Zambruni A, Bracci E, Benazzi B, Zappoli P, Berzigotti A et al."Torsade de pointes" during amiodarone infusion in a cirrhotic woman with a prolonged QT interval *Dig. Liver Dis.* 2009;41(7):535-8

[64] Buchi KN, Rollins, DE, Tolman KG, Achari R, Drissel D, Hulse JD. Pharmacokinetics of esmolol in hepatic disease. *J. Clin. Pharmacol.* 1987;27(11):880-4

[65] Wiest D. Esmolol. A review of its therapeutic efficacy and pharmacokinetic characteristics. *Clin. Pharmacokinet.* 1995;28(3):190-202.

[66] Hogue CW, Creswell LL, Gutterman, DD, Fleisher LA. Epidemiology Mechanisms, and risks. *2005 Chest* 2005;128:9S-16S

[67] Amar D. Strategies for perioperative arrhythmias. *Best Practice and Research Clinical Anesthesiology* 2004;4:565-77

[68] Amar D. Prevention and Management of perioperative arrhythmias in the thoracic surgical population. *Anesthesiolgy Clin.* 2008;26:325-35

[69] Sanchez-Quinones J, Marin F, Roldan V, Lip GYH.The impact of statin use on atrial fibrillation. *Q J. Med.* 2008;101:845-861

[70] Segev DL, Sozio SM, Shin EJ, Nazarian SM, Nathan H, Thuluvath PJ et al.Steroid avoidance in liver transplantation: meta-analysis and meta-regression of randomized trials. *Liver Transpl.* 2008;14(4):512-25

[71] Sgourakis G, Radtke A, Fouzas I, Mylona S, Goumas K, Gockel I et al. Corticosteroid-free immunosuppression in liver transplantation: a meta-analysis and meta-regression of outcomes. *Transpl. Int.* 2009;22(9): 892-905

[72] Chui, AK; Shi, L; Tanaka, K; Rao, AR; Wang, LS; Bookallil, M; Mayr, M; Chiu, E; Verran, DJ; Mears, D; Sheil, AG. Postreperfusion syndrome in orthotopic liver transplantation. *Transplant. Proc.* 2000, 32, 2116-7

[73] Acosta F, Sansano T, Contreras RF, Reche M, Beltran R, Roques V et al. Atropine prophylaxis *Transplant. Proc.* 1999 ;31(6):2394-5

[74] Ramsay, M. The reperfusion syndrome *Liver Transpl.* 2008, 14, 412-4.

[75] Findlay, JY; Keegan, MT; Pellikka, PP; Rosen, CB; Plevak, DJ. Preoperative dobutamine stress *Transplant Proc* .2005, 37, 2209-13.

[76] Gwak, MS; Kim JA; Kim, GS; Choi, SJ; Ahn, H; Lee, AH; Lee, JJ; Lee, S; Kim, M. Incidence of severe ventricular arrhythmias during pulmonary artery catheterization in liver transplant recipients. *Liver Transpl* .2007, 13, 1451-54.

Chapter IV

Valvular Heart Disease and Liver Transplantation

Andrew I. Gardner and Neville M. Gibbs[*]
Department of Anaesthesia, Sir Charles Gairdner Hospital
Nedlands, Australia

Abstract

The implications of valvular heart disease for the liver transplant candidate depend on the valvular lesion, its severity, and its natural history if untreated. There is extensive overlap in the symptoms and signs of both diseases, making clinical estimation of the severity of valvular disease difficult. Moreover, the presence of one of these diseases may influence the symptomatology and progression of the other. There is little information available on the risks of transplantation in patients with valvular heart disease, so most decisions must be based on first principles. This chapter outlines the aetiology, pathophysiology, and natural history of the most common valvular lesions, and describes the medical and surgical options that must be considered prior to liver transplantation. An algorithm for triage of patients with valvular heart disease is presented, and strategies for perioperative management are described.

Introduction

The presence of valvular heart disease as a co-morbidity in patients presenting for liver transplantation has several implications for the transplant anaesthetist. First, in some cases the natural history of the valvular disease may mean that liver transplantation cannot be considered; second, potentially treatable valvular conditions may require intervention before transplantation; third, the pathophysiological changes of valvular disease may influence

---

[*] Correspondence: Neville M Gibbs, Department of Anaesthesia, Sir Charles Gairdner Hospital, Hospital Avenue, Nedlands WA 6009, Australia, E-mail: nmg@cyllene.uwa.edu.au.

anaesthetic techniques; and fourth, the valvular disease may increase the risk of the procedure - in some cases to unacceptable levels.

The indication for liver transplantation must also be considered as part of the assessment process and balance of risks. This is because liver transplantation may occasionally be undertaken for symptomatic rather than prognostic reasons. Some pathologies, such as carcinoid disease, may cause both liver and valvular heart disease [1]. In these cases, the impact of transplantation on the progression of the valvular disease should also be considered.

There is little experience with liver transplantation in patients with moderate or severe valvular heart disease. This may be because the perioperative risks may have previously been considered too great. This means that there is little empirical evidence to guide decision making or management. Therefore, the assessment decisions and management must be based mostly on first principles, relying on a thorough knowledge of the valvular heart disease itself, and the likely pathophysiological consequences of the disease during liver transplantation. This chapter will review the basic principles related to liver transplantation in patients with valvular heart disease, and discuss the limited literature available on this topic. The focus will be on patients with uncorrected valvular heart disease, although the issues related to managing patients with previous valvular repairs or replacement will also be covered.

Pre-Operative Assessment

The main assessment issues of concern are listed in Table 1.

Table 1. Assessment of the liver transplant candidate with valvular heart disease

• Assessment of the severity of the valvular disease and its natural history
• Assessment of the natural history of the liver disease with transplantation
• Assessment of the natural history of the liver disease without transplantation
• Consideration of pre-transplant surgical correction of the valvular disease, including its risk
• Assessment of the impact of medical optimisation or surgical correction on the progression of the liver disease
• Estimation of the overall risk of liver transplantation in the setting of corrected or uncorrected valvular disease

Signs and Symptoms

Patients will fall into one of two groups: those with known or incidental findings of valvular disease, and those with previous surgically treated disease. Symptoms and signs of valvular disease may overlap with symptoms and signs of severe liver disease, making it difficult to estimate the severity of symptoms and signs related to valvular pathology. Examples include ascites that may be present from severe liver disease or right heart failure, and dyspnoea that may be a result of either left heart failure or hepatopulmonary syndrome [2]. In addition, exercise tolerance may be limited in patients with symptoms and signs of liver disease as a result of ascites, dyspnoea, reduced muscle mass and early hepatic encephalopathy, making it more difficult to assess the symptoms related directly to valvular disease.

Patients with severe chronic liver disease, especially those with cirrhotic disease, frequently have hyperdynamic circulations with markedly increased cardiac output and low systemic vascular resistance [2]. In these patients an ejection systolic murmur may be heard as a result of increased flow across a structurally normal valve. In this situation, structurally significant valvular pathology needs to be excluded.

The involvement of other systems in liver disease such as the development of pulmonary hypertension may also make the clinical assessment of the significance of valvular lesions difficult.

In patients with a history of previous surgical treatment of valvular disease, information regarding the date and type of procedure performed should be obtained, given that previous repairs and replacements may deteriorate over time, especially if bioprosthetic valves have been used.

Assessment of the Severity of Valvular Disease

With all patients, in addition to the usual detailed history, examination and special investigations, further specific assessment of valvular pathology and left ventricular function by echocardiography is required. Although electrocardiography is useful in showing changes consistent with prior ischaemic heart disease or left ventricular hypertrophy and confirmation of cardiac rhythm, it adds little to assessment of the severity of valvular disease. The most important role of echocardiography will be to confirm the diagnosis and determine the severity of the valvular disease (i.e. mild, moderate or severe) [3, 4]. This will have implications for the natural history of the valvular lesion, the options for medical management or surgical correction, and the risks of haemodynamic compromise during the transplantation procedure. The assessment of severity is made on relatively objective criteria based on valve areas, pressure gradients, and regurgitant fractions [3, 4]. Echocardiography will also provide information on potential complications, associated pathology, or evidence of end organ damage. For example, it may be possible to estimate pulmonary artery pressures, and detect the presence of thrombus in patients with established or paroxysmal atrial fibrillation. In the case of rheumatic heart disease, it will identify or exclude the involvement of other valves.

In most cases transthoracic echocardiography (TTE) will be sufficient. Transoesophageal echocardiography (TOE) allows for better assessment of the mitral valve. However, the risk of TOE must be considered in the presence of oesophageal varices. While echocardiography may estimate the severity of pulmonary hypertension, right heart catheterisation and direct measurement of pulmonary artery pressures may be required for confirmation or quantification.

Pre-Operative Optimisation

In assessing and preparing patients with valvular heart disease for transplantation, the opinion of both cardiologists and cardiac surgeons will be required.

With valvular heart disease, the decision to persist with medical therapy or to proceed to surgical correction is based on both symptomatic and prognostic grounds. While it is relatively easy to estimate symptomatic improvement, it is less easy to estimate differences in prognosis between operative and non-operative management. In considering the natural history of non-surgically treated valvular disease, it is worth noting that this prognostic information is often based on patients who were treated prior to the development of modern pharmacological agents, or who may have been considered too unwell, or at too high a risk to be considered for surgery. It may be that with more advanced medical management, the progression to severe morbidity and mortality is delayed, and the prognosis without surgery is improved.

Medical Management

There may be overlap in the medical therapy of liver disease and valvular disease. Medical treatment of valvular disease includes the use of angiotensin converting enzyme (ACE) inhibitors or angiotensin II receptor antagonists, beta-blockers, calcium channel blockers, diuretics, and digoxin. Angiotensin converting enzyme inhibitors may concurrently delay the progression of fibrotic liver disease, so their use is not contraindicated in patients with severe liver disease. Non-selective beta-blockers are frequently used in patients with severe liver disease to decrease portal pressure and reduce oesophageal variceal bleeding. Calcium channel blockers are extensively metabolised by the liver, and may be associated with elevations in serum transaminases and alkaline phosphatase. In contrast, digoxin is mainly excreted renally, with minimal metabolism by the liver. Diuretics are frequently prescribed to patients with liver disease to minimise fluid retention in ascites.

It is possible that the presence of some valvular lesions worsens or exacerbates the symptoms and signs of liver disease (e.g. fluid overload), or adversely affects liver function (e.g. increased venous pressures). Under these circumstances, identification and treatment of the valvular disease may improve the symptoms or progression of the liver disease. In other words, optimisation of the patient's cardiac function may have beneficial effects on liver function by increasing cardiac output, increasing hepatic blood flow, and reducing venous pressures.

Pre-Transplant Cardiac Surgical Options and Risks

Preoperative repair or replacement of diseased valves raises several issues. Patients with severe liver disease who are admitted to intensive care units have a high mortality and a poor prognosis. In patients undergoing open-heart surgery, this increased mortality has been linked to increased susceptibility to infections such as mediastinitis and septicaemia, as well as gastrointestinal complications and bleeding. There is also increased postoperative fluid retention, ascites, pleural effusions, and pericardial effusions [5, 6, 7]. Prolonged cardiopulmonary bypass (CPB) times have also been associated with a worsening of hepatic failure. Although there are several scoring systems to predict peri-operative mortality in patients undergoing heart surgery with CPB, there is no system that includes liver disease as a risk factor. Given the relatively small number of patients with severe liver disease who undergo heart surgery with CPB, it would be difficult to develop and validate a risk rating for these patients. One study of 24 patients suggests that patients with a Child-Pugh score of ≥ 8 have an overall mortality rate of 25%, with postoperative mortality rates of 6, 67, and 100% for Child-Pugh classes A, B, and C, respectively [6]. This study also identified preoperative serum total bilirubin and serum cholinesterase levels as predictors to differentiate between survivors and non-survivors.

Patients with Previous Valvular Surgical Correction

Mechanical heart valves have traditionally been inserted in younger patients as they have a longer therapeutic lifespan; however, these valves require lifelong anticoagulation. This may be difficult to manage in patients with severe liver disease, as many patients may have concurrent altered coagulation, low platelets, and already be at increased risk from bleeding complications (e.g. from oesophageal varices). Warfarin remains the most frequently used drug to anti-coagulate patients with mechanical heart valves; however, the direct thrombin inhibitor dabigatran may be a suitable alternative [8]. Although metabolised by esterases, one study has shown that dabigatran's pharmacokinetics and pharmacodynamics are not affected by moderate hepatic impairment (Child-Pugh B) [9]. Anticoagulation will need to be reversed prior to liver transplantation, and recommenced as soon as feasible post transplantation [10]. While warfarin may be reversed with vitamin K, plasma, and prothrombin complex concentrates, there is no reversal agent for dabigatran. Most dabigatran dosing regimens consist of twice daily administration, and for most elective surgery, a delay of 12 hours post last dose is sufficient for coagulation to return to near normal.

When not anticoagulated, patients with mechanical heart valves have an increased risk of thromboembolic events, with mechanical mitral valves presenting a higher risk than mechanical aortic valves. With aortic mechanical valves, the annual embolic risk is in the order of 10-20%, or a risk of 0.08-0.16% over a three day period; it is not known what the actual risk is for mitral valves, although it is considered to be considerably higher [11]. Surgery itself will increase the risk of thrombosis. Therefore, it is likely that there will be periods of both impaired coagulation and increased thrombotic risk peri-operatively.

While bioprosthetic valves offer the advantage of not requiring anticoagulation beyond a three month post-operative period, they have a limited lifespan requiring replacement in approximately 30% of patients within 10 years, and up to 50% within 15 years [12]. There is some evidence to suggest that newer bioprosthetic valves may have lifespans in excess of 20 years.

In liver transplant recipients, there is a higher incidence of bacterial and non-bacterial endocarditis on native valves, with one review estimating the mortality rate in these patients to be greater than 50%, with 58% of cases being diagnosed post mortem [13]. In developed countries in non-transplant patients, infective endocarditis of prosthetic valves accounts for between 7 and 25% of patients [13, 14].

Valvular Pathologies

In discussing the various valvular conditions, only chronic disease is considered, as patients with acute disease are unlikely to be considered for liver transplantation.

Aortic Stenosis

Assessment and Pathophysiology

Aortic stenosis is prevalent in 3% of patients over 65, as a result of degenerative aortic stenosis, calcification of a congenital bicuspid valve, or rheumatic heart disease [15]. 80% of patients are male. The risk factors for atherosclerosis are all risk factors for the development of aortic valve calcification. Symptoms of aortic stenosis due to degenerative disease occur in the seventh and eighth decade, those secondary to congenital bicuspid valves in the third and fourth decades, and those secondary to rheumatic heart disease tend to occur between 10 and 20 years after the acute rheumatic fever. Although in the majority of patients aortic stenosis is due to degenerative disease, in the younger populations being assessed for liver transplantation, the prevalence of other causes will be relatively increased. Other rarer conditions such as subvalvular or supravalvular stenosis may mimic the symptoms and signs of aortic stenosis, and should be excluded on echocardiography [15, 16].

Chronic obstruction to left ventricular outflow with aortic stenosis results in the development of concentric left ventricular hypertrophy, and in severe aortic stenosis this may progress to a reduction in left ventricular function and dilatation. In most patients with severe aortic stenosis, there will be ECG changes consistent with left ventricular hypertrophy, which may accompanied by signs of left ventricular strain. With left ventricular hypertrophy, there is an increased contribution of atrial contraction to left ventricular filling, which is lost in atrial fibrillation; this situation may lead to rapid progression of heart failure. There is alteration in the supply and demand balance of oxygen to the heart, with an increased demand caused by the hypertrophied left ventricle, and a reduction in supply secondary to in the increased intraventricular wall pressure.

The symptoms of aortic stenosis may include the symptoms of angina (even in the presence of normal coronary arteries), syncope, and heart failure.

There are different systems for grading the severity of aortic stenosis, with an aortic jet velocity of >4 m/s, a mean gradient of >40 mmHg or an aortic valve area of <1 cm^2 being considered as severe aortic stenosis [16].

The natural history of aortic stenosis determined from autopsy studies prior to the availability of surgical therapies is a mean survival of four years after the development of angina pectoris, three years after the development of syncope, and two years after the development of dyspnoea [15].

Medical Management

Medical treatment of aortic stenosis includes the use of beta-blockers and ACE inhibitors to treat angina and hypertension. The use of statins (HMG-Co A reductase inhibitors) may delay disease progression.

Surgical Management

Aortic valve replacement is indicated in patients with severe aortic stenosis who are symptomatic, have left ventricular dysfunction (ejection fraction <50%) or have other cardiac lesions requiring operative treatment. The predicted peri-operative mortality for isolated aortic valve replacement in a patient with no significant co-morbidities may be as low as 1.5%, with average published mortalities approximately 2.8%. Recent developments in percutaneous aortic valve replacement may reduce the need for CPB in patients with severe liver disease, but as these have been used mainly in patients previously considered unsuitable for standard aortic valve replacement (through a sternotomy with CPB), it is difficult to estimate the short and long term outcomes after these procedures [17].

Intraoperative Haemodynamic Management

The left ventricular hypertrophy occurring in severe aortic stenosis provides challenges to the anaesthetist should these patients present for liver transplantation. These patients require maintenance of afterload and avoidance of tachycardia to ensure adequate myocardial perfusion and to avoid myocardial ischaemia (Table 2) [18]. There is altered compliance of the left ventricle with higher pressures required to maintain adequate preload. This is of particular relevance during inferior vena cava cross clamping, which may be associated with hypotension requiring vasopressors and fluids. Although there has been an increasing trend away from using veno-veno bypass (VVB) in liver transplantation, if trial of clamping demonstrates a significant drop in afterload and other haemodynamic indices, its use should be considered to maintain normal haemodynamics as well as to reduce portal pressures.

Table 2. Preferred haemodynamic conditions in patients with common cardiac valvular diseases. In all cases normal contractility should be supported

	Heart Rate	Preload (Left ventricle)	Systemic vascular Resistance
Aortic Stenosis	Normal or below	High	Normal or above
Aortic Regurgitation	Normal or above	High	Normal or below
Mitral Stenosis	Normal or below	High	Normal or above
Mitral Regurgitation	Normal or above	Normal*	Normal or below

*Poorly tolerates increases or decreases in preload.

Aortic Regurgitation

Assessment and Pathophysiology

Aortic regurgitation may be a result of primary aortic valvular disease in approximately 50% of cases, or as a result of primary aortic root disease in the other 50% [15]. Primary valvular aortic regurgitation is most commonly due to rheumatic heart disease (often with a latency period of 10 to 15 years) or a congenital bicuspid valve, and predominantly occurs in males. Primary aortic root disease is idiopathic in most cases, but other conditions such as Marfan's syndrome, ankylosing spondylitis and syphilis should be excluded [15]. In patients with primary valvular disease, dilatation of the aortic annulus may occur and further increase regurgitation.

In aortic regurgitation, the stroke volume is increased; however, this includes the regurgitant volume that passes back through the incompetent valve. As disease progresses, there is an increase in left ventricular end-diastolic volume, and dilatation and hypertrophy of the left ventricle occur to compensate for the regurgitant fraction. As the regurgitation worsens, there is further dilatation of the left ventricle, a decrease in ejection fraction, and deterioration in left ventricular function. Patients with severe aortic regurgitation may not tolerate atrial arrhythmias, as they have an increased reliance on atrial contraction to ensure adequate ventricular filling.

The earliest symptom of aortic regurgitation is awareness of heartbeat followed by the development of exertional dyspnoea. However, most patients do not become symptomatic until after myocardial dysfunction has occurred. As the disease progresses, symptoms of heart failure including orthopnoea and paroxysmal nocturnal dyspnoea occur. Angina may occur secondary to left ventricular hypertrophy. As the disease further progresses, congestive hepatomegaly and peripheral oedema may develop. After diagnosis, the natural history of aortic regurgitation is approximately 75% survival at 5 years, and 50% at 10 years [15].

Medical Management

Medical treatment consists of diuretics and vasodilators, with control of hypertension.

Surgical Management

Surgical treatment should be considered before left ventricular dysfunction is so severe that normal function would not return after valve replacement, as in these cases there is a significant ongoing mortality despite surgery [15]. It should therefore be undertaken once there is evidence of left ventricular dysfunction, even if patients are asymptomatic. The overall perioperative mortality for a patient with an isolated aortic valve replacement is approximately 3%. Patients with dilated aortas may also require aortic repair at the time of valve replacement, with these complex procedures having a higher perioperative mortality.

Intraoperative Haemodynamic Management

In the liver transplant setting, anaesthesia goals are the maintenance of sinus rhythm, avoidance of bradycardia (to decrease the time for regurgitation to occur), and reduction of afterload to increase forward flow during systole (Table 2) [18].

Mitral Stenosis

Assessment and Pathophysiology

Mitral stenosis is most commonly caused by rheumatic fever. Other rare causes include congenital abnormalities, cardiac masses and previous endocarditis [19]. As the most common cause is rheumatic fever, other co-existing valve conditions should be excluded. In rheumatic disease there may be a long latency between the disease and development of severe valvular pathology.

Symptoms of mitral valve stenosis include dyspnoea, cough, and the development of severe cardiac failure. As disease progresses and atrial enlargement occurs, there is increased risk of the onset of atrial fibrillation, which is associated with further deterioration in symptoms, and the risk of development of left heart thrombi.

The normal mitral valve area is 4 to 6 cm^2 with severe mitral valve stenosis occurring when the mitral valve area is <1 cm^2 or a transvalvular gradient of >10 mmHg [15]. The elevated atrial pressure required to generate blood flow across the stenosed valve eventually results in increased pulmonary venous pressures, the development of pulmonary hypertension, and the development of right ventricular failure.

The natural history of severe mitral stenosis with medical therapy alone is 44% five year survival, and 32% 10 year survival [15, 19].

Medical Management

Medical treatment includes diuretics and restriction of sodium intake. Where atrial fibrillation is present and chronic and irreversible, the use of digoxin, beta-blockers and calcium channel blockers may be used to slow ventricular rate, and the patient is anticoagulated with warfarin.

Surgical Management

Surgical treatment consists of either mitral valvotomy or mitral valve replacement. Mitral valvotomy may be performed percutaneously, with results being similar to open valvotomy [19]. This offers the advantage in patients with liver disease of not requiring CPB. Approximately 50% of patients who undergo valvotomy will require re-operation within ten years [15].

Mitral valve replacement is indicated in the presence of mixed mitral valve disease, or in patients in whom valvotomy has been unsuccessful. The overall perioperative mortality for isolated mitral valve replacement is approximately 5%, and the 10 year survival of surgical survivors is approximately 70% [15].

As severe mitral stenosis is associated with pulmonary hypertension, which is a risk factor for perioperative mortality for liver transplantation, it is unlikely that patients with uncorrected mitral stenosis would be activated for liver transplantation.

Intraoperative Haemodynamic Management

Patients with mitral stenosis require adequate left atrial filling and pressures to ensure flow through the stenotic valve into the left ventricle. Tachycardia should be avoided where possible to allow adequate time for flow across the valve in diastole. Maintenance of sinus rhythm allows for the atrial kick to improve ventricular filling. Fluid requirements should be a balance between increased filling pressures required for the left atrium, and the potential to overload causing congestive heart failure (Table 2) [18].

Mitral Regurgitation

Assessment and Pathophysiology

The causes of chronic mitral regurgitation include rheumatic disease, dilation of the mitral valve annulus, mitral valve prolapse, secondary to ischaemia, and less commonly dilated cardiomyopathies and hypertrophic obstructive cardiomyopathy [15]. Mitral regurgitation can also occur secondary to pathophysiological changes relating to aortic valve disease.

Pathophysiological changes in severe mitral regurgitation include left atrial dilatation with increased left atrial pressures, and increased pulmonary venous and arterial pressures, and the onset of atrial fibrillation.

Patients with mitral regurgitation normally become symptomatic only when the disease becomes severe, as they develop fatigue and symptoms of left, and then right heart failure.

The natural history of asymptomatic mitral regurgitation is a five year mortality of 22%, and with severe mitral regurgitation one study indicating a 67% mortality at eight years [20]. On the basis of the natural history of asymptomatic disease, patients with mild or asymptomatic mitral regurgitation who undergo liver transplantation should undergo regular cardiology review after transplant.

Medical Management

Medical treatment of severe mitral regurgitation includes the use of beta-blockers, ACE inhibitors, diuretics, and digoxin. In the presence of atrial fibrillation, warfarin is introduced if there are no contraindications.

Surgical Management

Mitral valve repair or replacement is indicated once there are severe symptoms, or if patients have deteriorating left ventricular function despite being asymptomatic [20]. Repair offers the advantage that in patients who are in sinus rhythm, long-term anticoagulation is not required. In patients with atrial fibrillation, procedures to reduce atrial fibrillation such as pulmonary vein isolation may be performed to reduce the requirement for anticoagulation.

Intraoperative Haemodynamic Management

In patients with moderate mitral regurgitation, the heart rate should be kept in the upper range of normal to reduce the period of time in diastole when left ventricular distension may occur. Maintenance of sinus rhythm offers the advantage of the atrial contraction contribution to ventricular filling. Afterload reduction will enable increased forward ventricular ejection (Table 2) [18].

Tricuspid Valve Disease

Tricuspid stenosis is almost always secondary to rheumatic heart disease and may occur in up to 10% of patients with severe mitral stenosis [15]. If severe, patients develop symptoms and signs of right heart failure. Patients with tricuspid stenosis frequently have tricuspid regurgitation. Isolated tricuspid regurgitation is normally secondary to other cardiac pathologies. Surgical options include valve repair, annuloplasty, or valve replacement. However, tricuspid valve replacements are associated with an increased incidence of thromboembolic events.

The elevated venous pressures that occur with tricuspid disease have the potential to worsen chronic liver disease. Severe right-sided heart failure may result in chronic liver inflammation and increased cirrhosis.

Pulmonary Valve Disease

Pulmonary valve disease is relatively rare in comparison to other valvular pathologies. In cases of pulmonary valve disease, as with tricuspid disease, carcinoid syndrome should be excluded.

Patient Triage

Once the patient's condition has been reviewed, taking into account the natural and treated history of liver disease, the patient's current liver and cardiac function, and the natural and treated history of the valvular disease, patients may be triaged into one of three categories (Figure 1).

- Suitable to proceed with transplantation
- Require further medical or surgical optimisation
- Unsuitable for transplantation based on high peri-operative risk, or poor cardiac prognosis.

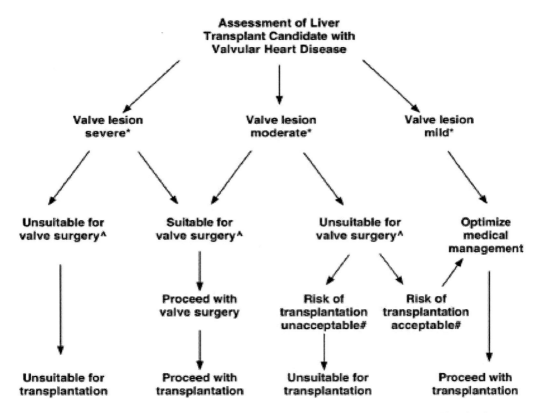

*Assessment of valve lesion severity based on cardiology opinion and echocardiographic criteria.
^Suitability for valve surgery based on cardiothoracic surgical opinion and extent and nature of liver disease (ie. Child-Pugh class) and other co-morbidities.
#Assessment of transplantation risk based on anaesthetic, cardiology, and hepatology opinions.
This flowchart assumes that there are no other contraindications to transplantation.

Figure 1. A possible algorithm for triage of liver transplant candidates with uncorrected valvular heart disease.

Perioperative Management

The surgical procedure for liver transplantation involves the potential for large fluid shifts and rapidly altering cardiovascular conditions with the application and release of inferior vena cava cross clamps, and these should be considered with the pathophysiology of each valvular condition [21].

Preoperative Management

While waiting transplantation, patients with valvular disease should be reviewed regularly, and have repeated echocardiography to ensure that there has been no further progression of disease and that their haemodynamic management remains optimised. In patients who are anticoagulated, pre-operative partial or full reversal of anticoagulation may be required.

Pre-Anhepatic Phase

In all patients with valvular disease or previous valve replacements, the peri-operative antibiotic regimen should include adequate prophylaxis to reduce the risk of infective endocarditis.

In addition to routine monitors, the use of TOE and the insertion of a pulmonary artery catheter should be considered. Transoesophageal echocardiography offers the advantages of being able to continually assess ventricular function in the presence of cardiac filling changes, to estimate cardiac output, and to assess the changes in valvular function that may occur with fluid shifts. In order to obtain maximal information, the presence of a person trained and skilled in TOE is required. In patients with severe oesophageal varices, TOE may be contraindicated. A thermodilution pulmonary artery catheter allows for measurement of cardiac output as well as pulmonary artery and pulmonary artery occlusion pressures. The calculated haemodynamic indices may be of use in guiding therapy. The pulmonary artery catheter offers another advantage in that it can used for continued haemodynamic monitoring in the intensive care unit. Other less invasive cardiac output monitors may also be suitable [21].

As the pre-anhepatic phase involves surgical dissection to expose and mobilise the liver, there is the potential for large blood loss, especially in patients with cirrhotic disease, portal hypertension, and coagulopathy. The release of ascites may also be associated with hypotension. Manipulation of the liver during this phase may result in sudden decreases in venous return.

Anhepatic Phase

The anhepatic phase is associated a decreased venous return, decreased cardiac output, and decreased arterial pressure. The use of a piggyback technique to allow some flow through the vena cava during the anhepatic phase should be discussed with the surgical team preoperatively. If a trial of inferior vena cava clamping indicates that adequate filling and arterial pressure cannot be maintained, VVB should be instituted. Vasopressors and fluids will be normally be required to maintain adequate blood pressure and cardiac output, particularly if VVB is not used. However, large volumes of fluid may have the propensity to cause cardiac failure in patients with valvular heart disease.

This phase is often associated with the development of acidosis and hypocalcaemia. Although the normal heart may tolerate a mild reduction in contractility associated with these biochemical disturbances, the presence of valvular disease may increase the likelihood of decompensation and the development of cardiac failure.

Post-Anhepatic Phase

In addition to the usual correction of electrolyte abnormalities, inotropes should be prepared to maintain myocardial function should this be adversely affected on reperfusion. Immediately post-reperfusion there is usually a transient physiological insult to the myocardium, the extent of which depends on the preservation of the liver, the flushing of potassium from the liver, and the delivery of relatively cool blood into the coronary circulation. While in most patients this is transitory, it may be more significant or prolonged in patients with underlying valvular heart disease.

In this period, there is also the potential for further blood loss. Fluid therapy and inotrope requirement should be titrated to echocardiography findings, pulmonary artery, or other indices of cardiac function.

Post-Operative Management

In patients with valvular heart disease, the particular concerns in the postoperative period include the reinstitution of anticoagulation where required and continued antibiotic prophylaxis. Regular cardiac medications and their side effects should be reviewed with respect to the changes that occur as the hyperdynamic circulation resolves towards normal, and hepatic metabolism is improved.

Conclusion

Patients presenting for liver transplantation with valvular heart disease provide challenges to all members of the transplant team. In order to minimise the perioperative risk, appropriate triage and pre-operative optimisation of patients with valvular heart disease is required. Intraoperative haemodynamic management requires a thorough understanding of the pathophysiology of the various valvular lesions and the particular stresses associated with liver transplantation. Irrespective of the extent of preoperative preparation, the intraoperative management of the valvular heart disease, and the anaesthetists's skills will have a major role in ensuring a successful outcome.

References

[1] Prasad MK, Rozario CJ, Arrowsmith JE. Anesthetic management of the patient with carcinoid heart disease. In: Arrowsmith JE, Simpson J. Problems in Anesthesia: Cardiothoracic Surgery. London: Martin Dunitz. 2002. pp 293-299.

[2] Moller S, Dumcke CW, Krag A. The heart and the liver. *Expert Rev. Gastroenterol Hepatol* 2009; 3: 51-64.

[3] Matyal R, Mahmood F. Assessment of valvular function and abnormalities with TEE. *Int Anesthesiol Clin* 2008; 46:63-81.

[4] Perrino AC, Reeves ST. A practical approach to transesophageal echocardiography. 2nd ed. Philadelphia, Lippincott Williams and Wilkins, 2008.

[5] Fisouli F, Salzberg SP, Rahmanian PB, et al. Early and late outcome of cardiac surgery in patients with liver cirrhosis. *Liver Transpl* 2007; 13:990-995.

[6] An Y, Xiao YB, and Zhong QJ. Open-heart surgery in patients with liver cirrhosis: indications, risk factors, and clinical outcomes. *Eur Surg Res* 2007; 39:67-74.

[7] Pollard RJ, Sid A, Gibby GL. Aortic stenosis with end-stage liver disease: prioritizing surgical and anesthetic therapies. *J Clin Anesth* 1998 10:253-261.

[8] Sun JCJ, Davidson MJ, Lamy A, Eikelboom JW. Antithrombotic management of patients with prosthetic heart valves: current evidence and future trends. *Lancet* 2009; (374):565-576.

[9] Stangier J, Stahle H, Rathgen, Roth W, Shaker-Nejad K. Pharmacokinetics and pharmacodynamics of dabigatran etexilate, an oral direct thrombin inhibitor, are not effected by moderate hepatic impairment. *J Clin Pharmacol* 2008; 48:1411-1419.

[10] Watts SA, Gibbs NM Outpatient management of the chronically anticoagulated patient for elective surgery. *Anaesth Intensive Care* 2003; 31:145–154.

[11] Shlebak A, Malik I. Managing heparin anticoagulation in patients with prosthetic cardiac valves: balancing the risk. *Heart* 2009; 95:1643-1645.

[12] Vongpatanasin W, Hillis LD, Lange RA. Prosthetic heart valves. *N Eng J Med* 1996; 335; 407-416.

[13] Paterson DL, Dominquez EA, Chang FY, Snydman DR, Singh N. Infective endocarditis in solid organ transplant recipients. *Clin Infect Dis* 1998; 26:689-694.

[14] Mylonakis E, Calderwood SB. Infective endocarditis in adults. *N Eng J Med* 2001; 345; 1318-1330.

[15] O'Gara P, Braunwald E. Valvular Heart Disease. In: Kasper DL, Braunwald E, Fauci AS, Hauser SL, Longo DL, Jameson JL et al, eds. Harrison's principles 17th ed, New York, McGraw-Hill, 2008.

[16] Zigelman CZ. Edelstein PM. Aortic valve stenosis. *Anesthesiol. Clin* 2009; 27: 519-532.

[17] Grube E, Schuler G, Buellesfeld L, et al. Percutaneous aortic valve replacement for severe aortic stenosis in high-risk patients using the second and third generation self-expanding core valve prosthesis: device success and 30-day clinical outcome. *J Am Col Cardiol* 2007; 50: 69-76.

[18] Sukernik MR, Martin DM. Anesthetic management for the surgical treatment of valvular heart disease. In Hensley R, Martin D, Gravlee GP, eds. A practical approach

to cardiac anesthesia. 4th Ed, New York, Lippincott Williams and Wilkins. 2008, pp 198-229.
[19] Chandrashekhar Y, Westaby S, Narula J. Mitral stenosis. *Lancet* 2009; 375: 1271-1283.
[20] Otto CM, Salerno CT. Timing of surgery in symptomatic mitral regurgitation. *N Eng J Med* 2005; 352: 928-929.
[21] Fabbroni D, Bellamy M. Anaesthesia for hepatic transplantation. *Continuing Education in Anaesthesia, Critical Care and Pain* 2006; 6: 171-175.

Chapter V

Pulmonary Hypertension and Liver Transplantation

*Michael Ramsay**
Chairman, Department of Anesthesiology, Baylor University Medical Centre
Dallas Texas 75240, USA

Abstract

Portopulmonary hypertension is found in 5-6% of patients with portal hypertension. This may or may not be associated with liver cirrhosis. If cirrhosis is present the severity of the liver cirrhosis does not correlate with the degree of pulmonary hypertension. The diagnosis of portopulmonary hypertension includes a mean pulmonary artery pressure of greater than 25 mm Hg at rest and a pulmonary vascular resistance of greater than 240 dynes.s.cm^{-5} and the presence of portal hypertension. Approximately 20% of patients with liver cirrhosis presenting for liver transplantation will have increased pulmonary artery pressures, but in the majority of patients this is the result of intravascular volume overload, together with a high flow state that is typically seen in patients with liver cirrhosis and this may be further affected by the presence of a cirrhotic cardiomyopathy. However the key differentiator of these causes of pulmonary hypertension from true portopulmonary hypertension is that in this group the pulmonary vascular resistance is normal or low.

The etiology of portopulmonary hypertension is not well understood. Initially endothelial dysfunction in the pulmonary arterioles may occur as the result of sheer stress forces from the high velocity circulation and the toxic effects of inflammatory molecules that are either not cleared by the liver or are released by the diseased liver.

The clinical symptoms may be minimal in the early phases of the disease but as it progresses shortness of breath, chest pain, fatigue, palpitations and syncope may present. However these symptoms are not distinct from those of progressive liver disease, therefore all liver transplant candidates should be screened for portopulmonary hypertension. The current screening tool is the trans-thoracic Doppler echocardiogram. If

---

* Correspondence: Michael Ramsay, MD, FRCA, Chairman, Department of Anesthesiology, Baylor University Medical Centre, Dallas Texas 75240, USA, Tel: +1-214-820-3296, E-mail: docram@baylorhealth.edu.

the right ventricular systolic pressure is 50 mm Hg or greater a right heart catheterization should be performed and the pulmonary vascular resistance calculated. Once the diagnosis of portopulmonary hypertension has been made a careful assessment of right ventricular function is required by echocardiography. Liver transplantation will treat many of these patients but not all, and it cannot be predicted which patients will respond to transplantation. The risks of liver transplantation increase with the severity of the pulmonary hypertension and those patients with evidence of right heart dysfunction should undergo pulmonary vasodilator therapy prior to consideration for transplant.

Introduction

Portal hypertension with and without liver cirrhosis has been associated with pulmonary complications [1]. One of these complications is pulmonary artery hypertension and when this is associated with portal hypertension it is termed portopulmonary hypertension (POPH). This is a very serious complication for the patient, as the right heart ventricle (RV) is well designed to pump volume but only at low pressures and low after load. The RV does not have the muscle power to handle the increased workload if a significant increase in pulmonary vascular resistance (PVR) occurs unless this increase in after load is gradual and hypertrophy of the ventricle muscle can take place. If this increase in RV wall strength does not occur the right heart will become dilated and dysfunctional resulting in venous congestion of the liver. Eventually as the POPH progresses right heart failure will occur and eventual patient demise. If liver transplantation is contemplated in a patient with POPH, then the state of the right ventricle must be carefully assessed as any dysfunction of the RV will cause liver graft congestion and possible failure and this may result in the loss of the graft and the patient.

Portopulmonary Hypertension

Portopulmonary hypertension is defined as pulmonary hypertension associated with portal hypertension. The diagnostic criteria for POPH include a mean pulmonary artery pressure (mPAP) of greater than 25 mmHg at rest together with a PVR greater than 240 dynes.s.cm^{-5} and a transpulmonary gradient of greater than 12 mmHg. [2] The pulmonary artery oclusion pressure (PAOP) of less than 15 mmHg is usually included in the definition but in many of the patients with end-stage liver disease there is a very hyperdynamic circulation, volume overload and in some patients a significant cirrhotic cardiomyopathy. These complications may cause an elevation in the pulmonary artery occlusion pressure in addition to the patient having an elevated PVR. Therefore the PAOP of less than 15 mm Hg may exclude patients with true POPH that have these confounding factors. The transpulmonary gradient (TPG) (mPAP-PAOP) is a measure of the obstruction to blood flow across the pulmonary circulation and distinguishes the contribution of volume from PVR to the increases in mPAP [3]. This is important as approximately 20% of patients with end-stage liver disease presenting for liver transplantation will have elevated pulmonary artery pressures but this is the result of pulmonary venous hypertension and the PVR is normal or low. True POPH with an elevated PVR occurs in approximately 5-6% of liver transplant patients and is caused by pathological changes in the pulmonary arterioles that increase the resistance to blood flow and the work of the RV. It is a progressive disease with a life expectancy of approximately 2 years without liver transplantation [4]. More recent reports have shown some improvement in these survival numbers and may reflect better vasodilator therapy [5,6]. Portopulmonary hypertension may be ameliorated temporarily by pulmonary vasodilator therapy and this should be used to optimize patients for liver transplantation. Many patients will have their POPH reversed with liver transplantation but in some patients the POPH will continue after liver transplantation and in other patients POPH may develop *de novo* after a successful liver transplant. [7,8]

Pathophysiology

The etiology of POPH has not been clearly defined but the histological changes are very similar to those changes found in primary pulmonary hypertension. The pulmonary arteriole vascular wall may exhibit medial hypertrophy, plexiform lesions, intimal proliferation and adventitial fibrosis. It is possible that in the group of patients that fail to respond to liver transplantation some of the patients may have true primary pulmonary hypertension and not POPH. The condition is progressive and when it reaches the fibrosis stage it is very unlikely that it can be repaired and perhaps if this stage could be identified a combined double-lung liver transplant may be considered.

The increased blood flow in the pulmonary arterioles is associated with the typical high cardiac output state that occurs with portal hypertension and liver cirrhosis. This creates stress sheer forces on the vascular endothelium and may well be the cause of endothelial dysfunction [9,10]. The vascular endothelium is the modulator of hemodynamics and as it becomes dysfunctional it can no longer maintain this role. Increased levels of endothelin-1, a potent vasoconstrictor produced by the endothelium are found in POPH, and also reports of increased levels of other vasoactive molecules and inflammatory molecules such as angiotensin 1, thromboxane B2, and prostaglandin $F_2\alpha$. [11, 12] Vasodilator substances such as nitric oxide and prostacyclin synthase may be reduced or in some areas of the pulmonary circulation produced in excess. The result of this is that sometimes hepatopulmonary syndrome (HPS) may be found, caused by the vascular dilatations producing effective pulmonary shunts. HPS may co-exist with POPH in the same patient, with one or the other pathological states predominating [13]. On top of theses pathological changes, the dysfunctional endothelium may not produce adequate thrombomodulin and microthrombosis may occur causing an acute increase in PVR, mPAP and acute RV dysfunction [14]. In the early stages the vasoconstriction is reversible with pulmonary vasodilator therapy. There have also been some genetic links to the cause of pulmonary hypertension and biomarkers have been sought by investigators for the etiology of POPH. Mutation in the gene that codes bone morphogenic protein receptor type 11 has been associated with primary pulmonary hypertension but has not yet been identified in patients with POPH. Other possible risk factors for developing POPH have been identified as the female sex and autoimmune hepatitis [12]. Other studies have implicated genetic variation in estrogen signaling and cell growth regulators as being potential risk factors[15 - 17].

Presentation

The clinical presentation of POPH maybe masked by the symptoms of the underlying liver disease and portal hypertension. Dyspnea on exertion, fatigue, weakness and orthopnea are frequently seen. Moderate hypoxemia and a decreased arterial partial pressure of carbon dioxide have been reported [18]. The electrocardiogram may show a right heart strain pattern including a right bundle branch block. Serum B-type natriuretic peptide may be found to be elevated [19].

If patients are not screened for POPH at initial assessment for liver transplantation, it may not be discovered until the time of transplantation. At this time a careful evaluation made under the pressure of a donor graft being present on ice, must be made. The correct decision on whether to go forward with liver transplantation is crucial as both the graft and the patient's outcome are at risk.

Screening

Every patient presenting with for liver transplantation, with portal hypertension should be screened by two-dimensional Doppler trans-thoracic echocardiography (TTE) to detect possible pulmonary hypertension [20-23]. The TTE allows the estimation of right ventricular systolic pressure (RVSP) provided there is a tricuspid regurgitant jet present. The RVSP is calculated from the peak tricuspid regurgitant jet velocity (TRV) using the modified Bernoulli equation and estimating the right atrial pressure (RAP): $RVSP = 4(TRV)^2 + RAP$. This evaluation, if it can be made has a 97% sensitivity and 77% specificity for diagnosing moderate and severe POPH. [22] If the RSVP is found to be greater than 50 mm Hg a right heart catheterization is indicated to fully characterize the hemodynamic data. Recently a potentially more accurate screening test has been reported utilizing the ratio of peak TVR to the right ventricular outflow tract velocity time integral. This value provides an accurate test for identifying a PVR of more than 120 $dyne.s.cm^{-5}$ [23]. The sensitivity and negative predictive value of this test was reported as 100%. It is also vital that both right and left ventricular anatomy and function are well characterized, taking in to account that the typical patient with cirrhosis has an elevated cardiac output and low systemic vascular resistance. This may give the impression of a dynamic functioning heart and mask significant cirrhotic cardiomyopathy that has been reported to occur in 100% of patients with liver cirrhosis [24]. Any dilation of the right heart chambers must be noted as the risk to undergoing liver transplantation is right heart dysfunction or failure with graft congestion and subsequent graft loss and potential loss of the recipient. The RV that has reduced contractility is very sensitive to increases in workload and will become dysfunctional and fail [25].

Most patients that have pulmonary hypertension presenting for liver transplantation do not have true POPH. On close examination of the pulmonary hemodynamics, most of these patients will have a normal or low PVR and are suffering from volume overload, high output failure or cardiomyopathy with ventricular dysfunction, or a combination of all of these factors. True POPH is only found in 5-6% of transplant candidates and is the result of pathological changes in the pulmonary vasculature. [4]. However true POPH can also exist complicated by volume overload, high output failure and cardiomyopathy, so guidelines on management must be tempered by these possible confounding pathologies. It is also the reason that a normal PAOP does not always fit in the definition of POPH. An elevated PAOP is very compatible and is frequently seen with true POPH. The critical factors are the elevated TPG > 12 mm HG and a PVR > 240 dyne.s.cm^{-5} which have to be determined by right heart catheterization.

If pulmonary hypertension is identified some centers perform a vasodilator challenge to test the potential pulmonary vascular reactivity to give an indication of possible reversibility. This may help with the decision to transplant or not as after liver transplantation the POPH may resolve if it will reverse with drug therapy. If an acute rise in POPH occurs in the perioperative period this may also give a strategy on how to treat it. Possibly vasoreactivity gives an indication that a fixed pathology such as fibrosis in the pulmonary arterioles has not occurred giving hope that a liver transplant may reverse the pathology. However this hypothesis has not yet been tested with a randomized controlled clinical trial. In one vasoreactivity trial, inhaled nitric oxide has been compared to intravenous epoprostenol and oral isosorbide-5-mononitrate in patients with POPH and the results have demonstrated variable reductions in pulmonary hemodynamics [26].

Pharmacotherapy

Once diagnosed with POPH the patient should be treated to optimize the PVR and RV function for potential liver transplantation. Unlike HPS that is reversed by liver transplantation POPH may not reverse immediately and may require prolonged vasodilator therapy. In a few patients undergoing liver transplantation the POPH will not reverse and these patients cannot be predicted ahead of time.

The institution of diuretic therapy can reduce the hypervolemia that may be a significant component of the presentation of an elevated mPAP, and can certainly reduce the CVP and chamber dilatation.

The use of calcium channel blockers are contraindicated in the treatment of POPH as they have been demonstrated to increase the hepatic venous gradient and portal vein flow in cirrhotic patients [27]. Beta-blockers have also been demonstrated to adversely affect hemodynamics [28].

Epoprostenol an analogue of prostaglandin I$_2$ is a potent pulmonary arteriole vasodilator. It is an intravenous agent that because of its short half-life requires a continuous infusion via an indwelling catheter. This poses a potential infection risk over the long term that it frequently needed. Epoprostenol is also an inhibitor of platelet function; causes splenomegaly and these both may have a significant negative impact on the effect of the existing thrombocytopenia usually found in the cirrhotic patient[29]. Other side effects associated with long-term intravenous epoprostenol include jaw pain, headache, flushing, nausea and other unpleasant symptoms. However therapy with epoprostenol has been shown to be effective in some patients by improving the pulmonary hemodynamics and allowing time for RV function to improve, mPAP to ameliorate and allow successful liver transplantation[30-32]. Sudden cessation of the epoprostenol infusion may result in rebound vasoconstriction, severe pulmonary hypertension and potential death and so must be avoided.

Other prostacyclin analogues have been trialed in clinical case series with some positive outcomes. Iloprost may be administered intravenously but has the advantage that it can be delivered via an inhaler. The length of action is short and requires frequent administration, up to 6 to 9 times a day but it does avoid the need for an indwelling catheter [33, 34]. In an experimental animal model inhaled iloprost was shown to improve global hemodynamics [35]. Intravenous iloprost has been used as a bridge to liver transplantation in patients with POPH [36].

Treprostinil has been administered over the long term subcutaneously with some positive results [37]; treprostinil also may be administered intravenously.

Endothelin receptor antagonists block the vasoconstrictive action of endothelin-1 on the pulmonary vasculature. They have the advantage that they may be given orally. Bosentan is a dual endothelin receptor antagonist blocking both endothelin A and B receptors so that endothelin-1 cannot bind and cause vasoconstriction. Bosentan has been associated with an increase in hepatic enzymes in a small percentage of patients on initiation of therapy [38,39]. However, in a group of patients with severe POPH bosentan and iloprost were shown to be safe and the bosentan group had better long-term survival [34]. Ambrisentan is another endothelin-1 receptor blocker that has just been approved for the treatment of primary pulmonary hypertension with no reported hepatic adverse effects and this may be a more suitable agent for treating POPH [40].

The phosphodiesterase 5 inhibitor, sildenafil is another oral drug that has shown efficacy in treating POPH. [41,42] The cyclic guanosine monophosphatase-specific phosphodiesterase type 5 enzymes that are found in the pulmonary vascular endothelium are selectively inhibited. This prolongs the effects of nitric oxide (NO) mediated vasodilatation in the endothelium [43].

Inhaled milrinone, a phosphodiesterase-3 inhibitor, has been used as a selective pulmonary vasodilator, when delivered via a nebulizer system, in cardiac surgery and may have a role in the treatment of decompensated pulmonary hypertension in liver transplantation. When administered as an inhalant milrinone does not cause systemic hypotension [44].

Chronic inhalation of NO has been used in the treatment of primary pulmonary hypertension and also to reverse acute elevations in mPAP during liver transplantation. [45,46}

Combination therapies of these drugs have been used with some success [47].

New antiproliferative therapies that block the platelet-derived growth factor receptor may allow a reversal of the vascular remodeling and cause a reduction in POPH are under review [48]. For more details about pharmacotherapy see chapter 15.

Staging of POPH: Risk Management

The risk of undergoing liver transplantation in the patient with POPH has been assessed based on the mPAP and an experience based on case reports, case series, local databases and a small national database. However mixed pathologies may exist in this patient group including volume overload, high cardiac output and cirrhotic cardiomyopathy that will alter the risks of going ahead with transplantation. The key factors to survival rest with the RV function and the level of fixed resistance to the outflow of the RV, which is a function of the

PVR more than the actual value of the mPAP. However it is a good starting point to trigger a risk evaluation.

A patient who has compensated well to an increase in PVR by a strengthening of the RV may successfully undergo a liver transplant with a high mPAP ulike a patient who has poorly compensated and has a low mPAP.

As a guide, in patients with an elevated PVR, an mPAP of 25 mmHg to 35 mm Hg is termed mild POPH and does not have an increased risk for transplantation. Moderate POPH is an mPAP of 35 to 45 mm Hg and this has a significantly increased mortality of up to 50%. Severe POPH, an mPAP of greater than 45 mm Hg has up to 100% mortality. [49] The critical factor in each patient undergoing liver transplantation is whether the RV is able to handle the increases in mPAP caused by increases in volume, and significant increases in cardiac output against a potentially fixed resistance to flow. Therefore in the preoperative assessment the acute response to vasodilator therapy may give good information on how the patient will respond intraoperatively. A challenge with volume and a dobutamine infusion to increase cardiac output while observing RV function by echocardiography may also be helpful in assessing how the patient may tolerate transplantation.

The speed of onset of POPH is not known. However whenever endothelial dysfunction occurs there is the possibility of pulmonary microthrombosis and an acute rise in PVR and mPAP. Patients who are diagnosed with POPH should be started on vasodilator therapy and periodically undergo reassessment for suitability for liver transplantation. The screening for POPH and the aggressive treatment with pulmonary vasodilator therapy to reverse the process and optimize the patient for liver transplantation has improved the outcomes of this patient group [50-54].

A POPH Risk Assessment Algorithm is presented on Table 1.

Perioperative Management

If POPH is first diagnosed on the operating table immediately prior to liver transplantation a careful assessment of the pulmonary hemodynamics and RV function must be made with a right heart catheterization and trans-esophageal echocardiograph (TEE). If mPAP < 35 mm Hg and RV good then consider going ahead with transplant as long as CVP is normal. Otherwise defer transplant until pulmonary hemodynamics and RV can be optimized.

If the patient has known POPH and has been treated then a careful reassessment has to be made to be sure that there has been no deterioration in RV function. As the patient may have had deterioration in renal function with resulting volume overload continuous veno-venous hemodialysis may be necessary if the vascular filling pressures are elevated. This can easily be instituted in the operating room at the time of surgery.

Table 1. Portopulmonary hypertension risk assessment algorithm

1. All liver transplant candidates screened by TTE. If RVSP > than 50mm Hg perform right heart catheterization
2. mPAP < 35 mm Hg and PVR 250 – 300 dyne/s/cm^{-5}, good RV function: start on vasodilator therapy and place on transplant waiting list. Reassess every 6 months or if clinical deterioration. At time of transplant recheck with right heart catheter and TEE in the operating room prior to starting surgery.
3. mPAP 35 to 45 mm Hg and PVR 250 to 350 dyne/s/cm^{-5}, test reversibility, assess RV function, start on vasodilator therapy. If RV function good, stress with volume and dobutamine. If RV fails test or function is reduced defer surgery and monitor effect of chronic vasodilator therapy. If RV function excellent consider going ahead with transplant.
4. mPAP > 45 mm Hg and PVR t greater than 250 dyne/s/cm^{-5} treat with vasodilator therapy and defer transplant until mPAP improved and RV function good.
5. Following transplant continue to treat mPAP and PVR until values normalized.

The intraoperative management of the patient requires both right heart catheterization and TTE monitoring to manage the perturbations of the procedure. The key strategies to optimal management include reducing PVR and preventing acute rises in PVR and maintain good RV function. Monitor for early signs of RV decompensation so that early interventions can be made before the patient or the new graft become compromised. Systemic perfusion pressure must be maintained to prevent right ventricular ischemia and sinus rhythm should be maintained to allow adequate RV filling. Maintenance of normocapnia, and avoidance of hypoxia with the early treatment of acidosis and hypothermia are essential in preventing a rise in PVR [55]. These considerations also apply postoperatively in the critical care unit and early weaning from mechanical ventilation and tracheal extubation should not be considered in this very high acuity group of patients.

Acute Decompensated Pulmonary Hypertension

A strategy must be in place before starting the liver transplant on how to manage an acute decompensation in RV function caused by an elevation in mPAP. The new graft will quickly become congested and fail unless urgent effective therapy is undertaken to rapidly reduce mPAP and PVR. The period of highest risk is at the time of reperfusion of the graft. This is when an increase in cardiac output may occur up to 300% of the baseline value [3]. This massive increase in flow facing a fixed resistance in the pulmonary vasculature may cause a very large and rapid increase in mPAP. **Figure 1**

The effect of an ischemia/reperfusion injury on the vascular endothelium may compound the deleterious effects of this critical event [56,57]. Inotropic therapy to assist the RV contractility may be required such as dobutamine or inhaled milrinone. Early initiation of pulmonary vasodilators is essential. Inhaled nitric oxide has been shown to be effective in some instances [46]. Figure 2 Inhaled iloprost is another therapy that may be effective but the nebulizer and the administration tools for these agents must be immediately available. Vasopressin may have a role in maintaining systemic pressure as under experimental conditions it produces pulmonary vasodilatation and systemic vasoconstriction, but this has not been confirmed consistently in the clinical environment [58].

Other potential therapies include the use of an intra-aortic balloon pump to maintain left ventricular function, a right ventricular assist device and even a balloon septoplasty to create an atrial septal defect to decompress the right heart.

Postoperative Care

These patients can be expected to have a prolonged and critical recovery period. All the intraoperative measures need to be maintained to prevent a rebound of pulmonary hypertension during this period.

The role of liver transplantation in the treatment of POPH is not well defined. There are case reports of complete reversal of POPH after liver transplantation but there are other case series where pulmonary vasodilator has had to be continued for the long term [59-64]. There are other reports of progression of POPH after transplantation and eventual demise of the patient [65]. There may be a window of opportunity for carefully assessed patients who respond to vasodilator therapy to undergo early transplantation. The United Network for Organ Sharing (UNOS) is considering making an exception for those patients diagnosed with POPH and responds effectively to vasodilator therapy [66].

A therapeutic option for the patient with a fixed PVR and moderate to severe POPH maybe a combined lung and liver transplant [67]. The overall survival in one case series of 10 patients who underwent a double lung and liver transplant was at 1, 3and 5 years: 69, 62 and 49% respectively.

Conclusion

The etiology of POPH has not been fully elucidated. The effect of portal hypertension is to cause endothelial dysfunction in the pulmonary arterioles. This may result in a vasodilatation process HPS, or a proliferative process POPH or both entities may exist together. Which patients with portal hypertension will develop POPH is unknown. The key to understanding which patients with POPH will tolerate liver transplantation is the RV function. Impaired RV function will cause graft congestion with possible loss of graft and potential patient demise. Therefore those patients that do not respond to vasodilator therapy with a reduction in PVR and mPAP and with improvement in RV function are a relative contraindication to liver transplantation. Other factors to be considered are the impact of volume overload, high cardiac output and cirrhotic cardiomyopathy.

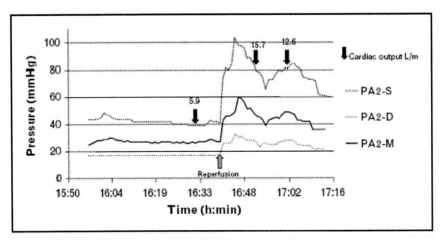

PA2-S, pulmonary artery pressure-systolic; PA2-D, pulmonary artery pressure – diastolic; PA2-M, pulmonary artery pressure – mean.
Reprinted from .[3] with permission.

Figure 1 Increase in cardiac output with concomitant increase in pulmonary artery pressures at reperfusion of the liver graft.

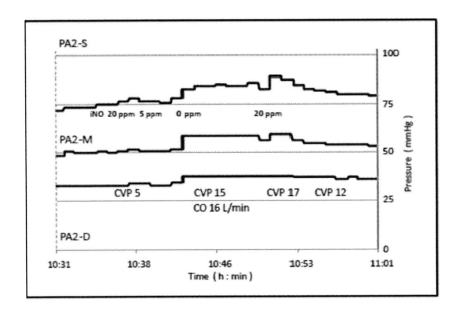

PA2-S, pulmonary artery pressure-systolic; PA2-D, pulmonary artery pressure – diastolic; PA2-M, pulmonary artery pressure – mean. CVP, central venous pressure,
CO, cardiac output.

Figure 2. The effect of withdrawing inhaled nitric oxide on right heart function following liver transplantation. Note the rise in CVP from 5 mm Hg to 17 mm Hg and then reducing to 12 mm Hg on restarting the nitric oxide.

Transplantation has been successful in patients who have responded to vasodilator therapy and many patients have been able to be weaned off therapy in the months post transplantation. However there are reports that even a successful liver transplant in this patient group does not guarantee a reversal of the pathological process. Careful assessment and optimization of the patient with POPH is necessary to delineate the risks of undergoing liver transplantation and whether this is the right therapy for the patient.

References

[1] Mantz FA, Craig E. Portal axis thrombosis with spontaneous portacaval shunt and resultant cor pulmonale. *Arch Pathol Lab Med* 1951; 52:91-7.
[2] Rodriguez-Roisin R, Krowka M, Hervé P, Fallon M. ERS Task Force Pulmonary-Hepatic Vascular Disorders (PHD) Scientific CommitTTE. Pulmonary-Hepatic Vascular Disorders. *Eur Respir J* 2004; 24:861-80.
[3] Ramsay M. Portopulmonary hypertension and right heart failure in patients with Cirrhosis. *Curr Opin Anaesthesiol* 2010; 23:145-50.
[4] Herve P, Lebrec D, Brenot F, Simonneau G, Humbert M, Sitbon O, Duroux P. Pulmonary vascular disorders in portal hypertension. *Eur Resp J* 1998; 11:1153-66.
[5] Kawut SM, Krowka MJ, Trotter JF, Roberts KE, Benza RL, Badesch DB et al. Pulmonary Vascular Complications of Liver Disease Study Group. Clinical risk factors for portopulmonary hypertension. *Hepatology* 2008; 48:196-203.
[6] Le Pavec J, Souza R, Herve P, Lebrec D, Savale L, Tcherakian C et al. Portopulmonary hypertension: Survival and prognostic factors. *Am J Respir Crit Care Med* 2008; 178:637-43.
[7] Koch DG, Caplan M, Reuben A. Pulmonary hypertension after liver transplantation: Case presentation and review of the literature. *Liver Transpl* 2009; 15:407-12.
[8] Ramsay M. Liver transplantation and pulmonary hypertension: pathophysiology and management strategies. *Curr Opin Organ Transplant* 2007; 12:274-80.
[9] Schroeder RA, Ewing CA, Sitzman JV, Kuo PC.. Pulmonary expression of iNOS and HO-1 protein is upregulated in a rat model of prehepatic portal hypertension. *Dig Dis Sci* 2000; 45:2405-10
[10] Ramsay M. Portopulmonary hypertension and hepatopulmonary syndrome and liver transplantation. *Int Anesthesiol Clin* 2006; 44:69-82.
[11] Bernardi M, Gulberg V, Colantoni A, Trevisani F, Gasbarrini A, Gerbes AL. Plasma endothelin-1 and 3 in cirrhosis: relationship with systemic hemodynamics, renal function and neurohumeral systems. *J Hepatol* 1996, 24: 161-8.
[12] Maruyama T, Ohsaki K, Shimoda S, Kaii Y, Harada M.. Thromboxane-dependent portopulmonary hypertension. *Am J Med* 2005; 118: 93-4.
[13] Kaspar MD, Ramsay MA, Shuey CB Jr, Levy MF, Klintmalm GG. Severe pulmonary hypertension and amelioration of hepatopulmonary syndrome after liver transplantation. *Liver Transpl Surg* 1998; 4:177-9
[14] Newman JH. Pulmonary hypertension. *Am J Respir Care Med* 2005; 172:1072-7
[15] Roberts KE, Fallon MB, Krowka MD, Brown RS, Trotter JF, Peter I et al. Pulmonary Vascular Complications of Liver Disease Study Group*et.* Genetic risk factors for portopulmonary hypertension in patients with advanced liver disease. *Am J Respir Crit Care Med* 2009; 179:835-42.

[16] Roberts KE, Fallon MB, Krowka MJ, Benza RL, Knowles JA, Badesch DB et al. Pulmonary Vascular Complications of Liver Disease Study Group Serotonin transporter polymorphisms in patients with portopulmonary hypertension. *Chest* 2009; 135:1470-5.

[17] Peng T, Zamanian R, Krowka MJ, Benza RL, Roberts KE, Taichman DB et al. Pulmonary Vascular Complications of Liver Disease Study Group. *Biomarkers* 2009;14 :156-60.

[18] Swanson KL, Krowka MJ. Arterial oxygenation associated with portopulmonary hypertension. *Chest* 2002;121:1869-75

[19] Bernal V, Pascual I, Esquivias P, García-Gil A, Mateo JM, Lacambra I et al. N-Terminal brain natriuretic peptide as a diagnostic test in cirrhotic patients with pulmonary arterial hypertension. *Transplant Proc* 2009; 41:987-8.

[20] Colle IO, Moreau R, Godinho E, Belghiti J, Ettori F, Cohen-Solal A et al. Diagnosis of portopulmonary hypertension in candidates for liver transplantation. *Hepatology* 2003; 37: 401-9.

[21] Murray KF, Carithers RL Jr. AASLD practice guidelines: evaluation of the patient for liver transplantation. *Hepatology* 2005;41:1407-32.

[22] Kim W, Krowka M, Plevak D, Lec J, Rettke SR, Frantz RP, Wiesner RH. Accuracy of Doppler echocardiography in the assessment of pulmonary hypertension in liver transplant candidates. *Liver Transpl* 2000;6:453-8.

[23] Farzaneh-Far R, McKeown BH, Dang D, Roberts J, Schiller NB, Foster E. Accuracy of Doppler-estimated pulmonary vascular resistance in patients before liver transplantation. *Am J Cardiol* 2008; 101:259-62.

[24] Alqahtani SA, Fouad TR, Lee SS. Cirrhotic cardiomyopathy. *Semin Liver Dis* 2008;28:59-69

[25] Afifi S, Shayan S, Al-Qamari A. Pulmonary hypertension and right ventricular function: interdependence in pathophysiology and management. *Int Anesthesiol Clin* 2009;47:97-120

[26] Ricci GL, Melgosa MT, Burgos F, Valera JL, Pizarro S, Roca J et al. Assessment of acute pulmonary vascular reactivity in portopulmonary hypertension. *Liver Transpl* 2007; 13:1506-14.

[27] Ota K, Shijo H, Kokawa H, Kubara K, Kim T, Akiyoshi N et al. Effects of nifedipine on hepatic venous pressure gradient and portal vein blood flow in patients with cirrhosis. *J Gastroenterol Hepatol* 1995; 10: 198-204.

[28] Provencher S, Herve P, Jais X, Lebrec D, Humbert M, Simonneau G, Sitbon O. Deleterious effect of beta-blockers on exercise capacity and hemodynamics in patients with portopulmonary hypertension. *Gastroenterology* 2006; 130:120-6.

[29] Findlay JY, Plevak DJ, Krowka MJ, Sack EM, Porayko MK. Progressive splenomegaly after epoprostenol therapy in portopulmonary hypertension. *Liver Transpl Surg* 1999; 5: 362-5.

[30] Fix OK, Bass NM, De Marco T, Merriman RB. Long-term follow-up of portopulmonary hypertension: effect of treatment with epoprostenol. *Liver Transpl* 2007; 13: 875-85.

[31] Krowka MJ, Frantz RP, McGoon MD, Severson C, Plevak DJ, Weisner RH. Improvement in pulmonary hemodynamics during intravenous epoprostenol (prostacyclin): a study of 15 patients with moderate to severe portopulmonary hypertension. *Hepatology* 1999; 30: 641-48.

[32] Kuo PC, Johnson LB, Plotkin JS, Howell CD, Bartlett ST, Rubin LJ. Continuous intravenous infusion of epoprostenol for the treatment of portopulmonary hypertension. *Transplantation* 1997; 63: 604-6.

[33] Krug S, Sablotzki A, Hammerschmidt S, Wirtz H, Sevfarth HJ. Inhaled iloprost for the control of pulmonary hypertension. *Vasc Health and Risk Management* 2009; 5: 465-74.

[34] Hoeper M, Seyfarth H, Hoeffken G, Wirtz H, Spiekerkoetter E, Pletz MW et al. Experience with inhaled iloprost and bosentan in portopulmonary hypertension. *Eur Respir J* 2007; 30: 1096-102.

[35] Rex S, Missant C, Claus P, Buhre W, Wouters PF. Effects of inhaled iloprost on right ventricular contractility, right ventriculo-vascular coupling and ventricular interdependence: a randomized placebo-controlled trial in an experimental model of acute pulmonary hypertension. *Crit Care* 2008, 12: 1-13.

[36] Minder S, Fischler M, Muelhaupt B, Zalunardo MP, Jenni R, Clavien PA, Speich R. Intravenous iloprost bridging to orthotopic liver transplantation in portopulmonary hypertension. *Eur Respir J* 2004; 24:703-7.

[37] Benza RL, Rayburn BK, Tallaj JA, Pamboukian SV, Bourge RC. Treprostinil-based therapy in the treatment of moderate-to-severe pulmonary arterial hypertension: long-term efficacy and combination with bosentan. *Chest* 2008;134(1):139-45

[38] Rubin LJ, Badesch DB, Barst RJ, Galie N, Black CM, Keogh A et al. Bosentan therapy for pulmonary artery hypertension . *N Engl J Med* 2002;346:896-903.

[39] Galiè N, Rubin Lj, Hoeper M, Jansa P, Al-Hiti H, Meyer G et al. Treatment of patients with mildly symptomatic pulmonary arterial hypertension with bosentan (EARLY study): a double-blind, randomised controlled trial. *Lancet* 2008;371(9630):2093-100

[40] McGoon MD, Frost AE, Oudiz RJ, Badesch DB, Galie N, Olschewski H et al. Ambrisentan therapy in patients with pulmonary arterial hypertension who discontinued bosentan or sitaxsentan due to liver function test abnormalities. *Chest* 2009 ;135(1):122-9.

[41] Gough M, White J. Sildenafil therapy is associated with improved hemodynamics in liver transplantation candidates with pulmonary artery hypertension. *Liver Transpl* 2009;15: 30-36.

[42] Hemnes A, Robbins I. Sildenafil monotherapy in portopulmonary hypertension can facilitate liver transplantation. *Liver Transpl* 2009;15:15-19.

[43] Montani D, Chaumais MC, Savale L, Natali D, Price LC, Jaïs X et al. Phosphodiesterase type 5 inhibitors in pulmonary arterial hypertension. *Adv Ther* 2009;26(9):813-25.

[44] Wang H, Gong M, Bin Z, Dai A. Comparison of inhaled and intravenous milrinone in patients with pulmonary hypertension undergoing mitral valve surgery. *Adv Ther* 2009; 26:462-8.

[45] Findlay JY, Harrison BA, Plevak DJ, Krowka MJ. Inhaled nitric oxide reduces pulmonary artery pressures in portopulmonary hypertension. *Liver Transpl Surg* 1999; 5:381-7

[46] Ramsay MAE, Spikes C, East CA, et al. The perioperative management of portopulmonary hypertension with nitric oxide and epoprostenol. *Anesthesiology* 1999; 90:299-301.

[47] Austin MJ, McDougall NI, Wendon JA, Sizer E, Knisely AS, Rela M et al. Safety and efficacy of combined use of sildenafil, bosentan, and iloprost before and after liver transplantation in severe portopulmonary hypertension. *Liver Transpl* 2008;14:287-91.

[48] Tapper E, Knowles D, Heffron T, Lawrence EC, Csete M. Portopulmonary hypertension: imatinib as a novel treatment and the Emory experience with this condition. *Transpl Proc* 2009; 1:1969-71.

[49] Swanson KL, Wiesner RH, Nyberg SL, Rosen CB, Krowka MJ. Survival in portopulmonary hypertension: Mayo Clinic experience categorized by treatment subgroups. *Am J Transplant* 2008; 8:2445-53.

[50] Swanson KL, Krowka MJ. Screen for portopulmonary hypertension, especially in liver transplant candidates. *Cleve Clin J Med* 2008;75:121-36.

[51] Ashfaq M, Chinnakotla S, Rodgers L.Ausloos K, Saadeh S, Klintmalm GB et al. The impact of treatment of portopulmonary hypertension on survival following liver transplantation. *Am J Transpl* 2007; 7:1258-64.

[52] Krowka M, Mandell M, Ramsay M, Kawut SM, Fallon MB, Manzarbeitia C et al. Hepatopulmonary syndrome and portopulmonary hypertension: a report of the multicenter liver transplant database. *Liver Transpl* 2004; 10:174-82.

[53] Naeije R, Huez S. Expert opinion on available options treating pulmonary arterial hypertension. *Expert Opin Pharmacother* 2007; 8: 2247-65.

[54] Porres-Aguilar M, ZuckermanM, Figueroa-Casas J, Krowka M. Portopulmonary hypertension: state of the art. *Ann Hepatol* 2008; 7: 321-30.

[55] Zamanian RT, Haddad F, Doyle RL, Weinacker A. Management strategies for patients with pulmonary hypertension in the intensive care unit. *Crit Care Med* 2007;35:2037-50

[56] Ramsay M. The reperfusion syndrome: have we made any progress? *Liver Transpl* 2008; 14: 412-4.

[57] Paugam-Burtz C, Kavafyan J, Merckx P, Dahmani S, Sommacale D, Ramsay M et al. Postreperfusion syndrome during liver transplantation for cirrhosis: outcome and predictors. *Liver Transpl* 2009; 15: 522-9

[58] Braun EB, Palin CA, Hogue CW. Vasopressin during spinal anesthesia in a patient with primary pulmonary hypertension treated with intravenous epoprostenol. *Anesth Analg* 2004; 99:36-37.

[59] Sugimachi K, Soejima Y, Morita S, Ueda S, Fukuhara T, Nagata S et al. Rapid normalization of portopulmonary hypertension after living donor liver transplantation. *Transpl Proc* 2009; 41:1976-8.

[60] Umeda N, Kamath P. Hepatopulmonary syndrome and portopulmonary hypertension. *Hepatol Res* 2009;39:1020-2.

[61] Swanson K, Wiesner R, Nyberg S. Rosen CB, Krowka MJ. Survival in portopulmonary hypertension: Mayo Clinic experience categorized by treatment subgroups. *Am J Transpl* 2008;8:2445-53.

[62] Singh C, Sager J. Pulmonary complications of cirrhosis. *Med Clin N Am* 2009; 95:871-83.

[63] Yeshua H, Blendis L, Oren R. Pulmonary manifestations of liver diseases. *Sem Cardiothorac Vasc Anesth* 2009;13:60-9.

[64] Golbin J, Krowka M. Portopulmonary hypertension. *Clin Chest Med* 2007; 28: 203-18.

[65] Krowka MJ, Mandell MS, Ramsay MA, Kawut SM, Fallon MB, Manzarbeitia C et al. Hepatopulmonary syndrome and portopulmonary hypertension: a report of the multicenter liver transplant database. *Liver Transpl* 2004;10(2):174-82.

[66] Krowka M, Fallon M, Mulligan D, Gish RG. Model for end-stage liver disease (MELD) exception for portopulmonary hypertension. *Liver Transpl* 2006;12: S114-S116.

[67] Grannas G, NeippM, Hoeper M, Gottlieb J, Luck R, Becker T.et al. Indications for and outcomes after combined lung and liver transplantation: a single center experience on 13 consecutive cases. *Transplantation* 2008; 85 (4):524-31.

In: Cardiovascular Diseases and Liver Transplantation
Editor: Zoka Milan, pp. 99-111
ISBN: 978-1-61122-910-3
© 2011 Nova Science Publishers, Inc.

Chapter VI

Hypertrophic Obstructive Cardiomypathy in Liver Transplant Patients

Paco E. Bravo[1] and Fadi G. Hage[2, 3]

[1]The Russell H Morgan, Department of Radiology and Radiological Sciences, Johns Hopkins University, Baltimore, MD, USA
[2]Division of Cardiovascular Diseases, University of Alabama at Birmingham, Birmingham, AL, USA
[3]Section of Cardiology, Birmingham Veteran's Administration Medical Center, Birmingham, AL, USA

Abstract

Hypertrophic obstructive cardiomyopathy (HOCM) is a complex cardiovascular disorder affecting patients with varying degrees of cardiac manifestations. The optimal treatment strategy for patients with HOCM and end-stage liver disease (ESLD) undergoing evaluation for orthotopic liver transplantation (OLT) is not well defined. Although medical management is the accepted first-line treatment, symptomatic patients with severe left ventricular outflow tract (LVOT) obstruction unresponsive to medications may require further interventions prior to surgery. Perioperative cardiovascular adverse effects in HOCM patients during non-cardiac surgery are relatively high. The anesthetic management of HOCM patients can be challenging and involves understanding the many factors that can be expected to aggravate the dynamic LVOT obstruction during OLT.

---

* Correspondence: Fadi G. Hage, MD, Zeigler Research Building 1024, 1530 3rd AVE S, Birmingham AL 35294-0006, USA, Tel: +205-934-0406, Fax: +205-934-0424, E-mail: fhage@cardmail.dom.uab.edu.

Introduction

Hypertrophic cardiomyopathy (HCM) is a complex genetic cardiac disease, diagnosed principally with trans-thoracic echocardiography (TEE) by demonstrating left ventricular (LV) hypertrophy with wall thickness of at least 15 mm in adults, typically asymmetric, in the absence of another cardiac or systemic disease capable of producing a similar degree of hypertrophy, such as hypertension or aortic stenosis [1]. HCM is characterized by a heterogeneous clinical expression, affecting patients of all ages and a diverse clinical course, where some individuals remain asymptomatic throughout life while others develop severe symptoms of heart failure (HF), angina or syncope, and a minority present with sudden cardiac death.

Hypertrophic obstructive cardiomyopathy (HOCM), a subset of HCM, refers to the presence of dynamic (in contradistinction to the fixed obstruction seen with aortic stenosis and membranous subaortic stenosis) LV outflow tract (OT) obstruction usually caused by systolic anterior motion (SAM) of the anterior mitral valve leaflet and projection of the hypertrophied interventricular septum into the LVOT in systole, leading to the creation of a gradient between the LV cavity and aorta (Figure 1 and Figure 2). The LVOT gradient is an independent predictor of HOCM-related death (approximately two-fold increased risk of death in HOCM vs. HCM without LVOT obstruction), progression to New York Heart Association (NYHA) class III or IV HF, and for death from HF or stroke when it exceeds 30 mm Hg [2].

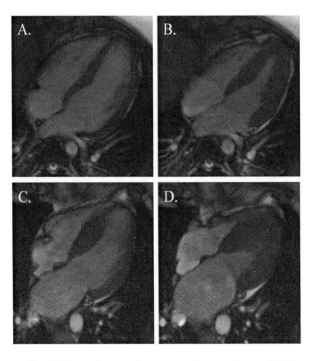

Figure 1. Four-chamber cardiac MRI cine image of a patient with normal septal thickness (A, B) compared to a HOCM patient with septal hypertrophy (C, D) during end of diastole (A, C) and systole (B, D). Please note the left ventricular end-systolic cavity obliteration (D) in HOCM.

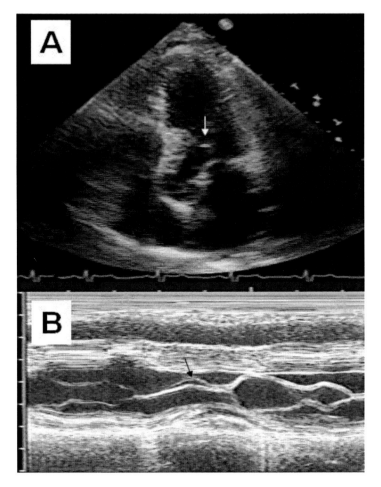

Figure 2. Trans-thoracic echocardiography of a patient with ESLD and HOCM. A. 5-chamber view showing hypertrophied interventricular septum and SAM of the anterior mitral valve leaflet (white arrow). B. M-Mode across the mitral valve showing SAM of the anterior mitral valve leaflet (black arrow). Reprinted with permission from [25]

HOCM General Management

The management of HOCM patients is aimed at alleviating symptoms of HF, angina and syncope on one hand, and preventing sudden death in high-risk individuals on the other. Medical therapy is the first line of treatment and consists of beta-blockers, calcium channel antagonists and disopyramide, solely or in combination. Surgical septal myectomy, and more recently alcohol septal ablation (ASA), is recommended for the small subgroup of patients (5%) who have both a large outflow gradient (usually > 50 mmHg at rest or on provocation) and moderate to severe HF or angina symptoms unresponsive to maximal medical therapy. Some advocate that young asymptomatic or mildly symptomatic patients with significantly marked outflow obstruction (75 to 100 mm Hg at rest) may also be considered for prophylactic surgical treatment [1].

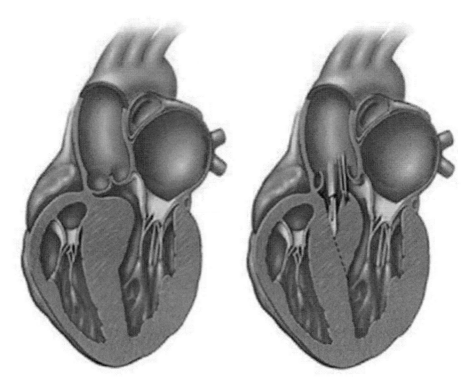

Figure 3. The septum is exposed through an oblique aortotomy and then a relatively small amount of muscle is excised from the proximal septum. This Figure is reproduced from www.mayoclinoc.org by permission of Mayo Foundation for Medical Education and Research. All rights reserved.

During surgical myectomy, the septum is approached through the aortic valve via an aortotomy, followed by resection of a relatively small amount of muscle from the proximal septum (approximately 3 to 12 g) extending from near the base of the aortic valve to beyond the distal margins of mitral leaflets, thereby eliminating, or significantly reducing the LVOT gradient and SAM (Figure 3) [3].

In contrast, ASA consists of the infusion of 1 to 3 ml of absolute alcohol into the first septal perforating branch of the left anterior descending coronary artery through an angioplasty catheter, inducing a myocardial infarction of approximately 20% of the septum (Figure 4). In order to avoid leakage of alcohol to the main coronary artery and excessive damage to the LV, the alcohol is infused distally to a fully expanded intravascular balloon which is kept inflated for 5 minutes after the infusion of alcohol [4]. Furthermore, this procedure should be guided in real-time by contrast echocardiography which can help define the target area and safely determine the septal artery that has to be infused in order to increase the success rate and decrease the chances of ablating essential areas of the myocardium [5]. The resulting scarring leads to progressive thinning and restricted excursion of the ventricular septum, and ultimately to reduction of LVOT and mitral regurgitation, thereby mimicking the LV remodeling that results from surgical myectomy [1, 6].

Historically, septal myectomy has been the "gold standard" treatment for HOCM patients refractory to medical therapy, perhaps due to more than 40 years of experience with this procedure, a relatively low perioperative mortality rate ~ 1–3%, high success rate with clinical improvement reported in ~ 90% of patients, and excellent long-term survival [7].

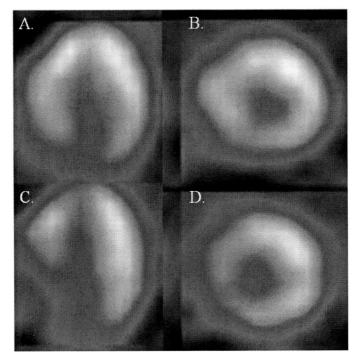

Figure 4. Imaging of ASA in HOCM. Single photon emission computed tomography myocardial perfusion imaging with Tc-99m sestamibi before (A, B) and after (C, D) ASA. Septal hypertrophy is seen at baseline and there is an area of decreased perfusion in the septum after ASA. Shown are horizontal long axis (A, C) and short axis (B, D) cross sections through the LV.

ASA emerged in 1995 [8] as an alternative procedure to surgery and has since grown quickly in popularity to the point that it is estimated that more ASAs have been performed since its introduction than the total number of surgical myectomies performed during the last 45 years [7]. Studies have shown that ASA is as effective as surgery in improving symptoms and reducing LVOT gradient in the short- and intermediate-term [9], and emerging data suggest long-term safety and effectiveness thereby countering a main argument of its detractors, namely the absence of long-term data with ASA [10-12]. Data from our group suggest that ASA improves diastolic function in addition to lowering LVOT gradients [13]. Concern has also been raised with regards to the risk of LV remodeling and ventricular arrhythmias at the site of myocardial necrosis after ASA. Studies using serial myocardial perfusion imaging after ASA have surprisingly shown that the infarct size decreases with time without an increase in LVOT obstruction or recurrence of symptoms, and that symptomatic ventricular arrhythmias are rare after ASA [14]. At present, there is no general agreement between cardiologists and surgeons regarding which procedure should be the first-line intervention for most HOCM patients after medical treatment failure. Patients with advanced age or significant comorbidities and/or relative contraindications to surgery are often considered good candidates for ASA.

Permanent dual-chamber pacing is an alternative therapeutic method that has been associated with a substantial decrease in outflow gradient, as well as amelioration of symptoms in patients with severe outflow obstruction and refractory symptoms, although the response in most patients is not as dramatic as initially thought [1, 15]. The mechanism for improvement is unclear but it seems related to a short term effect of LVOT gradient reduction by dyssynchronous contraction of the septum caused by right ventricular pacing and more long-term effect of ventricular remodeling [15, 16].

Risk of Non-Cardiac Surgery in HOCM Patients

HOCM individuals demonstrate dynamic LVOT gradient, which may exist at baseline or be latent and manifest only upon provocation by a number of physiologic changes such as reductions in preload and afterload or increases in contractility. It is notable that these physiological conditions are prevalent in the peri-operative period, which may flag a high-risk situation for patients with HOCM therefore necessitating extra vigilance and proactive strategies to avoid complications.

There are very few studies available addressing the risk of anesthesia and non-cardiac surgery in patients with HOCM. The incidence of adverse perioperative cardiovascular events varied from 16% to 40% in the studies reviewed [17-19], with a low rate of perioperative death (no events reported) and myocardial infarction (< 3%) in HOCM patients undergoing non-cardiac surgery. For instance Thompson et al. [17] evaluated 35 HOCM patients who underwent one or more non-cardiac surgical procedures. In 22 individuals who had catheterization prior to surgery, the average resting and peak (after provocation) LVOT gradients were 30 (range 0 – 150 mmHg) and 81 mm Hg (range 50-250 mm Hg), respectively. No perioperative cardiac deaths were reported, and only one patient developed myocardial infarction and HF following surgery. The most common complications were atrial arrhythmias (14%) and hypotension (14%) both requiring intervention. Similarly, Haering and colleagues [18] studied 77 HOCM patients, of whom 39% had a resting LVOT gradient > 10 mmHg (mean 31 mmHg, range 10-100 mmHg). No perioperative cardiac deaths were observed, only one patient had a myocardial infarction, and 14% became transiently hypotensive. In contrast a higher proportion of perioperative HF (16%) and non-life threatening arrhythmic episodes (25%) were described. The type of surgery (major vs. minor), duration of surgery, and intensity of monitoring were important predictors of adverse outcome. Surprisingly, in this report, the magnitude of resting LVOT gradient, SAM, and severity of mitral regurgitation, were not related to the occurrence of adverse cardiac events [18].

In conclusion, HOCM patients undergoing noncardiac surgery have a high incidence of adverse cardiac events. However, irreversible cardiac morbidity and mortality seem to be extremely low, based on the limited data available, to prohibit surgery, with the caveat that published literature may be biased towards better outcomes. Important independent risk factors for adverse outcome include major surgery and increasing duration of surgery.

HOCM Patients Undergoing Liver Transplantation

The optimal treatment strategy for patients with HOCM and end-stage liver disease (ESLD) is not well defined. HOCM per se is not a contraindication for orthotopic liver transplantation (OLT). There are a handful of reports in the literature of HOCM patients undergoing successful OLT without major perioperative cardiovascular complications (Table 1) [20-25].

Table 1. Summary of case reports on HOCM patients undergoing successful OLT

Study	Age	Gender	ESLD Etiology	Rest LVOT gradient by TTE (mmHg)	Attributed HOCM Symptoms	Treatment prior to OLT
Lim 1995 [20]	50	Male	Cryp-togenic	130	DOE, near syncope	BB
Harley 1996 [21]	46	Male	Alcohol	36	None	N/A
Harley 1996 [21]	32	Female	Auto-immune Hepatitis	60	None	N/A
Paramesh 2005 [22]	53	Male	Hepatitis C	100*	Progressive weakness	CCA + ASA
Cywinski 2005 [23]	53	Male	Alcohol and Hepatitis C	Normal **	None	N/A
Hage 2008 [25]	58	Female	Auto-immune Hepatitis	91	None	BB
Hage 2008 [25]	51	Male	Alcohol and Hepatitis C	64	CP, DOE, near syncope	BB + ASA
Chin 2009 [24]	58	Female	N/A	N/A	N/A	N/A

*Rest LVOT gradient measured during cardiac catheterization
**LVOT gradient was normal at rest but abnormal on provocation (155 - 189 mmHg)
ESLD: End stage liver disease. LVOT: Left ventricular outflow tract. TTE: Trans-thoracic echocardiography.
HOCM: Hypertrophic obstructive cardiomyopathy. OLT: Orthotopic liver transplant. DOE: Dyspnea on exertion. BB: Beta-blockers. N/A: Not available. CCA: Calcium channel antagonists. ASA: Alcohol septal ablation. CP: Chest pain.

Pre-Operative Evaluation and Management

Many HOCM patients are asymptomatic and only diagnosed during the screening process when a loud systolic ejection murmur prompts further evaluation with echocardiography. These patients may demonstrate high resting or provokable LVOT gradients in spite of the relative absence of symptoms (Table 1) [21, 23, 25].

A smaller proportion of patients, on the other hand, may experience moderate to severe limiting symptoms attributed to HOCM as well as high resting or inducible LVOT obstruction by the time of the pre-op evaluation [20, 22, 25]. This represents a special situation since this subgroup of HOCM patients is considered to be at high risk to undergo OLT without further intervention. There are a couple of case reports of such patients in the literature, where the treating medical group opted for ASA as a bridge to OLT [22, 25].

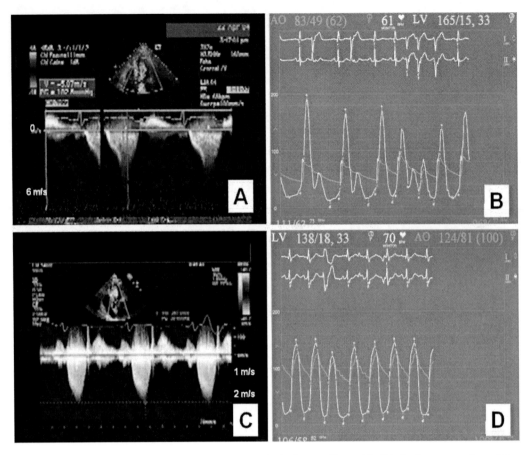

Figure 5. A 51 year old man with ESLD secondary to alcoholism and hepatitis C infection was evaluated for liver transplantation after he quit alcohol use. During his evaluation he was found to have symptomatic HOCM that was refractory to medical therapy. He was deemed at high risk for OLT secondary to his HOCM and at high risk for surgical myectomy secondary to his ESLD. He underwent ASA by injection of 4cc of absolute alcohol into the first septal artery. His LVOT gradient showed significant improvement from before (A, B) to after (C, D) ASA using Doppler echocardiography (A, C) and cardiac catheterization (B, D). LV pressure tracing in yellow color and aortic pressure tracing in pink. Reprinted with permission from [25].

ESLD patients have a high operative risk for surgical myectomy [26, 27]; therefore ASA emerges as a good alternative to septal myectomy in these patients. On both case reports, ASA resulted in improvement of symptoms and resting LVOT gradient and successful OLT followed an average of 15 months after ASA (Figure 5). Another approach was used in a HOCM patient with significant dyspnea on exertion, near syncopal episodes, and very high resting LVOT gradient (130 mmHg) undergoing successful OLT, after his symptoms and gradient (65 mmHg) improved with beta-blockage therapy [20]. However, these patients need to be followed up closely after OLT as their disease may progress to an extent that requires intervention (Figure 6).

The decision whether or not to continue with surgery should be individualized. In our opinion, rather than basing this decision solely on the severity of LVOT gradient severity, the assessment should take into account the severity of cardiovascular symptoms as well as the presence and severity of an LVOT obstruction and other comorbidities.

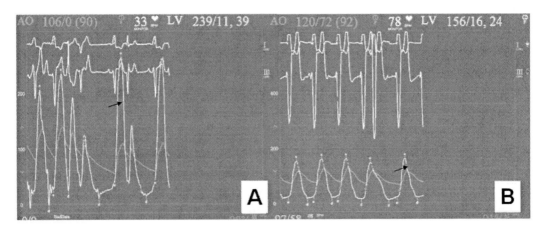

Figure 6. A 58 year old woman with ESLD secondary to autoimmune hepatitis and HOCM had a significant 91mmHg LVOT gradient at rest during evaluation for OLT but her symptoms were stable on beta-blocker therapy. She underwent OLT with no adverse cardiovascular events, but within a year of OLT her LVOT gradient increased further and she developed symptoms refractory to medical therapy. She underwent ASA by infusing 3cc of absolute alcohol into the first and second septal arteries under myocardial contrast echocardiography and fluoroscopic guidance. The LVOT gradient decreased from 100mmHg at rest and 200mmHg after a premature ventricular contraction (arrow) at baseline (A) to 10mmHg and 30mmHg at rest and after a premature ventricular contraction (arrow), respectively, post-ablation (B). The patient became symptom free after ASA an echocardiogram done 1 year later showed reduction in her LV wall thickness, a preserved LV systolic function and no detectable LVOT gradient. Reprinted with permission from [25].

It is reasonable to continue beta-blockers, or calcium channel antagonists, until the time of surgery and to start such therapy in patients not already on treatment since these medications can reduce the LVOT gradient as well as improve symptoms prior to OLT. If such treatment is to be started in the perioperative period in patients naive to these medications, it is better to start therapy several weeks before surgery and to titrate the medications slowly to allow for hemodynamic alterations as well as to ensure tolerance and absence of significant side-effects.

Intra-operative challenges in HOCM patients undergoing liver transplantation.

Anesthetic recommendations are based on data from a handful of case reports [20, 21, 23, 24], and derived from the described physiologic characteristics of HOCM or from anesthetic experience with HOCM patients undergoing cardiac surgery [28] or during pregnancy and delivery [29, 30].

Anesthetic management of HOCM involves understanding the many factors that can be expected to aggravate or have a negative impact on the dynamic LVOT obstruction during OLT. Conditions generally considered desirable include depressed myocardial contractility, and normal or increased systemic vascular resistance (SVR) and LV diastolic volume.

Anhepatic Phase

ESLD patients have a hyperdynamic circulation characterized by a high cardiac output and low SVR. The anesthetic management goals include maintenance of adequate preload and SVR as well as avoidance of marked increases in ventricular contractility. In this regard, continuous intraoperative transesophageal echocardiography (TEE) monitoring plays an important role in the management of HOCM patients during OLT. TEE is effective in rapidly disclosing new information and monitoring during periods of hemodynamic instability, and may have a significant impact on intraoperative patient management during OLT. Additionally, TEE is well tolerated by patients, and is generally considered a low-risk procedure [31].

LVOT obstruction in HOCM is largely due to contraction of the subaortic musculature. As a result, drugs and interventions associated with enhanced myocardial contractility should be avoided, as they may potentially increase LVOT obstruction. In this respect, all volatile anesthetic drugs have varying degrees of negative inotropic and chronotropic effects; isoflurane, desflurane, and sevoflurane produce less pronounced reductions in myocardial contractility and greater decreases in SVR than halothane or enflurane [32]. Therefore the hemodynamic properties of halothane and enflurane have been considered to be advantageous in HOCM patients undergoing non-cardiac surgery including OLT. In fact, halothane was the most frequent primary anesthetic used in a case series of non-cardiac surgery [17] as well as in case reports of HOCM patients undergoing OLT [21, 23]. Cywinski and colleagues advocate further reduction of both heart rate and contractility during the anhepatic stage by means of the infusion of a short acting selective beta-blocker, such as esmolol, before and during allograft reperfusion [23].

Venodilation, hypovolemia, and blood loss are common causes of LV end-diastolic volume reduction during OLT, all of which act to augment the LVOT gradient if not detected and corrected promptly. Intraoperative TEE can be vital to the management of the hemodynamic status of these patients, as it can detect in real time a rise in the severity of LVOT obstruction manifested by a relative empty LV cavity, worsening SAM, and/or mitral regurgitation as well as direct measurement of the LVOT gradient with the use of Doppler echocardiography [20, 21, 23]. Prompt recognition with TEE will facilitate targeted therapy with volume and/or vasoconstrictors (phenylephrine) in case of reductions in LV end-diastolic volumes and/or SVR respectively. Moreover, the presence of significant mitral regurgitation can confound the interpretation of the pulmonary artery wedge pressure recordings from the pulmonary artery catheter, where increased severity of regurgitation can result in elevated pressures despite the need for more volume replacement [20, 21].

Reperfusion Phase

Postreperfusion syndrome (PRS) refers to a series of hemodynamic changes, primarily hypotension, immediately after reperfusion of the grafted liver, but also bradyarrhythmia, decrease in cardiac output, increases in pulmonary artery wedge pressure, and decrease in SVR. Most patients undergoing OLT develop some degree of PRS, but only a few develop clinically significant hypotension which seems to be associated with acute decrease in SVR caused by unknown vasoactive substances [33]. Avoidance of a decrease in afterload is extremely important to prevent reflex tachycardia and subsequent increased contractility, which can ultimately translate in worsening LVOT obstruction.

During the anhepatic or reperfusion phase, increases in SVR can be achieved with infusion of phenylephrine, a pure alpha receptor agonist with no inotropic or chronotropic effect. The use of epinephrine may be contraindicated since it induces tachycardia and increases contractility, thus enhancing LVOT obstruction. Treatment of the PRS in HOCM patients should be guided by invasive monitoring devices and intraoperative TEE findings as described above. Administration of large volumes of intravenous fluids during these periods of hemodynamic instability may be necessary during OLT surgery. Since HOCM also results in varying degrees of diastolic dysfunction, overly aggressive fluid resuscitation may lead to perioperative congestive HF and caution and moderation should be exercised in this regard.

Finally, if hypotension, worsening LVOT obstruction, and SAM result in intraoperative OLT myocardial ischemia, management should be aimed at increasing the preload with fluids and in the presence of hypotension, phenylephrine to sustain the blood pressure. A beta-blocker may be initiated once the patient is hemodynamically stable in order to decrease contractility and heart rate [34].

Conclusion

Perioperative mortality and MI rates seem to be low but other cardiovascular complications relatively high in HOCM patients undergoing non-cardiac surgery, including OLT. Perioperative cardiovascular compromise is the main concern of performing a major surgery, such as OLT, in HOCM patients. Limited literature suggests that most of these complications are transitory and treatable, and studies have failed to document increased postsurgical mortality rates in these individuals. HOCM patients with significant limiting symptoms and high LVOT obstruction gradients represent a subset of patients who may benefit from ASA as a bridge to OLT in order to avoid these reported perioperative complications, with the downside of delaying surgery for several months. Finally, anesthetic management of HOCM involves understanding the many factors that can be expected to aggravate or have a negative impact on the dynamic LVOT obstruction during OLT.

References

[1] Maron BJ, McKenna WJ, Danielson GK, Kappenberger LJ, Kuhn HJ, Seidman CE, et al. American College of Cardiology/European Society of Cardiology clinical expert consensus document on hypertrophic cardiomyopathy. A report of the American College of Cardiology Foundation Task Force on Clinical Expert Consensus Documents and the European Society of Cardiology Committee for Practice Guidelines. *J. Am. Coll .Cardiol.* 2003; 42(9):1687-713.

[2] Maron MS, Olivotto I, Betocchi S, Casey SA, Lesser JR, Losi MA et al. Effect of left ventricular outflow tract obstruction on clinical outcome in hypertrophic cardiomyopathy. *N. Engl. J. Med.* 2003 23;348(4):295-303.

[3] Sellke, FW. Sabiston and Spencer's Surgery of the Chest. 8th Edition. Philadelphia: Saunders Elsevier 2009.

[4] Hage FG; Aqel R, Aljaroudi W, Heo J, Pothineni K, Hansalia S, et al. Correlation between serum cardiac markers and myocardial infarct size quantified by myocardial perfusion imaging in patients with hypertrophic cardiomyopathy after alcohol septal ablation. *The American Journal of Cardiology* 2010;105(2):261-6.

[5] Aqel RA, Hage FG, Cogar B, Burri M, Wells B, Allison S, et al. Trans-thoracic echocardiography guided procedures in the catheterization laboratory. *Echocardiography* 2007; 24(9):1000-7.

[6] Libby P. Braunwald's Heart Disease: A Textbook of Cardiovascular Medicine. 8th Edition. Philadelphia: Saunders Elsevier; 2007.

[7] Maron., BJ, Dearani JA, Ommen SR, Maron MS, Schaff HV, Gersh BJ et al. The case for surgery in obstructive hypertrophic cardiomyopathy. *J. Am. Coll. Cardiol.* 2004 16;44(10):2044-53.

[8] Sigwart U. Non-surgical myocardial reduction for hypertrophic obstructive cardiomyopathy. *Lancet* 1995; 22:346(8969):211-4.

[9] Alam M, Dokainish H, Lakkis N. Alcohol septal ablation for hypertrophic obstructive cardiomyopathy: a systematic review of published studies. *J. Interv. Cardio* 2006; 19(4):319-27.

[10] Fernandes VL, Nielsen C, Nagueh SF, Herrin AE, Slifka C, Franklin J et al. Follow-up of alcohol septal ablation for symptomatic hypertrophic obstructive cardiomyopathy the Baylor and Medical University of South Carolina experience 1996 to 2007. *JACC Cardiovasc Interv* 2008 ;1(5):561-70.

[11] Kwon DH, Kapadia SR, Tuzcu EM, Halley CM, Gorodeski EZ, Curtin RJ, et al. Long-term outcomes in high-risk symptomatic patients with hypertrophic cardiomyopathy undergoing alcohol septal ablation. *JACC Cardiovasc. Interv* .2008; 1(4):432-8.

[12] Agarwal S, Tuzcu EM, Desai MY, Smedira N, Lever HM, Lytle BW, et al. Updated meta-analysis of septal alcohol ablation versus myectomy for hypertrophic cardiomyopathy. *J. Am. Coll. Cardiol* .2010; 23;55(8):823-34.

[13] Hage FG, Karakus G, Luke WD, Jr,; Suwanjutah T, Burri MV, Nanda NC et al. Effect of alcohol-induced septal ablation on left atrial volume and ejection fraction assessed by real time three-dimensional trans-thoracic echocardiography in patients with hypertrophic cardiomyopathy. *Echocardiography* 2008;25(7):784-9.

[14] Aqel RA, Hage FG, Zohgbi GJ, Tabereaux PB, Lawson D, Heo J et al. Serial evaluations of myocardial infarct size after alcohol septal ablation in hypertrophic cardiomyopathy and effects of the changes on clinical status and left ventricular outflow pressure gradients. *Am. J. Cardiol* .2008;101(9):1328-33.

[15] Nishimura RA, Trusty JM, Hayes DL, Ilstrup DM, Larson DR, Hayes SN et al. Dual-chamber pacing for hypertrophic cardiomyopathy: a randomized, double-blind, crossover trial. *J. Am. Coll. Cardiol.* 1997;29(2):435-41.

[16] Fananapazir L; Epstein ND, Curiel RV, Panza JA, Tripodi D, McAreavey D. Long-term results of dual-chamber (DDD) pacing in obstructive hypertrophic cardiomyopathy. Evidence for progressive symptomatic and hemodynamic improvement and reduction of left ventricular hypertrophy. *Circulation* 1994;90(6):2731-42.

[17] Thompson RC, Liberthson RR, Lowenstein E. Perioperative anesthetic risk of noncardiac surgery in hypertrophic obstructive cardiomyopathy. *JAMA* 1985;254(17):2419-21.

[18] Haering JM, Comunale ME, Parker RA, Lowenstein E, Douglas PS, Krumholz HM et al. Cardiac risk of noncardiac surgery in patients with asymmetric septal hypertrophy. *Anesthesiology* 1996;85(2):254-9.

[19] Chang, KH, Sano E, Saitoh Y, Hanaoka K. Anesthetic management of patients with hypertrophic obstructive cardiomyopathy undergoing non-cardiac surgery. *Masui* 2004 ;53(8):934-42.

[20] Lim YC, Doblar DD, Frenette L, Fan PH, Poplawski S, Nanda NC. Intraoperative transesophageal echocardiography in orthotopic liver transplantation in a patient with hypertrophic cardiomyopathy. *J Clin Anesth* 1995;7(3):245-9.

[21] Harley ID, Jones EF, Liu G, McCall PR, McNicol PL. Orthotopic liver transplantation in two patients with hypertrophic obstructive cardiomyopathy. *Br. J. Anaesth.* 1996;77(5):675-7.

[22] Paramesh AS, Fairchild RB, Quinn TM, Leya F, George M, Van Thiel DH. Amelioration of hypertrophic cardiomyopathy using nonsurgical septal ablation in a cirrhotic patient prior to liver transplantation. *Liver Transpl* 2005;11(2):236-8.

[23] Cywinski JB, Argalious M, Marks TN, Parker BM. Dynamic left ventricular outflow tract obstruction in an orthotopic liver transplant recipient. *Liver Transp.* 2005;11 (6):692-5.

[24] Chin JH, Kim YK, Choi DK, Shin WJ, Hwang GS. Aggravation of mitral regurgitation by calcium administration in a patient with hypertrophic cardiomyopathy during liver transplantation: a case report. *Transplant. Proc* .2009;41(5):1979-81.

[25] Hage FG, Bravo PE, Zoghbi GJ, Bynon JS, Aqel RA. Hypertrophic obstructive cardiomyopathy in liver transplant patients. *Cardiol. J* .2008;15(1):74-9.

[26] Hayashida N, Shoujima T, Teshima H, Yokokura Y, Takagi K, Tomoeda H et al. Clinical outcome after cardiac operations in patients with cirrhosis. *Ann. Thorac. Surg.* 2004;77(2):500-5.

[27] Suman A, Barnes DS, Zein NN, Levinthal GN, Connor JT, Carey WD. Predicting outcome after cardiac surgery in patients with cirrhosis: a comparison of Child-Pugh and MELD scores. *Clin. Gastroenterol. Hepatol.* .2004;2(8):719-23.

[28] Cregg N, Cheng DC, Karski JM, Williams WG, Webb G, Wigle ED. Morbidity outcome in patients with hypertrophic obstructive cardiomyopathy undergoing cardiac septal myectomy: early-extubation anesthesia versus high-dose opioid anesthesia technique. *J. Cardiothorac. Vasc. Anesth* .1999;13(1):47-52.

[29] Matthews, T; Dickinson JE. Considerations for delivery in pregnancies complicated by maternal hypertrophic obstructive cardiomyopathy. *Aust. N Z J. Obstet. Gynaecology* 2005;45(6):526-8.

[30] Pitton MA, Petolillo M, Munegato E, Ciccarese AA, Visentin S, Paternoster DM. Hypertrophic obstructive cardiomyopathy and pregnancy: anesthesiological observations and clinical series. *Minerva Anestesiol* .2007;73(5):313-8.

[31] Suriani RJ, Cutrone A, Feierman D, Konstadt S. Intraoperative transesophageal echocardiography during liver transplantation. *J. Cardiothorac. Vasc. Anesth.* 1996 ;10(6):699-707.

[32] Miller, RD. Miller's Anesthesia. 7th Edition. Churchill Livingstone. 2009.

[33] Aggarwal S, Kang Y, Freeman JA, Fortunato FL Jr., Pinsky MR. Postreperfusion syndrome: hypotension after reperfusion of the transplanted liver. *J. Crit. Care* 1993; 8(3):154-60.

[34] Popescu WM, Perrino AC, Jr. Critical cardiac decompensation during laparoscopic surgery. *J. Am. Soc. Echocardiogr* .2006;19(8):1074 e5-6.

Chapter VII

Obesity and Liver Transplantation

Paul J. Thuluvath[*]
Department of Surgery and Medicine
Georgetown University School of Medicine, Washington DC, USA
Institute for Health and Liver Disease, Mercy Medical Center, Baltimore, MD, USA

Abstract

Obesity is common among liver transplant recipients, and about 10% of liver transplant recipients have severe or morbid obesity. Registry data indicate that there was more than 40% increase in severe or morbid obesity in the past decade among liver transplant recipients. Patients with severe or morbid obesity often have many there co-morbidities including occult cardiovascular diseases, diabetes, hyperlipidemia, cancer and restrictive lung disease. Severe or morbid obesity increases both short and long-term post-transplant morbidity and mortality. Infections, wound dehiscence, increased ventilator dependency and increased intensive care stay are the most common complications in morbidly obese patients, and these complications increase the transplant costs significantly. Cardiovascular complications are the main causes of increased mortality. Patients with preexisting diabetes or coronary artery disease are approximately 40% more likely to die within 5 years from transplantation compared to non-diabetics or those without coronary artery disease with an additive effect with more than one risk factor. Severely or morbidly obese patients, if considered for liver transplantation, should undergo more rigorous cardiovascular screening. Patients with diffuse coronary artery disease or those with significant coronary artery disease that is not amenable to coronary stenting should not be waitlisted. Other contraindications include patients with renal failure who are not eligible for combined liver/kidney transplantation, and those with one or more other serious co-morbidities such as uncontrolled hypertension and micro and macro vascular complications including stroke. To improve outcomes, patients with

---

[*] Correspondence: Paul J. Thuluvath, MD, FRCP, Professor of Surgery (Transplantation) and Medicine, The Georgetown University School of Medicine, Washington, DC; Director, Center for Liver and Biliary Diseases, Mercy Medical Center, #718, 301 St. Paul's Street, Baltimore, MD 21202, Tel: 410 332 7308, E-mail: thuluvath@gmail.com.

severe or morbid obesity should undergo careful surveillance and health maintenance programs before and after liver transplantation.

Introduction

The prevalence of obesity in general population is increasing all over the world, and its impact on morbidity, mortality and utilization of health resources continues to escalate in a significant manner [1-5]. According to the most recent report from the World Health Organization, a third of the population are obese (defined as Body Mass Index or BMI $\geq$30 kg/m^2) in many countries including Egypt, Saudi Arabia and United States of America (USA). Many other countries including the United Kingdom (22.7%), Mexico (23.6%) and South Africa (21.6%) are not far behind. While 87% of the population in Thailand has normal BMI (18.5-24.99 kg/m^2), only 35.7% of the US population has normal BMI suggesting that there are significant geographic variations in the prevalence of obesity.

The dramatic increase in the prevalence of obesity in the general population in the past two decades is also reflected in the liver transplant (LT) recipients in the USA and elsewhere [6,7]. In the USA, within a decade, the prevalence of obesity increased by 93% among LT recipients [6, 7]. In 1999, only 7.8% of LT recipients had severe (BMI $\geq$ 35 kg/m^2) or morbid obesity (BMI $\geq$ 40 kg/m^2), but by 2008, 11% had severe or morbid obesity [8]. These data indicate that there was 41% increase in severe or morbid obesity among liver transplant recipients in the past decade. It is possible that fluid overload may have overestimated the prevalence of obesity in this population, but it is unlikely that this factor has changed in the past decade [9].

Other co-morbidities such as type II diabetes mellitus (DM) and hyperlipidemia, often associated with obesity, have also increased in the past decade among transplant recipients. Between 1999 and 2008, prevalence of type II DM among transplant recipients increased by 44%, from 14.9% in 1999 to 21.5% in 2008[8]. In addition to the pre-existing DM, new onset of DM (NODM) was seen in 26.4% of transplant recipients (UNOS data) after a median follow up of 685 days; in this population, obesity has been shown to be one of the important risk factors for the development NODM [10]. Similar observations have been made in lung transplant recipients also; in one study 35.4% (34 of 94 patients) developed NODM and BMI was significantly higher in the group that developed NODM [11]. In another study from Egypt, NODM was seen 18.2 % of living donor renal transplant recipients [12]. In this study, NODM showed a significant correlation with obesity, and moreover, post-transplant DM was a significant factor for the development of coronary artery disease (CAD) and lower long-term graft (43.5% vs. 53.6%) and patient (79.9% vs. 86.1%) survival [12].

To our knowledge, there are no studies that have critically analyzed the prevalence of hyperlipidemia and its relationship to obesity in liver transplant recipients. Centers for Disease Control and Prevention had analyzed the prevalence of hyperlipidemia among youths using National Health and Nutrition Examination Survey (NHANES) for 1999-2006 and found a very strong relationship between hyperlipidemia and BMI [13]. In this study, hyperlipidemia was seen 14.2% of youths with normal weight, 22.3% of those with overweight and 42.9% of those with obesity. It is more than likely that this relationship exists among transplant recipients as well.

Obese patients usually have multiple risk factors for cardiovascular diseases including type II DM or insulin resistance, hyperlipidemia and hypertension. The relationship between obesity and cardiac complications has been examined in more detail among renal transplant recipients. In one study, cumulative post-transplant incidence of cardiovascular complications in patients with obesity was compared to those without obesity [14]. The 5-year cumulative incidence of any cardiac diagnosis increased from 8.7% to 29.4% across the lowest to highest BMI quartiles. More importantly, BMI independently predicted cardiac events in patients with non-diabetic renal failure [14]. Cardiovascular disease is one of the main causes of death in LT recipients with functional grafts. Obesity has shown to exaggerate the negative impact of other risk factors such as donor graft cold ischemia time on graft survival [15]. Additionally, obesity may also increase cancer risks in LT recipients.

Impact of Obesity on Morbidity and Mortality

The impact of obesity on renal transplantation has been studied more extensively than liver transplantation [16,17]. An analysis of 51,927 renal transplant recipients showed that extremes of BMI (< 18 and > 36) were associated with worse graft and patient survival [16]. In addition, higher BMI was associated with delayed graft function and chronic graft failure. Registry data (from 1987 to 2002) on 6,658 children aged 2 to 17 years who received renal transplantation showed that BMI >95 percentile (9.7% of the study population) for age was associated with a higher risk of death (relative risk 2.9 for cadaver and 3.7 for living donor) and graft loss (19% vs. 10% for non-obese) due to thrombosis [18]. Obesity has also been described as a negative predictor of morbidity and mortality after combined kidney/pancreas, pancreas alone, lung and heart transplantation [19-22].

Single center studies on liver transplantation have shown inconsistent results mainly because of the differences in the definition of obesity, sample size, reporting and selection bias [23-28]. These studies, however, showed a trend towards higher post-operative complications, length of hospital stay and hospital costs for obese recipients [25,27,28]. Wound infections or dehiscence, increased ventilator dependency and increased intensive care stay were more common in morbidly obese patients. In many of the above single center studies, patients with BMI $\geq$ 30 kg/m^2 were grouped together and therefore, the impact of severe or morbid obesity on sold organ transplantation could not be assessed independently. Moreover, the sample size of these studies was inadequate to assess the independent effect of severe or morbid obesity on liver transplant outcomes.

There are many confounding factors that determine the outcome of liver transplant recipients, and therefore, it is important to have a large sample size to adjust for these variables to determine the independent effect of obesity. The United Network for Organ Sharing (UNOS) database has many limitations, but it provides a large unselected patient population to examine hard endpoints such as death. Nair et al examined UNOS datasets from 1988 to 1996 and reported that liver transplant recipients with severe (BMI 35-39.9 kg/m^2, n=911) or morbid (BMI $\geq$ 40 kg/m^2, n=355) obesity are more likely to have a higher mortality compared to others [6]. Those who were overweight (BMI 25.1- 30kg/m^2, n=5,913) and obese (BMI 30-34.9kg/m^2, n=2,611) had similar outcomes as those who were non-obese (BMI < 25kg/m^2, n=8,382). In this study, immediate, 1-year and 2-year survival rates were lower for severely and morbidly obese patients. Five-year mortality was significantly higher for both severely (51%) and morbidly obese patients (57% vs. 44-47%), mostly as a result of adverse cardiovascular events (28% vs. 16-22%). When adjusted for other co-morbidities, however, only morbid obesity was an independent predictor of mortality. Another analysis of UNOS data from 1987 to 2007 confirmed lower survival after LT at the extremes of body weight (BMI <18.5 kg/m^2 or BMI $\geq$ 40 kg/m^2) [29]. Multivariate analysis confirmed that underweight and very severe obesity were independent predictors of death. In this analysis, infections and cancer events leading to death were common in morbidly obese patients.

In both renal and liver transplant recipients, cardiovascular complications were the main cause of increased mortality [6,17]. Previous studies have shown that LT recipients with diabetes or coronary artery disease (CAD), both commonly associated with obesity, were approximately 40% more likely to die within 5 years from LT compared to non-diabetics or those without CAD [30,31]. Presence of both diseases had a far more negative impact than either disease alone [31].

In the above studies, the risk associated with obesity was assessed in a retrospective manner using datasets that were not specifically designed to assess these risks. These results, therefore, need to be treated with caution and moreover, the observed mortality, like all clinical situations, may not be applicable to an individual patient.

Should We Offer Liver Transplantation to Morbidly Obese Patients?

In a previous study, Pelletier et al, using Scientific Registry of Transplant Recipients (SRTR) database, examined the association between BMI and liver transplant survival benefit in a retrospective cohort of liver transplant candidates who were initially wait-listed for liver transplantation between 2001 and 2004 [7]. The unadjusted rate of removal from the waitlist for reasons other than transplant or death was similar to those with normal BMI for severely obese group, but it was lower for morbidly obese group. Crude mortality rates after transplant were higher for morbidly obese group and those who were underweight (BMI <20). However, when the covariate adjusted relative risk of death for post-transplant recipients was compared to those on the waitlist (post-transplantation vs. waitlist mortality), there were survival advantages for all BMI categories including those who were malnourished.

Based on the above study, Pelletier and colleagues argued that there are survival benefits in severely and morbidly obese patients with advanced liver disease [7]. This conclusion was based on the assumption that those who were transplanted, irrespective of their BMI, would do better than those who are waitlisted, but not transplanted. There will not be any disagreement with this conclusion by the strict definition of 'survival benefit'. One could intuitively agree that any patient with advanced cirrhosis (Child C or high MELD scores) or even very advanced liver cancer (even those who are outside San Francisco criteria) would live longer than a comparable group that did not receive LT. The important question that we should be asking is not whether morbidly obese patients with end stage liver diseases are better off with LT than without LT, but whether we could use the donor organs more effectively by transplanting into those who are likely to have better long-term outcomes. On the same token, one could argue that it is unfair to deny LT to patients just because they are morbidly obese.

The practical question is whether we should offer LT irrespective of BMI based on 'survival benefit' or select only those who are likely to have better outcomes based on other surrogate markers of risks other than BMI. If that is the approach we want to adopt for the sake of fairness, what objective criteria do we use for the selection process? To answer these questions, we need to understand why patients with morbid obesity do poorly after organ transplantation.

Cardiovascular Risk Factors and Complications in Morbidly Obese Recipients

Morbid obesity is often associated with other co-morbidities such as cardiovascular diseases, diabetes, hyperlipidemia, cancer and restrictive lung disease. In obese renal and liver transplant recipients, cardiovascular (CV) complications are the main cause of increased mortality [6, 16, 17]. In one study, as discussed earlier, post-transplant cardiac complications (congestive heart failure, atrial fibrillation and myocardial infarction) were assessed in 1,102 renal allograft recipients stratified by BMI quartiles [14]. Cardiac complications increased from 8.7% to 29.4% across the lowest to highest BMI quartiles. Each 5 unit BMI increase predicted 25% higher cardiac complications. As in most studies, heart failure and atrial fibrillation were the most common cardiovascular complications after renal transplantation. Coronary artery calcification is a marker of coronary artery disease. In one study, coronary artery calcification was found to correlate with metabolic syndrome in renal transplant recipients [32]. In this study, coronary artery calcification scores were significantly higher at baseline and at follow up in patients with metabolic syndrome. Coronary artery calcification scores could also be used as a non-invasive test to assess cardiovascular risk in liver transplant candidates with obesity and other risk factors.

In liver transplant recipients, CV disease is the third most common cause of death after LT, only behind recurrence of primary disease/chronic rejection and malignancy [33-38]. It has been shown that between 2% and 21% of patients will die of a CV event if they survive greater than one year after LT [33-35]. Even more patients (up to 24%) will have a non-fatal CV event after LT [38]. Those with preexisting diabetes or CAD are approximately 40% more likely to die within 5 years from transplantation compared to non-diabetics or those without CAD [31]. Presence of both diseases has a far more negative impact than either disease alone indicating the additive effects of cardiovascular risk factors [31].

The prevalence of CV risk factors, including hyperlipidemia, hypertension, obesity and DM are likely to increase after liver transplantation [39-45]. About a third of patients undergoing LT are obese prior to LT [6-8], and additional 25% of non-obese patients will become obese within 3 years after LT [40]. In one series, post-transplant metabolic syndrome was present in 58% in transplant recipients, with an increased risk of CV complications in the post-transplant metabolic syndrome group (30% vs. 8% respectively, $p = 0.003$) as compared to the non-metabolic syndrome group [41]. When compared with non-diabetic post-LT patients, the development of new onset DM after transplant is associated with an increased risk of cardiac (47.8% vs. 23.9%) and vascular complications (15.2% vs. 5.4%) [39]. The accelerated rate of macrovascular complications in patients after LT probably is multifactorial. Patients with morbid obesity often have many risk factors and these confounding risk factors add up resulting in significant morbidity, mortality and higher transplant related costs.

Evaluation and Follow-Up of Severely or Morbidly Obese Transplant Candidates

Population based epidemiological studies have shown that obesity is an independent predictor of mortality [1,2,3, 5]. Collective outcome data from liver and renal transplantation also suggest that morbidly obese patients have an increased morbidity and mortality compared to less obese patients. These cumulative data mandates that morbidly obese patients were carefully evaluated for other serious co-morbid illnesses before listing. UNOS registry data suggest that there is a reluctance to transplant morbidly obese patients in the USA [46]. This is justified based on the current data supporting increased post-operative complications, costs and mortality. Nevertheless, single center studies indicate that some of these patients have acceptable outcomes, and it is more likely a reflection of better selection process [23,25,27,28,47].

Before wait listing, severely obese patients and those who have metabolic syndrome should undergo rigorous cardiovascular screening including carotid duplex, adequate dobutamine stress echo, coronary calcium score, coronary computed tomography (CT) angiography and/or cardiac catheterization. A significant proportion of patients, especially in the MELD era, have renal insufficiency that precludes the use of contrast agents, and this is a major limiting factor for routine CT angiography or cardiac catheterization in high-risk patients. Coronary calcium score could be potentially used as a non-invasive marker of CAD, and this may help to select patients for more invasive procedures [32]. Our group had examined the utility of insulin resistance and microalbuminuria as surrogate markers of cardiovascular disease in 143 liver transplant candidates [48]. Insulin resistance was assessed by homeostatic model of insulin resistance (HOMA-IR). Microvascular disease was present in 40.5% patients; it was more common in those with DM when compared to non-diabetics (62.5% vs. 18.3%). Significant microalbuminuria had a sensitivity of 85%, a specificity of 100% and a positive predictive value of 100% for the presence of microalbuminuria. If these observations are confirmed by other groups, microalbuminuria could be used as another surrogate marker for risk stratification.

Although there are no absolute, theoretical contraindications, morbidly obese patients with significant CAD that is not amenable to stenting, or those with renal failures who are not eligible for combined liver/kidney transplantation should not be listed for liver transplantation. Similarly, morbidly obese patients with one or more other serious co-morbidities such as uncontrolled hypertension, micro and macro vascular complications, diffuse CAD or strokes should not be offered liver transplantation. The decision not to transplant a patient should be based on sound clinical judgment and the 'expected' outcome used only for guidance [49-50]. There are many variables that predict the outcomes of liver transplantation, and it is therefore important to consider all variables during the selection process [51]. One of the important functions of the LT selection process is to determine whether the recipient can withstand a transplant operation and emerges with an acceptable quality of life and outcomes. Transplant community has not yet defined the 'acceptable outcomes'. It has been suggested that if the predicted patient survival is less than 50% at 1-year, LT should not be offered. So far, no one has attempted to define the acceptable survival at 3 or 5-years. If morbidity and mortality associated with transplantation outweigh that of the chronic liver disease, then clearly LT is not in the best interest of the patient. From society's point of view, given the limited number of organs, it is preferable to allocate organ to patients who will benefit to the greatest extent. These competing viewpoints should be taken into consideration during the selection process.

Once listed, patients with severe obesity should undergo careful surveillance and health maintenance programs to improve the outcomes. Hypertension, diabetes and hyperlipidemia should be well controlled prior to transplantation. In one study, a structured weight management program has been shown to reduce mean body weight by 7.1% in 32 patients with chronic kidney disease over a period of 12 months allowing 9 of 32 patients, previously excluded from renal transplantation, to be enrolled into the transplant waiting list [52]. A similar process may allow us to offer liver transplant in a 'selective' manner to some morbidly obese patients, and thereby assuring a lower morbidity and a better long-term survival.

Post-Transplant Management

For the reasons discussed earlier, obese patients should be carefully managed after liver transplantation to minimize the morbidity and mortality. Co-morbid conditions such as DM, hypertension and hyperlipidemia should be carefully managed. Transplant recipients should be encouraged to lose weight by active participation in weight management program. A recent meta-analysis has shown that steroid avoidance may cause statistically significant decreases in cholesterol levels and may reduce the risk of diabetes [53]. Calcineurin-inhibitors sparing immunosuppressive regimens may be considered in patients who have difficulty controlling their diabetes or hypertension. Patients should be screened regularly for the presence of microalbuminuria, and those with diabetes should be carefully assessed for other microvascular complications. Even in the absence of cardiac symptoms, it is reasonable to do routine cardiovascular screening including cardiac stress tests periodically (frequency to be individualized) in all high-risk recipients. Cancer is an important cause of long-term morbidity and mortality after liver transplantation [29, 54]. Both obesity and type-2 DM increase the risks for a variety of cancers (1.5 to 3.5 fold increase), including esophageal, colorectal, pancreatic, breast and endometrial cancer, and these associations should be taken into consideration during the post-transplant surveillance [55-59]. Possible mechanisms for increased cancer risk in patients with obesity and type-2 DM include hyperinsulinemia, insulin like growth factors, adipocytokines, or increased bioavailability of steroid hormones.

The role of bariatric surgery in transplant recipients is undefined. One study examined bariatric surgery among renal transplant candidates and recipients using Medicare billing claims within USRDS registry data from 1991-2004 [60]. Of 188 cases, 72 were performed pre-listing, 29 on the waitlist and 87 post-transplant. Thirty-day mortality of bariatric surgery was higher (3.5%) on the waitlist and post-transplant patients compared to reported mortality rates in patients without renal disease. Weight loss after bariatric surgery in this group was comparable to those without kidney disease. In the absence of randomized controlled trials, the role of bariatric surgery could be better defined in this population by carefully conducted case-control studies assessing long-term outcomes and quality of life. Bariatric surgery is going to be technically more difficult in liver transplant recipients. Nevertheless, this option should be explored in liver transplant recipients.

Conclusion

The presence of morbid obesity, and to some extent severe obesity, increases post-liver transplant complications, costs and mortality significantly. Morbidly obese patients, if considered for liver transplantation, should undergo rigorous cardiovascular testing before listed, and should undergo close monitoring and management before and after liver transplantation. This process may allow us to offer liver transplantation in a 'selective manner' to some morbidly obese patients, thereby assuring a lower morbidity and a better long-term survival.

References

[1] Allison DB, Fontaine KR, Manson JE, Stevens J, VanItallie TB. Annual deaths attributable to obesity in the United States. *JAMA* 1999;282:1530-8.

[2] Lee IM, Manson JE, Hennekens CH, Paffenbarger RS, Jr. Body weight and mortality. A 27-year follow-up of middle-aged men. *JAMA* 1993;270:2823-8.

[3] McTigue K, Larson JC, Valoski A, Burke G, Kotchen J, Lewis CE et al. Mortality and cardiac and vascular outcomes in extremely obese women. *JAMA* 2006;296:79-86.

[4] Weil E, Wachterman M, McCarthy EP, Davis RB, O'Day B, Iezzoni LI, Wee CC. Obesity among adults with disabling conditions. *JAMA* 2002;288:1265-8.

[5] Yan LL, Daviglus ML, Liu K, Stamler J, Wang R, Pirzada A et al. Midlife body mass index and hospitalization and mortality in older age. *JAMA* 2006;295:190-8.

[6] Nair S, Verma S, Thuluvath PJ. Obesity and its effect on survival in patients undergoing orthotopic liver transplantation in the United States. *Hepatology* 2002;35:105-9.

[7] Pelletier SJ, Schaubel DE, Wei G, Englesbe MJ, Punch JD, Wolfe RA et al. Effect of body mass index on the survival benefit of liver transplantation. *Liver Transpl.* 2007;13:1678-83.

[8] Thuluvath PJ, Guidinger MK, Fung JJ, Johnson LB, Rayhill SC, Pelletier SJ. Liver transplantation in the United States, 1999-2008. *Am. J. Transplant* .2010;10:1003-19.

[9] Leonard J, Heimbach JK, Malinchoc M, Watt K, Charlton M. The impact of obesity on long-term outcomes in liver transplant recipients - results of the NIDDK liver transplant database. *Am. J. Transplant.* 2008;8:667-72.

[10] Kuo HT, Sampaio MS, Ye X, Reddy P, Martin P, Bunnapradist S. Risk factors for new onset diabetes mellitus in adult liver transplant recipients, an analysis of the Organ

Procurement and transplant Network/United Network for organ Sharing database. *Transplantation* 2010;89:1134-40.

[11] Ollech JE, Kramer MR, Peled N, Ollech A, Amital A, Medalion B et al. Post-transplant diabetes mellitus in lung transplant recipients: incidence and risk factors. *Eur. J. Cardiothoracic. Surg.* 2008;33:844-8.

[12] Elmagd MM, Bakr MA, Metwally AH, Wahab AM. Clinicpathologic study of posttransplant diabetes after living-donor renal transplant. *Exp. Clin. Transplant.* 2008;6:42-7.

[13] Prevalence of abnormal lipid levels among youth- United States, 1999-2006. MMWR *Morb. Mortal .Wkly. Rep.* 2010;59:78

[14] Lentine KL, Rocca-Rey LA, Bacchi G, Wasi N, Schmitz L, Salvalaggio PR, et al. Obesity and cardiac risk after kidney transplantation experience at one center and comprehensive literature review. *Transplantation* 2008;86:303-12.

[15] Segev DL, Kucirka LM, Nguyen GC, Cameron AM, Lock JE, Simpkins CE, Thuluvath PJ, et al. Effect modification in liver allografts with prolonged cold ischemia time. *Am. J Transplant.* 2008;8:658-66.

[16] Meier-Kriesche HU, Arndorfer JA, Kaplan B. The impact of body mass index on renal transplant outcomes: a significant independent risk factor for graft failure and patient death. *Transplantation* 2002;73:70-4.

[17] Jindal RM, Zawada ET, Jr. Obesity and kidney transplantation. *Am. J. Kidney Dis.* 2004;43:943-52.

[18] Hanevold CD, Ho PL, Talley L, Mitsnefes MM. Obesity and renal transplant outcome: a report of the North American Pediatric Renal Transplant Cooperative Study. *Pediatrics* 2005;115:352-6.

[19] Bumgardner GL, Henry ML, Elkhammas E, Wilson GA, Tso P, Davies E et al. Obesity as a risk factor after combined pancreas/kidney transplantation. *Transplantation* 1995;60:1426-30.

[20] Grady KL, Naftel D, Pamboukian SV, Frazier OH, Hauptman P, Herre J et al. Post-operative obesity and cachexia are risk factors for morbidity and mortality after heart transplant: multi-institutional study of post-operative weight change. *J. Heart Lung. Transplant.* 2005;24:1424-30.

[21] Kanasky WF, Jr., Anton SD, Rodrigue JR, Perri MG, Szwed T, Baz MA. Impact of body weight on long-term survival after lung transplantation. *Chest* 2002;121:401-6.

[22] Hanish SI, Petersen RP, Collins BH, Tuttle-Newhall J, Marroquin CE, Kuo PC et al. Obesity predicts increased overall complications following pancreas transplantation. *Transplant Proc* 2005;37:3564-6.

[23] Braunfeld MY, Chan S, Pregler J, Neelakanta G, Sopher MJ, Busuttil RW et al. Liver transplantation in the morbidly obese. *J. Clin. Anesth.* 1996;8:585-90.

[24] Hillingso JG, Wettergren A, Hyoudo M, Kirkegaard P. Obesity increases mortality in liver transplantation--the Danish experience. *Transpl. Int* .2005;18:1231-5.

[25] Nair S, Cohen DB, Cohen MP, Tan H, Maley W, Thuluvath PJ. Postoperative morbidity, mortality, costs, and long-term survival in severely obese patients undergoing orthotopic liver transplantation. *Am. J. Gastroenterol.* 2001;96:842-5.

[26] Sawyer RG, Pelletier SJ, Pruett TL. Increased early morbidity and mortality with acceptable long-term function in severely obese patients undergoing liver transplantation. *Clin. Transplant.* 1999;13:126-30.

[27] Keeffe EB, Gettys C, Esquivel CO. Liver transplantation in patients with severe obesity. *Transplantation* 1994;57:309-311.
[28] Schaeffer DF, Yoshida EM, Buczkowski AK, Chung SW, Steinbrecher UP, Erb SE, Scudamore CH. Surgical morbidity in severely obese liver transplant recipient - a single Canadian Center Experience. *Ann. Hepatol* .2009;8:38-40.
[29] Dick AA, Spitzer AL, Seifert CF, Deckert A, Carithers RL Jr, Reyes JD, Perkins JD. Liver transplantation at the extremes of body mass index. *Liver Transpl.* 2009; 15;968-77.
[30] John PR, Thuluvath PJ. Outcome of liver transplantation in patients with diabetes mellitus: a case-control study. *Hepatology* 2001;34:889-95.
[31] Yoo HY, Thuluvath PJ. The effect of insulin-dependent diabetes mellitus on outcome of liver transplantation. *Transplantation* 2002;74:1007-2.
[32] Adeseun GA, Rivera ME, Thota S, Joffe M, Rosas SE. Metabolic syndrome and coronary artery calcification in renal transplant recipients. *Transplantation* 2008;86:728-32.
[33] Asfar S, Metrakos P, Fryer J et al. An analysis of late deaths after liver transplantation. *Transplantation* 1996;61:1377-81.
[34] Pruthi J, Medkiff KA, Esrason KT et al. Analysis of causes of death in liver transplant recipients who survived more than 3 years. *Liver Transpl.* 2001;7:811-15.
[35] Johnston SD, Morris JK, Cramb R et al. Cardiovascular morbidity and mortality after orthotopic liver transplantation. *Transplantation* 2002;73:901-6.
[36] Abbasoglu O, Levy MF, Brkic BB et al. Ten years of liver transplantation: an evolving understanding of late graft loss. *Transplantation* 1997;64:1801-7.
[37] Ciccarelli O, Kaczmarek B, Roggen F et al. Long-term medical complications and quality of life in adult recipients surviving 10 years or more after liver transplantation. *Acta Gastroenterol. Belg.* 2005;68:323-30.
[38] Guckelberger O, Byram A, Klupp J et al. Coronary event rates in liver transplant recipients reflect the increased prevalence of cardiovascular risk-factors. *Transpl. Int.* 2005;18:967-74.
[39] John PR, Thuluvath PJ. Outcome of patients with new onset diabetes mellitus after liver transplantation compared with those without diabetes mellitus. *Liver Transpl.* 2002; 8:708-13.
[40] Richards J, Gunson B, Johnson J, Neuberger J. Weight gain and obesity after liver transplantation. *Transpl. Int.* 2005;18:461-66.
[41] Laryea M, Watt KD, Molinari M, Walsh MJ, McAllister VC, Marotta PJ et al. Metabolic syndrome in liver transplant recipients: prevalence and association with major vascular events. *Liver Transpl.* 2007;13;1109-14.
[42] Fernández-Miranda C, Sanz M, dela Calle A, et al. Cardiovascular risk factors in 116 patients 5 years or more after liver transplantation. *Transpl Int* 2002;15:556-62.
[43] McCaughan GW, O'Brien E, Sheil AG. A follow up of 53 adult patients alive beyond 2 years following liver transplantation. *J. Gastroenterol. Hepatol.* 1993;8:569-73.
[44] Stegall MD, Everson G, Schroter G et al. Metabolic complications after liver transplantation. Diabetes, hypercholesterolemia, hypertension, and obesity. *Transplantation* 1995;60:1057-60.
[45] Guckelberger O, Bechstein WO, Neuhaus R et al. Cardiovascular risk factors in long-term follow-up after orthotopic liver transplantation. *Clin Transplant* 1997;11:60-65.

[46] Segev DL, Thompson RE, Locke JE, Simpkins CE, Thuluvath PJ, Montgomery RA, Maley WR. prolonged waiting times for liver transplantation in obese patients. *Ann. Surg* .2008;248:863-70.

[47] Neal DA, Tom BD, Luan J, Wareham NJ et al. Is there disparity between risk and incidence of cardiovascular disease after liver transplant? *Transplantation* 2004;77:93-99.

[48] Krok KL, Milwala F, Maheshwari A, Rankin R, Thuluvath PJ. Insulin resistance and microalbuminuria are associated with microvascular disease in patients with cirrhosis. *Liver Transpl.* 2009;15:1036-42.

[49] Thuluvath PJ. When is diabetes mellitus a relative or absolute contraindication to liver transplantation? *Liver Transpl.* 2005;11:S25-29.

[50] Thuluvath PJ. Morbid obesity and gross malnutrition are both poor predictors of outcomes after liver transplantation: what can we do about it? *Liver Transpl.* 2009;15:838-41.

[51] Thuluvath PJ, Yoo HY, Thompson RE. A model to predict survival at one month, one year, and five years after liver transplantation based on pretransplant clinical characteristics. *Liver Transpl.* 2003;9:527-32.

[52] Cook SA, MacLaughlin H, Macdougall IC. A structured weight management programme can achieve improved functional ability and significant weight loss in obese patients with chronic kidney disease. *Nephrol. Dial. Transplant* .2008;23;263-8.

[53] Segev DL, Sozio SM, Shin EJ, Nazarian SM, Nathan H, Thuluvath PJ et al. *Liver Transpl* 2008;14;512-25.

[54] Sheiner PA, Magliocca JF, Bodian CA et al. Long-term medical complications in patients surviving >or = 5 years after liver transplant. Transplantation 2000;69:781-9.

[55] Pischon T, Nothlings U, Boeing H. Obesity and cancer. *Proc Nutr Soc* 2008;67:128-45.

[56] Percik R, Stumvoll M. Obesity and cancer. *Exp. Clin. Endocrinol.* Diabetes 2009;117:563-6.

[57] Grote VA, Becker S, Kaaks R. Diabetes mellitus type 2- an independent risk factor for cancer? *Exp Clin Endocrinol Diabetes* 2010;118:4-8.

[58] Nicolucci A. Epidemiological aspects of neoplasms in diabetes. *Acta Diabetol.* 2010: 47:87-95.

[59] Diabetes mellitus and risk of colorectal cancer: a meta-analysis. *J. Natl. Cancer Inst.* 2005;97:1679-87.

[60] Modanlou KA, Muthyala U, Xiao H, Schnitzier MA, Salvalaggio PR, Brennan DC et al Bariatric surgery among kidney transplant candidates and recipients: An analysis of the United States Renal Data System and literature review. *Transplantation* 2009;87:1167-73.

In: Cardiovascular Diseases and Liver Transplantation
Editor: Zoka Milan, pp. 125-137
ISBN: 978-1-61122-910-3
© 2011 Nova Science Publishers, Inc.

Chapter VIII

Liver Disease and Chronic Advanced Heart Failure

Jill M. Gellow[*1] *and Askay S. Dessai*[2]

[1]Division of cardiology, Oregon Health and Science University, Portland, Oregon
[2]Division of cardiology, Brigham and Women's Hospital, Boston, Massachusetts

Abstract

Chronic liver injury is common in patients with chronic heart failure. In this population, hepatic fibrosis and cirrhosis are thought to develop as a result of increased venous pressure, hypoxia and hepatocellular necrosis. In addition, advanced heart failure is associated with the up regulation of pro-inflammatory cytokines and increased oxidative stress, both of which may contribute to the development of hepatic fibrosis. The development of irreversible liver injury may be insidious in patients with advanced heart failure, given considerable overlap in the clinical presentations of advanced heart and liver disease. However, the presence of chronic liver disease has important implications for the management and prognosis of patients with heart failure, particularly patients with advanced heart failure undergoing evaluation for heart transplantation or mechanical circulatory support (MCS). We review here the clinico-pathologic spectrum of liver disease in heart failure patients, emphasizing the approach to diagnosis and prognostic implications.

Introduction

Nearly five million people in the United States are living with heart failure and each year approximately 550,000 new cases are diagnosed. Heart failure accounts for up to 15 million

---

[*] Correspondence: Jill M. Gelow, MD MPH, Oregon Health and Science University, Division of Cardiology, 3181 SW Sam Jackson Park Road, UHN 62, Portland, Oregon 97239, Tel: (503) 494-8750, Fax: (503) 494-8550, Email: gelowj@ohsu.edu.

office visits per year and is the most common reason for hospitalization among elderly adults. Despite advances in treatment, heart failure remains a morbid disease; the 10-year mortality following an initial diagnosis is 90% [1].

The development of heart failure is characteristically associated with elevated cardiac filling pressures and reduced forward cardiac output that may lead to secondary end-organ damage. Since hepatic congestion follows rapidly on elevation in systemic venous pressures, liver injury is particularly common. In this chapter, we describe the spectrum of liver pathology seen in patients with symptomatic heart failure and review the implications of chronic liver disease for the prognosis and management of heart failure.

The Spectrum of Liver Disease in Heart Failure

Reversible Hepatic Injury in Heart Failure

The spectrum of hepatic abnormalities in heart failure ranges from acute ischemic hepatitis, a consequence of acute, severe reduction in cardiac output, to more chronic changes including congestion, cholestasis, fibrosis, and cirrhosis [2-5].

Acute severe reduction of cardiac output, regardless of the presence of overt cardiogenic shock, can result in cardiogenic ischemic hepatitis. This disorder is characterized by a rapid and marked elevation of serum transaminase levels, between 10 to 20 times the upper limit of normal, followed by a more than 50% decrease within 72 hours after restoration of adequate cardiac output. Ischemic hepatitis is often associated with a consumptive coagulopathy. Usually the ischemic liver injury is self-limiting when it affects a normal liver. However, more serious changes may occur when the liver has been previously damaged [4].

Heart failure exacerbations in patients with normal cardiac output may also be associated with passive hepatic congestion and associated abnormalities of liver function tests, a condition sometimes referred to as "congestive hepatopathy". A range of abnormalities including elevations of aspartate aminotransferase (AST), alanine aminotransferase (ALT), alkaline phosphatase and total bilirubin may be seen, but hepatic synthetic function remains intact. In general, these liver function abnormalities resolve with treatment of heart failure and are not indicative of underlying hepatic disease [2-4].

Chronic Liver Injury in Heart Failure

Distinct from these acute, reversible changes, chronic heart failure may also lead to irreversible liver injury, specifically hepatic fibrosis and cirrhosis. The development of these changes is often insidious and clinically silent. In fact, advanced fibrosis can occur in the absence of abnormal serum liver chemistries, findings of portal hypertension or alterations of hepatic synthetic function. Further, when clinical abnormalities are present, it may be difficult to distinguish hepatic fibrosis or cirrhosis from transient, reversible hepatic congestion [2-5]. Since the presence of such advanced liver disease may have significant implications for the clinical management of patients with heart failure (particularly those who are candidates mechanical circulatory support and transplantation), the remainder of this chapter will focus on the pathophysiology of liver disease in the chronic heart failure population and the implications of chronic liver disease for the treatment of advanced heart failure patients.

Pathology and Pathophysiology of Chronic Liver Disease in Advanced Heart Failure

In patients with chronic heart failure, hepatic fibrosis and cirrhosis are thought to develop as a result of increased venous pressure, hypoxia and hepatocellular necrosis. In addition, advanced heart failure is associated with the up regulation of pro-inflammatory cytokines (e.g., tumor necrosis factor-α, interleukin-1β) and increased oxidative stress, both of which may contribute to the development of hepatic fibrosis [6-8].

Several autopsy studies have examined the histopathologic findings of liver disease in patients with heart failure, specifically chronic passive congestion and centrilobular necrosis [9-12]. In a study of 1000 consecutive adults with suspected cardiac disease undergoing autopsy from 1967 to 1977, centrilobular necrosis correlated significantly with the severity of sustained or episodic hypotension. In contrast, chronic passive congestion was associated with right-sided heart failure. Chronic passive congestion and centrilobular necrosis frequently occurred together, suggesting that chronic passive congestion may contribute to the development of centrilobular necrosis [9].

Autopsy studies have also demonstrated a role for thrombosis in the pathogenesis of liver disease in chronic heart failure. In patients with cardiac cirrhosis, the distribution of liver fibrosis correlates with the distribution of hepatic and portal vein obliteration caused by the organization of thrombus. Propagation of thrombosis into medium sized hepatic veins causes necrosis of the hepatic parenchyma and intensifies stasis in the hepatic sinusoids that in turn promotes sinusoidal thrombosis, fibroblast activation and collagen deposition [13]. Intrahepatic portal vein sclerosis is also more common in patients with severe heart failure compared to patients with other etiologies of liver disease [14].

Though autopsy studies have been immensely helpful in understanding hepatic disease in heart failure patients, additional insight regarding the etiology and prevalence of hepatic fibrosis and cirrhosis in heart failure has been provided by observational clinical studies. Meyers et al evaluated congestive hepatopathy in a diverse population of 83 patients with acute (n=12), chronic (n=53) and acute on chronic (n=18) heart disease [15]. Although cirrhosis was rare in this study (n=1), centrilobular fibrosis seen in 74% of patients, and fibrosis severe enough to distort the normal microscopic architecture was identified in 19%. Hepatic fibrosis did not correlate with systemic or hepatic hemodynamics [15]. More recently, we conducted a clinicopathologic correlation of advanced heart failure patients (n=61) undergoing evaluation for heart transplantation or mechanical circulatory support (MCS) implantation. The majority of patients had liver disease characterized by congestion, pericentral fibrosis and necrosis and sinusoidal dilation (Figure 1). Hepatic fibrosis was identified in 80% of those evaluated, with bridging fibrosis or cirrhosis occurring in 37% of patients (Figure 2) [16].

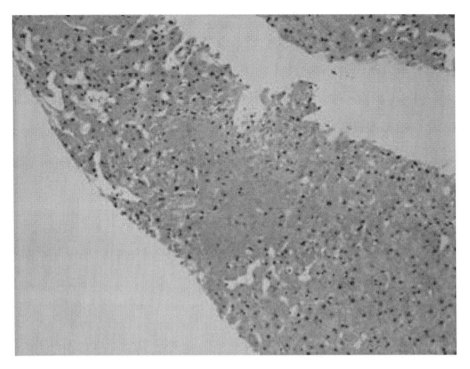

Figure 1. H&E stained liver biopsy with pericentral congestion, hepatocyte necrosis and sinusoidal dilatation.

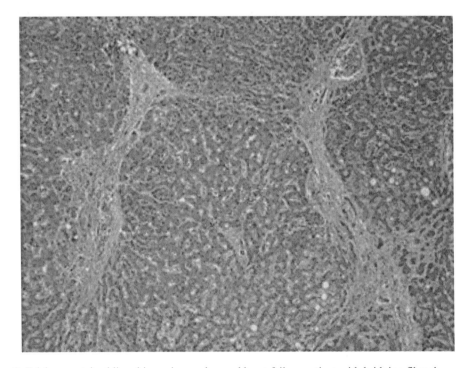

Figure 2. Trichrome stained liver biopsy in an advanced heart failure patient with bridging fibrosis.

Implications of Chronic Liver Disease in the Treatment of Advanced Heart Failure

Cardiac Surgery

Identification of chronic liver disease in the advanced heart failure population is important because it has significant implications for management. Patients with cirrhosis have worse outcomes following cardiac surgery [17-24]. Cardiac surgical morbidity and mortality is generally considered to be unacceptably high in patients with moderate to advanced cirrhosis (Child-Pugh Class B and C). Major complications occur in up to 80% of patients with Child Class B or C cirrhosis [21]. Cardiac surgical morbidity and mortality is acceptable in Child-Pugh Class A patients. In addition to Child-Pugh Class A, cardiac surgery can be performed with a more acceptable risk profile in patients with a Child-Pugh Score ≤7 or a Model of End Stage Liver Disease (MELD) score of ≤13 [22]. Perioperative morbidity and mortality in patients with cirrhosis is primarily due to bleeding, hepatic decompensation and infection [17, 19-21, 23]. Chest tube drainage and transfusion requirements are three times the average values, and bleeding requiring reoperation is common [17, 19-20, 23].

Cardiopulmonary bypass triggers the production and release of numerous vasoactive substances and cytokines that affect coagulopathy, vascular resistance, vascular permeability, fluid balance and major organ function. This complex inflammatory response contributes to the development of post-operative complications, including liver dysfunction [25]. Minimizing cardiopulmonary bypass times or performing off-pump cardiac surgery may reduce cardiac surgical risk in patients with liver disease [23, 26]. Normothermic cardiopulmonary bypass may be more adequate for supporting hepatic function than hypothermic cardiopulmonary bypass surgery [27].

Mechanical Circulatory Support (MCS)

The impact of liver disease on cardiac surgical morbidity and mortality is echoed in the MCS and cardiac transplantation literature. Advances in MCS have significantly improved the survival of patients awaiting cardiac transplantation (bridge-to-transplantation) and patients with end-state heart failure who are ineligible for heart transplant (destination therapy) [28-30]. First and second generation MCS devices are pulsatile pumps that have been successful in unloading the failing heart and preserving end-organ function [31, 32]. Their effectiveness, however, is limited by their large size and poor long-term durability. Newer generation continuous flow devices (axial or centrifugal) are smaller and more durable. They are technically easier to implant, are less prone to infection and have resulted in improved survival compared to pulsatile pumps [28]. The introduction of continuous flow MCS devices raised initial concern regarding the effect of non-pulsatile flow on end organ function. To date animal and clinical studies have shown no significant differences in hepatic function post MCS implantation in continuous flow devices compared to first and second-generation pulsatile flow devices [33-36].

Pre-implantation liver function is an important determinant of survival following MCS implantation. Patients with high pre-operative bilirubin, AST, ALT and LDH levels have a significantly higher likelihood of dying from liver failure following MCS implantation than those without elevated levels [37]. Low pre-operative direct bilirubin and total bilirubin have been shown to be the best predictors of post-operative survival [32]. Post-operative deterioration of hepatic function despite adequate device function in patients with pre-existing liver disease may in part be due to an augmented inflammatory response and altered hepatic microcirculation [38].

Bleeding is the most common postoperative complication after MCS implantation. The incidence of perioperative bleeding in all patients after device implantation remains significant and necessitates reoperation in up to 60% of implants, regardless of the type of device used [39]. Minimizing bleeding is particularly important following isolated left ventricular assist device (LVAD) implantation because high volume blood product resuscitation can lead to the development of right ventricular failure [39]. Right ventricular failure following LVAD implantation is associated with end-organ failure (including hepatic failure), increased hospital stay and high mortality [40-42].

After validating the ability of MELD scores to predict death in the Interagency Registry of Mechanical Circulatory Support (INTERMACS), Matthews, et al evaluated the risk of increasing MELD scores on operative death and bleeding in 211 patients undergoing MCS implantation at a single center from 1996-2007. Among these patients, the mean MELD score for operative deaths was 14 (25th % 11; 75th % 22) and the mean MELD score for survivors was 12 (25th % 9; 75th %15). Each five unit increase in MELD score increased the total perioperative blood product exposure by 15.1 ± 3.8 units (p < 0.001). A five unit increase in the unique component of MELD (not shared with its ability to predict bleeding) increased the odds of operative mortality by 60% and was predictive of post-operative renal replacement therapy and device infection [43]. Survival at 6 months for subjects with MELD scores ≥ 17 and < 17 was 74±6% and 88±3%, respectively (log rank p = 0.009). This was similar to the INTERMACS cohort, where 6 month survival for subjects with MELD score ≥ 17 was 67.5% compared with 82±3% in subjects with MELD scores< 17 (log rank p = 0.032) [43].

Orthotopic Heart Transplantation

Advanced heart failure patients with severe liver disease also have poor outcomes following heart transplantation. Preoperative hepatic insufficiency with prolongation of the prothrombin time or elevated serum levels of liver enzymes is an independent predictor of early death after heart transplantation [44].

Hsu et al reviewed twelve patients with cirrhosis who underwent heart transplantation between 1987 and 2007 at a single center. Causes of liver cirrhosis were alcoholism (n=2), cardiac (n=7) and unknown (n=3). The Child-Pugh Class was A in three patients, B in five patients and C in four patients. The hospital mortality rate was 50% and major in-hospital complications occurred in 75% of patients (n=9). Similar outcomes have been reported in advanced heart failure patients with extreme right heart failure and cardiac ascites [45-47]. These exceedingly poor outcomes have led many to consider the presence of cirrhosis, particularly in the advanced stages, an absolute contraindication to isolated cardiac transplantation.

Combined Heart Liver Transplantation

Given the poor outcomes for patients with cirrhosis following mechanical circulatory support and heart transplantation, the role of combined heart-liver transplantation has been increasingly considered. Several reports of single center combined heart-liver transplant experiences have been published, including patients with cardiac cirrhosis from restrictive cardiomyopathy, hypertrophic cardiomyopathy and congenital heart disease [48-54].

A total of 47 cases of combined heart-liver (n = 41) and heart-liver-kidney transplantation (n = 6) were reported to the United Network for Organ Sharing (UNOS) between October 1987 and December 2005. With a mean follow-up of 3.7 (range 0 to 12.6) years, patient, heart and liver graft survival rates were 84.8%, 84.8% and 82.4% at 1 year, and 75.6%, 75.6% and 73.5% at 5 years, respectively. Follow-up of patients who survived at least 6 months after transplantation (n = 39) showed that 28.2% of patients were on a single immunosuppressive agent [55].

Raichlin et al reviewed 15 combined heart-liver transplants at a single center from January 1992 and May 2007 [56]. Freedom from cardiac allograft rejection was 83% at 1 month and did not change with time. This rate was notably lower than that of cardiac allograft rejection in patients receiving isolated heart transplantation. The decrease in cardiac allograft rejection seen in patients receiving combined heart-liver transplantation is not unexpected, since additional data suggests that liver allografts are thought to enhance tolerance to other donor-specific allografts. Analysis of 133,416 UNOS patients showed that rejection rates for allografts co-transplanted with donor-specific primary liver, kidney, and heart allografts were significantly lower than rejection rates for allografts transplanted alone [57]. Despite these promising results, however, dual organ transplants remain a small proportion of the total number of cardiac transplants performed each year, and may be appropriate only for carefully selected patients at specialized centers with high volume.

Diagnosis of Liver Disease in Patients with Chronic Heart Failure

Physical Examination

Given the implications for clinical management, accurately determining the presence and severity of chronic liver disease in the advanced heart failure population is important. Unfortunately, the diagnosis of liver disease in patients with chronic heart failure is challenging in part due to considerable overlap in the physical examination findings of heart failure and liver disease. Hepatomegaly is a common manifestation of volume overload and decompensated heart failure. Signs of portal hypertension, including splenomegaly, jaundice, and ascites, may be apparent in patients with advanced heart failure even in the absence of cirrhosis. The triad of right heart failure, hepatomegaly and ascites, while suggestive of 'cardiac' cirrhosis, is neither sensitive nor specific for this diagnosis [4, 5]. Although liver disease is more prevalent in patients with advanced or end-stage heart failure, heart failure severity alone is a poor surrogate irreversible liver injury, as individual patients vary widely in their susceptibility to develop fibrosis [58].

Laboratory Findings

The liver biochemical profile also varies widely amongst heart failure patients, from a pattern of predominant intrahepatic cholestasis to a more 'mixed' picture with features of both inflammation and obstruction [16, 59-61]. The severity of abnormalities in the liver biochemical profile appear to correlate, at least in part, with the hemodynamic severity of heart failure. Levels of AST, ALT, lactate dehydrogenase (LDH) and total bilirubin are weakly correlated with the degree of elevation in right atrial pressure and pulmonary capillary wedge pressure as well as the degree of reduction in cardiac index [3]. Such abnormalities are also more prevalent in patients with more severe tricuspid valve regurgitation, perhaps due to reversal of flow in the hepatic veins and elevation in intrahepatic filling pressures during ventricular systole [59]. Although abnormalities of synthetic function (low serum cholesterol, low serum albumin, elevated prothrombin time) are more suggestive of advanced liver injury, these features are also nonspecific, and may also be seen in patients with cardiac cachexia due to advanced heart failure. Despite their limited utility for diagnosis of underlying liver disease, however, abnormalities in the liver biochemical profile do carry important prognostic implications in heart failure patients, with serum levels of AST and total bilirubin showing the strongest correlation with long-term survival in ambulatory heart failure patients [60].

Our own data suggest that relative to advanced heart failure patients without hepatic fibrosis on liver biopsy, those with hepatic fibrosis have worse renal function and are more likely to have moderate or severe tricuspid regurgitation and obstructive/cholestatic or mixed liver function abnormalities. However, in a referral population from a single transplant center, we found no association between the presence of hepatic fibrosis and gender, age, etiology of cardiomyopathy, duration of symptoms, prevalence of right or left ventricular dysfunction, cardiac filling pressures, type of biopsy or hepatitis C status, underscoring the challenge of identifying clinically relevant liver disease on the basis of clinical features or historical findings alone [16].

Hepatic Imaging

Given the challenges of clinical diagnosis, noninvasive imaging techniques are frequently used to evaluate liver disease severity in advanced heart failure patients. Ultrasound and computed tomography (CT) are frequently used for hepatic imaging in patient with heart failure because they are overall safe, readily available, and inexpensive [62, 63]. However, imaging with ultrasound or CT in this population may not be adequate to exclude hepatic fibrosis or cirrhosis [16]. We found that hepatic imaging with either CT or ultrasound had an extremely low sensitivity (30%) and poor negative predictive value (21%) for the diagnosis of hepatic fibrosis in an advanced heart failure population [16]. While MRI provides considerable advantages over CT and ultrasound, many advanced heart failure patient have implanted devices (pacemakers, defibrillators) which preclude this approach [63].

Liver stiffness measured by transient elastography is strongly associated with degree of liver fibrosis in a variety of liver diseases including viral hepatitis, alcoholic liver disease and primary biliary cirrhosis [64]. The role of transient elastography is uncertain in chronic heart failure patients. Liver stiffness was measured in ten patients with decompensated heart failure before and after treatment. Initial liver stiffness measurements were elevated in all patients and, in eight patients, measurements were elevated to a degree that suggested cirrhosis. After heart failure treatment, liver stiffness decreased in all ten patients [65]. Thus, liver congestion (elevated central venous filling pressures) must be excluded before liver stiffness can be used to assess hepatic fibrosis in heart failure populations. Additional studies are needed to confirm whether this modality could be a useful tool to noninvasively screen for hepatic fibrosis or cardiac cirrhosis in euvolemic heart failure patients [65].

Hepatic Biopsy

Given the limitations of noninvasive imaging studies, liver biopsy remains the gold standard for assessing hepatic fibrosis and cirrhosis [65]. Transjugular liver biopsy is particularly appealing in the advanced heart failure population because it can be performed simultaneously with pulmonary artery catheterization to assess intracardiac hemodynamics. Liver biopsy from this approach is generally safe, even in advanced heart failure patients; no complications have been reported in two small series [16, 66]. Despite well-known limitations including sampling error and susceptibility to variable interpretation, liver biopsy may be the only way to exclude irreversible damage. We have therefore proposed that this approach be considered for all patients with high risk features (prominent right heart failure, severe tricuspid regurgitation, findings of portal hypertension), undergoing evaluation for VAD or transplantation [16].

Conclusion

Liver dysfunction, including the development of hepatic fibrosis and cirrhosis, is common in patients with chronic heart failure. Patients with Child class B or C cirrhosis do poorly following cardiac surgery, including mechanical circulatory support implantation and cardiac transplantation. Clinical diagnosis of hepatic fibrosis is challenging and the utility of non-invasive imaging tests is limited. Transjugular liver biopsy should be considered in advanced heart failure patients undergoing evaluation for mechanical circulatory support implantation or heart transplantation since the presence of significant liver disease has important implications for management.

References:

[1] 2005 Writing Committee Members. 2009 Focused update incorporated into the ACC/AHA 2005 guidelines for the diagnosis and management of heart failure in adults. *Circulation* 2009; 119: e391-e470.

[2] Bynum TE, Boinott JK, Maddrey WC. Ischemic hepatitis. *Dig Dis Sci* 1979; 24: 129-35.

[3] Kubo C, Walter BA, John DHA, Clark M, Cody RJ. Liver function abnormalities in chronic heart failure. Influence of systemic hemodynamics. *Arch Intern Med* 1987; 147: 1227-30.

[4] Naschitz JE, Slobodin G, Lewis RJ, Zuckerman E, Yeshurun D. Heart diseases affecting the liver and liver diseases affecting the heart. *Am Heart J* 2000; 140: 111-20.

[5] Gaillourakis CC, Rosenberg PM, Friedman LS. The liver in heart failure. *Clin Liver Dis* 2002; 6: 947-67.
[6] Tilg H, Kaser A, Moschen AR. How to modulate inflammatory cytokines in liver diseases. *Liver Int* 2006; 26: 1029-9.
[7] Sawyer DB, Siwik DA, Xiao L, Pimentel DR, Singh K, Colucci WS. Role of oxidative stress in myocardial hypertrophy and failure. *J Mol Cell Cardiol* 2002; 34: 379-88.
[8] Parola M, Robino G. Oxidative stress-related molecules and liver fibrosis. *J Hepatol 2001;* 35: 297-306.
[9] Arcidi JM Jr., Moore GW, Hutchins GM. Hepatic morphology in cardiac dysfunction: a clinicopathology study of 1000 subjects at autopsy. *Am. J Pathol.*1981; 104: 159-66.
[10] Henrion J, luwaert R, Colin L, Schmitz A, Schapira M,Heller FR. Hypoxic hepatits: clinical and hemodynamic study in 142 consecutive cases. *Medicine* 2003; 82: 392-406.
[11] Henrion J, Luwaert R, Colin L, Schmitz A, Schapira M, Heller FR. Hypoxic hepatitis. Prospective clinical and hemodynamic study of 45 cases. *Gastroenterol Clin Biol* 1990; 14: 836-41.
[12] Seeto RK, Fenn B, Rockey DC. Ischemic hepatits: clinical presentation and pathogenesis. *Am J Med* 2000; 109: 1099-13.
[13] Wanless IR, Bernier V, Seger M. Intrahepatic portal vein sclerosis in patients without a history of liver disease. An autopsy study. *Am J Pathol* 1982; 106: 63-70.
[14] Wanless IR, Liu JJ, Butany J. Role of thrombosis in the pathogenesis of congestive hepatic fibrosis (cardiac cirrhosis). *Hepatology* 1995; 21: 1232-7.
[15] Meyers RP, Cerini R, Sayegh R, Moreau R, Degott C, Lebrec D, Lee SS. Cardiac Hepatopathy: Clinical, hemodynamic and histologic characteristics and correlations. *Hepatology* 2003; 37: 393-400.
[16] Gelow JM, Desai AS, Hochberg CP, Glickman JN, Givertz MM, Fang JC. Clinical predictors of hepatic fibrosis in chronic advanced heart failure. *Circ Heart Fail* 2010; 3: 59-64.
[17] Klemperer JD, Ko W, Krieger K, Connolly M, Rosengart TK, Altorki NK et al. Cardiac operations in patients with cirrhosis. *Ann Thorac Surg* 1998; 65: 85-7.
[18] Morisaki A, Hosono M, Sasak Y, Kubo S, Hirai H, Suehiro S, Shibata T. Risk factor analysis in patients with liver cirrhosis undergoing cardiovascular operations. *Ann Thorac Surg* 2010; 89: 811-8.
[19] Bizouarn P, Ausseur A, Desseigne P, Teurnier YL, Nougarede B, Train M, Luc Michaud J. Early and late outcomes after elective cardiac surgery in patients with cirrhosis. *Ann Thorac Surg* 1999; 67: 1334-9.
[20] Hayashida N, Shoujima T, Teshima H, Yokokura Y, Takagi K, Tomoeda H, Aoyagi S. Clinical outcomes after cardiac operations in patients with cirrhosis. *Ann Thorac Surg* 2004; 77: 500-5.
[21] Lin CH, Lin FY, Wang SS, Yu HY, Hsu RB. Cardiac surgery in patients with liver cirrhosis. *Ann Thorac Surg* 2005; 79: 1551-4.
[22] Suman A, Barnes DS, Zein NN, Levinthal GN, Connor JT, Careu WD. Predicting outcome after cardiac surgery in patients with cirrhosis: a comparison of Child-Pugh and MELD scores. *Clin Gastroenterol Hepatol.*2004; 2: 719-23.
[23] Kaplan M, Cimen S, Kut MS, Demirtas MM. Cardiac operations for patients with chronic liver disease. *Heart Surg. Forum* 2002; 5: 60-65.

[24] Murashita T, Komiya T, Tamura N, Sakaguchi G, Kobayashi T, Furukawa T et al. Preoperative evaluation of patients with liver cirrhosis undergoing open heart surgery. *Gen Thorac Cardiovasc Surg* 2009; 57: 293-97.

[25] Wan S, LeClerc JL, Vincent JL. Inflammatory response to cardiopulmonary bypass: Mechanisms involved and possible therapeutic strategies. *Chest* 1997; 112: 676-92.

[26] Onorati F, Rubino AS, Nucera S, Foti D, Sica V, Santini F et al. Off-pump coronary artery bypass surgery versus standard linear or pulsatile CPB; endothelial activation and inflammatory response. *Eur J Cardiothorac Surg*.2010; 37: 897-904.

[27] Hashimoto K, Sasaki T, Hachiya T, Onoguchi K, Takakura H, Oshiumoi M et al. Superior hepatic mitochondrial oxidation reduction state in normothermic cardiopulmonary bypass. *J Thorac Cardiovasc Surg* 2001; 121: 1179-86.

[28] Krishnamani R, DeNofrio D, Konstam M. Emerging ventricular assist devices for long-term cardiac support. *Nat Rev Cardiol* 2010; 7: 71-6.

[29] Rose EA, GA, Felijens AC, Moskowitz AJ, John R, Boyle AJ, Aaronson KD et al. Long-term use of a left ventricular assist device for end-stage heart failure. *N Engl J Med* 2001; 345: 1435-43.

[30] Miller LW, Pagani FD, Russel SD et al. Use of a continuous flow device in patients awaiting heart transplantation. *N Engl J Med* 2007; 357: 885-96.

[31] Farrar DJ, Hill JD. Recovery of major end organ function in patients awaiting heart transplantation with Thoratec ventricular assist devices. *J Heart Lung Transplant* 1994; 13: 1125-32.

[32] Frazier OH, Rose EA, Oz MC, Dembitsky W, McCarthy P, Radovancevic B et al. Multicenter clinical evaluation of the Heart Mate vented electric left ventricular assist system in patients awaiting heart transplantation. *J Thorac Cardiovasc Surg* 2001; 122: 1186-95.

[33] Letsou GV, Myers TJ, Gregoric ID, Delgado R, Shah N, Robertson K et al. Continuous axial-flow left ventricular assist device (Jarvik 2000) maintains kidney and liver perfusion for up to 6 months. *Ann Thorac Surg* 2003; 76: 1167-70.

[34] Saito S, Westaby S, Pittot D, Dudnikov S, Robson D, Catarino PA et al. End-organ function during chronic non-pulsatile circulation. *Ann Thorac Surg* 2002; 74: 1080-5.

[35] Radovancevic B, Vrtovec B, de Kort E, Radovancevic R, Gregoric ID, Frazier OH. End-organ function in patients on long-term circulatory support with continuous or pulsatile flow assist devices. *J Heart Lung Transplant* 2007; 26: 815-8.

[36] Kamdur F, Boyle A, Liao K, Colvin-Adams M, Joyce L, John R. Effects of centrifugal, axial and pulsatile left ventricular assist device support on end-organ function in heart failure patients. *J Heart Lung Transplant* 2009; 28: 352-9.

[37] Reinhartz O, Farrar DJ, Hershon JH, Avery GJ, Haeusslein EA, Hill JD. Importance of preoperative liver function as a predictor or survival in patients supported with Thoratec ventricular assist devices as a bridge to transplantation. *J Thorac Cardiovasc Surg* 1998; 116: 633-40.

[38] Masai T, Sawa Y, Ohtake S, Nishida T, Nishimura M, Fukushima N et al. Hepatic dysfunction after left ventricular mechanical assist in patients with end-stage heart failure: role of inflammatory response and hepatic microcirculation. *Ann Thorac Surg* 2002; 73: 549-55.

[39] Goldstein DJ, Beauford RB. Left ventricular assist devices and bleeding: Adding insult to injury. *Ann Thorac Surg* 2003; 75: S42-S47.

[40] Wadia Y, Etheridge W, Smart F, Wood P, Frazier OH. Pathophysiology of hepatic dysfunction and intrahepatic cholestasis in heart failure after left ventricular assist device. *J Heart Lung Transplant* .2005; 24: 361-70.

[41] Kavarna MN, Pessin-Minsley MS, Urtecho J, Catanses KA, Flannery M, Oz D. Right ventricular dysfunction and organ failure in left ventricular assist device recipients: a continuing problem. *Ann .Thorac Surg* 2002; 73: 745-50

[42] Kawai A, Kormos RI, Mandarino WA, Morita S, Griffith BP. Differential regional function of the right ventricle during the use of a left ventricular assist device. *ASAIO J* 1992; 38: M676-M678.

[43] Matthews JC, Pagani FD, Haft JW, Koelling TM, Naftel DC, Aaronson KD. Model for end-stage liver disease score predicts left ventricular assist device operative transfusion requirements, morbidity and mortality. *Circulation* 2010; 121: 214-20.

[44] Kirsh M, Baufreton C, Naftel DC, Benvenuti C, Loisance DY. Pretransplantation risk factors for death after heart transplantation: the Henri Mondor experience. *J. Heart Lung Transplant* 1998; 17: 268-77.

[45] Hsu RB, Chang CI, Lin FY, Chou NK, Chi NH, Wang SS, Chu SH. Heart transplantation in patients with liver cirrhosis. *Eur J Cardiothorac Surg* 2008; 34: 307-12.

[46] Hsu RB, Lin FY, Chou NK, Ko WJ, Chi NS, Wang SS. Heart transplantation in patients with extreme right ventricular failure. *Eur J Cardiothoac. Surg*.2007; 32: 457-61.

[47] Hsu RB. Heart transplantation in patients with end-stage heart failure and cardiac ascites. *Circ J* 2007; 71: 1744-8.

[48] Ahualli L, Stewart-Harris A, Bastianelli G, Radlovachi G, Bartolome A, Trigo PL et al. Combined cardiohepatic transplantation due to severe heterozygous familiar hypercholesteremia type II: first case in Argentina--a case report. *Transplant Proc* 2007; 39: 2449-53.

[49] Bernier PL, Grenon M, Ergina P, Schricker T, Chaudhury P, Metrakos P, Lachapelle K. Combined simultaneous heart and liver transplantation with complete cardiopulmonary bypass support. *Ann Thorac Surg* 2007; 83: 1544-5.

[50] Alkofer BJ, Chiche L, Khavat A, Deshayes JP, Lepage A, Saloux E, Reznik Y.Liver transplant combined with heart transplant in severe heterozygous hypercholesterolemia: report of the first case and review of the literature. *Transplant Proc* 2005; 37: 2250-62.

[51] 51.Nardo B, Beltempo P, Bertelli R, Montalti R, Vivarelli M, Cescon M et al. Combined heart and liver transplantation in four adults with familial amyloidosis: experience of a single center. *Transplant Proc* 2004; 36: 645-7.

[52] Haynes H, Farroni J. Successful combined heart-liver transplantation in a patient with hemochromatosis. *Prog Transplant* 2004; 14: 39-40.

[53] Eyraud D, Ben Menna M, Vaillant JC, Kitajima K, Lebray P, Pavie A et al. Perioperative management of combined heart-liver transplantation in patients with cirrhosis, renal insufficiency or pulmonary hypertension. *Clin Transplant*.2010 Mar 22, [Epub ahead of print].

[54] Hennessey T, Backman SB, Cecere R, Lachapelle K, de Varennes B, Ergina P, Metrakos P, Schricker T. Combined heart and liver transplantation on cardiopulmonary bypass: report of four cases. *Can J Anaesth*.2010; 57: 355-60.

[55] Te HS, Anderson AS, Millis JM, Jeevanandam V, Jensen DM. Current state of combined heart-liver transplantation in the United States. *J Heart Lung Transplant* 2008; 27: 753-9.

[56] Raichlin E, Daly RC, Rosen CB, McGregor CG, Charton MR, Frantz RP et al. Combined heart and liver transplantation: a single center experience. *Transplantation* 2009; 88: 219-25.

[57] Rana A, Robles S, Russo MJ, Halazun KJ, Woodland DC, Witkowski P, Ratner LE, Hardy MA. The combined organ effect: protective against rejection. *Ann Surg* 2008; 248: 871-9.

[58] Valla D. Cirrhosis of vascular origin. *Rev Prat* 1991; 41: 1170-3

[59] Lau GT, Tan HC and Kritharidea L. Type of liver dysfunction in heart failure and its relation to the severity of tricuspid regurgitation. *Am J Cardiol* 2002; 90: 1405-9.

[60] Batin P, Wickens M, McEntegart D, Fullwood L, Cowley AJ. The importance of abnormalities of liver function test in predicting mortality in chronic heart failure. *Eur Heart J* 1995; 16: 1613-18.

[61] Richman SM, Delman AJ, Grob D. Alteration in indices of liver function in congestive heart failure with particular reference to serum enzymes. *Am J Med* 1961; 30: 211-25.

[62] Sanford NL, Walsh P, Matis C, Baddeley H, Powell LW. Is ultrasonography useful in the assessment of diffuse parenchymal liver disease? *Gastroenterology* 1985; 89: 186-91.

[63] Bonekamp S, Kamel I, Solga S, Clark J. Can imaging modalities diagnose and stage hepatic fibrosis and cirrhosis accurately? *J Hepatol*.2009; 50: 17-35.

[64] Friedrich-Rust M, Ong MF, Martens S, Sarrazin C,Bojunga J, Zeuzem S et al. Performance of transient elastography for the staging of liver fibrosis: a meta analysis. *Gastroenterolgy* 2008; 134: 960-74.

[65] Millonig G, Friedrich S, Adolf S, Fonouni H, Golriz M, Mehrabi A et al. Liver stiffness is influenced by central venous pressure. *J Hepatol* 2010; 52: 206-10.

[66] Parera A, Banares R, Alvarez R, Casariego J, Carneros JA, Saicedo M, Palomo J, Cos E. The usefulness of transjugular hepatic biopsy in the evaluation of liver disease in candidates for heart transplantation. *Gastroenterol Hepatol* 1999; 22: 67-71.

In: Cardiovascular Diseases and Liver Transplantation
Editor: Zoka Milan, pp. 139-155
ISBN: 978-1-61122-910-3
© 2011 Nova Science Publishers, Inc.

Chapter IX

Combined Cardiac Surgery and Liver Transplantation

Eugenia Raichlin[*1], *Charles B. Rosen*[2,3], *Ioana Dumitru*[1], *Richard C. Daly*[2,4], *and Sudhir S. Kushwaha*[2]

[1]Department of Internal Medicine, Section of Cardiology, UNMC, Omaha, NE 68198, USA
[2]William J. Von Liebig Transplant Center, Mayo Clinic, Rochester, MN 55905, USA
[3]Department of Liver transplantation, Mayo Clinic, Rochester, MN 55905, USA
[4]Departments of Cardiothoracic Surgery, Mayo Clinic, Rochester, MN 55905, USA

Abstract

Liver transplantation (LT) is a viable treatment option for patients with end-stage liver disease (ESLD). However, the high incidence of advanced coronary atherosclerosis or severe valvular disease presents clinical dilemma in the treatment of liver transplant candidates. Combined simultaneous cardiac surgery and liver transplantation has been cautiously explored in this difficult patient population. Several small studies demonstrated that this is a feasible surgical option which can be performed safely, and morbidity is not prohibitive for success. Moreover, simultaneous combined heart and liver transplantation (CHLT) may be a lifesaving procedure for patients suffering from end-stage heart and liver diseases or several metabolic disorders.

Introduction

---

[*] Correspondence: Eugenia Raichlin, Assistant Professor, Department of Internal Medicine, Section of Cardiology, 982265 UNMC, Omaha, NE 68198-2265, USA, Tel: 402–559–5552, Fax: 402–559–8365, E-mail: eraichlin@unmc.edu.

Liver transplantation (LT) is a viable treatment option for patients with irreversible acute and chronic liver disease. The number of liver transplantations performed each year continues to increase and improvements in surgical and anesthetic techniques have allowed LT to be performed in older patients. The higher incidence of cardiac diseases, especially coronary artery disease (CAD) and aortic stenosis (AS), in older liver transplant candidates presents clinical dilemmas [1].

Advanced Coronary Atherosclerosis and End-Stage Liver Disease

The estimated prevalence of CAD in patients with ESLD is up to 27%, clearly exceeding the general health population [2]. CAD has been reported as the most common cause of complication and increases post LT mortality rate to 50% and the morbidity rate to the 81% [3].

There are no definitive recommendations and indications for the treatment of extensive CAD in patients with ESLD. In general, a staged procedure using percutaneous coronary intervention (PCI) prior to LT can be used if the patient can tolerate this approach and has appropriate anatomy [4]. However, the need for prolonged anti-platelet therapy along with the inability to predict the timing of LT, makes this a difficult option. Patients with significant CAD and lesions that are not amenable to PCI may require coronary artery bypass graft (CABG), but the mortality rates following CABG in patients with severe liver disease are relatively high [5, 6] and the application of CABG differs from patients with normal hepatic function [7]. Therefore, the presence of coexisting severe CAD and end stage liver disease (ESLD) may lead to certain clinical dilemmas: if the severity of CAD has a prohibitive operative risk, should these patients be excluded from LT? Can CABG be performed with reasonable risk-benefit consideration in patients who remain potential candidates for LT? What should be the timing of CABG? Which of these two procedures, CABG or LT, should be performed first or should they be performed simultaneously?[8]

Several studies have assessed outcomes of patients with cirrhosis undergoing cardiac surgery. In a prospective study of 12 patients with Child's class A or B cirrhosis who underwent elective cardiac surgery, postoperative morbidity and significant complications occurred in 58% of patients. In addition, both intensive care unit and total hospital stays were prolonged in these patients [5]. A retrospective study of 13 patients with cirrhosis who underwent cardiac surgery demonstrated 31% of overall perioperative mortality and 25% of major complications rates which occurred in 25% of patients with Child-Pugh's class A cirrhosis and 100% of patients with Child-Pugh's class B cirrhosis [6]. This is in marked contrast to mortality and morbidity rates of 1.8% and 8.4% in patients without cirrhosis undergoing cardiac surgery, respectively [9]. Csikesz et al demonstrated that patients with liver disease who underwent CABG have an 8-fold increase in the risk of death, and the risk increases to 22.7-fold if liver disease is complicated by pulmonary hypertension [10]. In patients with more advanced Child-Pugh's class B and C cirrhosis postoperative mortality after cardiac operations remains unacceptably high at 50 and 100 % respectively [11]. Thus, the role of CABG is a risk-benefit decision which very much depends on the severity of liver disease [12]. In patients with moderate ESLD, who survive CABG, this procedure may be carried out first and in the rare instance of rapid progression to liver failure, patients can be urgently transplanted. However, it is generally agreed that elective cardiac operations are contraindicated in patients with moderate and severe cirrhosis [6, 13]. The risk of surgery in patients with liver disease suggested a cut off MELD (Model for End-Stage Liver Disease) score of 13 for avoiding cardiac surgery [14]. Besides the Child-Pugh's classification and MELD score, lower preoperative levels of serum cholinesterase and higher preoperative bilirubin levels have been demonstrated to be an independent predictor of mortality in patients with liver dysfunction undergoing cardiac surgery [15].

It has been well documented that use of cardio-pulmonary bypass (CPB) in the patients with severe liver dysfunction is harmful and may result in the production and release of numerous vasoactive substances and cytotoxic chemicals that increase vascular resistance and affect vascular permeability [16]. CPB causes a decrease in the activity of endogenous atrial natriuretic peptides [17] and renal resistance to natriuretic action, which is similarly seen in patients with congestive heart failure.[18] Along with poor nutritional status and portopulmonary hypertension it may lead to water and sodium retention characterized by edema, ascites, pericardial effusion, and pleural effusion [5, 6, 18]. Exacerbation of preexisting coagulopathy may result in excessive mediastinal bleeding; hypothermia and hypoperfusion may increase susceptibility to infections [19]. In addition, patients with ESLD often have impaired renal function that can be compromised further by CPB [20]. The potential for further hepatic deterioration after prolonged surgery with CPB is also concerning [21].

Therefore, the avoidance of CPB may theoretically improve postoperative clinical outcome. Although the technique is not indicated in all patients requiring cardiac surgical interventions and the results of small studies are not conclusive, off-pump CABG is a potential alternative therapeutic strategy for patients with advanced cirrhosis requiring surgical revascularization [11]. Conversely, if LT undertaken as a first stage in patients with coexisting severe CAD the unavoidable major hemodynamic changes make this option very hazardous. Patients with ESLD have unique hemodynamics, namely, high resting cardiac outputs and low systemic vascular resistances [22, 23]. LT induces marked hemodynamic and hypercoagulability alterations such as elevation in systemic vascular resistance and a decrease in cardiac output, [24, 25] depression of protein C, protein S and antithrombin III levels [26]. All these could potentially adversely affect the outcome of patients and result in cardiac failure, one of the major causes of morbidity and mortality after LT [1, 27].

In this difficult patient population with advanced CAD and ESLD a simultaneous combined CABG and LT (CABG-LT) has been cautiously explored. This is done infrequently: only 17 combined CABG/LT procedures with significant high-risk coronary lesions, preserved left ventricular function and very advanced liver disease have been reported in the English language literature [8, 28-34].

In a single center series of 5 patients who underwent simultaneous combined CABG – LT procedure, Axelrod et al described the technical features associated with good outcome [30]. Donors were carefully selected to reduce the risk of primary liver allograft non-function or dysfunction. This would decrease the risk of significant hemorrhage and perioperative cardiac tamponade. In patients without malignancy, the cardiac procedure was performed first, while in the case of known malignancy, the abdomen was entered first to exclude metastatic disease. After drainage of ascitic fluid, the chest was entered through a median sternotomy incision and if not previously opened, the peritoneal cavity was not entered to avoid contamination of the bypass circuit by ascitic fluid. After heparinization, patients were placed on CPB and aortocoronary bypass was performed. Since prolonged use of CPB has been associated with significant intraoperative blood loss, all patients were weaned from CPB following construction of the proximal anastomoses and prior to initiation of recipient hepatectomy. The heparinization was reversed with protamine. Finally, the aortic cannula was removed and the right atrial cannula was left in place as outflow for porto-systemic venovenous bypass used during LT. Aprotinin was administered to 2 patients. The sternum and pericardial cradle were left open so that the mediastinum could be intermittently inspected to ensure hemostasis. The right atrial cannula was available for outflow from the veno-veno bypass circuit, and the surgical exposure was excellent even in the case of polycystic liver disease and massive hepatomegaly.

The abdomen was entered and the liver mobilized by dividing the ligamentous attachments. Next, the portal structures were dissected and the portal vein was mobilized to facilitate portal-sapheno-atrial bypass. The patients' left sapheno-femoral junction was identified and a heparin coated bypass cannula was inserted proximally. The portal vein was then cannulated and portal-systemic veno-venous bypass was initiated using the atrial cannula for outflow to provide maximum hemodynamic stability during the LT. The hepatectomy was completed, and the allograft was then anastomosed using either the standard technique or side-to-side-venacavaplasty. The same group has demonstrated that side-to-side venacavaplasty reduces warm and cold ischemic times, ease hepatectomy, and markedly reduced operative times [35]. The portal venous anastomosis was then constructed and the arterial anastomosis was performed after which the patient's hepatic coagulopathy was reversed using protamine and fresh frozen plasma. Finally, the biliary anastomosis was completed using a choledocho-choledochostomy without placement of a t-tube. At this point, the cardiac team returned to inspect for hemostasis and close the sternotomy using pleural and mediastinal drainage tubes. Next the abdominal incision was closed following the placement of drains as needed and the patient was transferred to the surgical intensive care unit. All patients were monitored with continuous transesophageal echocardiography (TEE) during their course on CPB and the LT [36].

Although CABG resulted in a minor increase in transaminases, there was no rejection or liver allograft loss. Despite the prolonged period with an open sternotomy, including manipulation of the biliary tree, there were no postoperative sternal wound infections. Transfusion volumes were high (12 units of packed red blood cells, 22 units of fresh frozen plasma, and 30 units of platelets) and 30% of patients required renal replacement therapy postoperatively [30]. The median duration of intubation was 2 days, and length of stay in the intensive care unit was 5.5 days,[37] overall, combined CABG-LT appears to be an effective procedure. From 17 reported patients undergoing combined CABG/LT procedures, [8, 28-34] the majority had a successful outcome: 2 intraoperative deaths have been reported resulting in intraoperative mortality of 11.8%. The 80% survival at 1 year is comparable with isolated LT [38]. Therefore, combined simultaneous CABG-LT is a consideration for selected patients with advanced liver and cardiac disease.

Cardiac Valvular Disease and End-Stage Liver Disease

Clinically significant valvular disease is rare in patients undergoing LT [39]. In a series of 69 patients (a subset of 4,823 patient examined) reported from Pittsburg the following types of valvular diseases were indicated: aortic valve (n=44, 64%), mitral valve (n=21, 30%), pulmonic valve (n=2, 3%), and tricuspid valve (n=2, 3%). The two most common diagnoses were aortic stenosis and post-endocarditis valvular insufficiency [40].

Performing liver transplantation in a patient with severe aortic stenosis carries a high risk, [41, 42] conversely, in the presence of cirrhosis; aortic valve replacement has a significant risk for mortality because of bleeding, renal and liver failure. A small series and a case report of patients with severe aortic valve stenosis and end-stage liver disease in which a staged procedure has been precluded has been reported [37, 41]. In the series of 4 patients requiring AVR-LT one patient died 14 hours postoperatively, because of acute severe pulmonary artery hypertension resulting in shock and refractory metabolic acidosis [37]. Since combining major cardiac surgery with a liver transplantation greatly increases the risk for severe fibrinolysis, a bioprosthetic valve was used in 3 from four reported cases to decrease the risk for postoperative bleeding by avoiding the need for systemic anticoagulation postoperatively. The availability of percutaneous and transapically delivered aortic valves in the last couple of years may make it easier to manage these patients and greatly decrease the operative mortality and morbidity in patients who are appropriate for the procedure [43]. Similarly, when feasible, percutaneous, or transapical mitral valve repair or replacement could be considered [44, 45] in this high risk group of patients.

Combined Heart and Liver Transplantation

Combined heart and liver transplantation (CHLT) is a lifesaving procedure for patients suffering from end-stage heart and liver diseases or several metabolic disorders. Following Shaw's initial description in 1985 [46] CHLT has become an accepted therapeutic solution in the treatment of this dual vital organ failure. However, in spite of reports of 1-year survival rates of 80% in the late 1990s for CHLT [47] and growing indications for this procedure, the world's experience with CHLT is small. The United Network for Organ Sharing (UNOS) reported that only 47 cases of combined heart-liver (n=41) and heart-liver-kidney transplantation (n=6) were performed in the United States from October 1987 to February 2007 at 15 transplant centers [48]. Recipients of CHLT represent only 1% of multiple organ transplants performed nationwide.

There have been several case reports and case series documenting the feasibility of performing either simultaneous or staged CHLT [47, 49-57].

The indications for CHLT are:

1. Combined end-stage heart and liver disease for unrelated causes. The most common example is end-stage liver disease with ischemic and non-ischemic dilated cardiomyopathy.

2. Combined end-stage heart and liver disease for related causes, including several well defined syndromes. Biliary atresia is often associated with cardiac abnormalities which may require a combined procedure.[58] Alagille syndrome may also be associated with cardiac abnormalities and the CHLT may be indicated because of poor survival following isolated liver transplantation (ILT). [59] Another group of disorders are iron deposition disorders such as a homozygous ß-thalassemia [60, 61] and genetic hemochromatosis [57, 59, 62, 63].
3. End-stage heart disease, the liver transplant being to correct underlying metabolic disorder [64] including homozygous familial hypercholesterolemia [46, 49, 63, 65, 66] and familial amyloidosis (FA) [50, 51, 53, 55].

As reported from the UNOS database for CHLT the most common indication for liver transplantation was amyloidosis (30%) following by genetic hemochromatosis (13%) and hepatitis C–related cirrhosis (13%), (Table 1) whereas those for a heart transplantation were congenital heart disease (13%) and idiopathic dilated cardiomyopathy(13%) [48]. (Table 2)

Table 1. Indications for Liver Transplantation

Indication	No. of cases
Amyloidosis	14 (30.4%)
Hepatitis C	6 (13%)
Hemochromatosis	6 (13%)
Cardiac cirrhosis	5 (10.8%)
Cryptogenic cirrhosis	4 (8.7%)
Alcoholic cirrhosis	3 (6.6%)
Primary biliary cirrhosis	2 (4.3%)
Glycogen storage disease	1 (2.2%)
α_1-anti-trypsin deficiency	1 (2.2%)
Autoimmune hepatitis	1 (2.2%)
Budd–Chiari syndrome	1 (2.2%)
Nodular regenerative hyperplasia	1 (2.2%)
Primary sclerosing cholangitis	1 (2.2%)

Based on OPTN data as of January 26, 2007.
Reproduced from [48] with permission.

Once a candidate has been listed for CHLT, allocation of the two organs is dictated by the listing priority of the specific organ that carries the most life-threatening risk. For many candidates, this risk is determined largely by the cardiac condition; however, in some cases with more symptomatic hepatic failure, a higher priority on the liver waiting list may permit the heart to be allocated along with the liver graft. The waiting list mortality rates for CHLT candidates in the pre-MELD and post-MELD eras have been studied by Porrett and colleagues.[67] In their analysis, patients with a moderate degree of liver failure (MELD scores of 20 to 29) and cardiac failure (Cardiac Status 2) demonstrated survival rates that approximated the waiting time for patients listed with Cardiac Status 1A/1B or patients with MELD scores 30. This study suggested that CHLT candidates are disadvantaged by the current allocation system and considered revision of the strategies to improve CHLT candidate's survival during waiting period.

Table 2. Indications for Heart Transplantation

Indication	No. of cases
Amyloidosis	14 (30.4%)
Congenital heart disease	6 (13%)
Idiopathic dilated cardiomyopathy	6 (13%)
Hemochromatosis	5 (10.9%)
Coronary artery disease[a]	3 (6.6%)
Alcoholic cardiomyopathy	3 (6.6%)
Valvular heart disease	2 (4.3%)
Viral dilated cardiomyopathy	2 (4.3%)
Glycogen storage disease	1 (2.2%)
Idiopathic restrictive cardiomyopathy	1 (2.2%)
Other[b]	3 (6.6%)

Based on OPTN data as of January 26, 2007.
Reproduced from [48] with permission.

Donors are matched for each recipient on the basis of ABO blood group identity. Preoperative panel-reactive antibody (PRA) levels are determined to assess the probability of sensitization. In contrast to the common practice of prospective HLA matching for isolated liver transplantation, CHLT recipients receive randomly HLA-matched organs in the same way as isolated heart recipients. This practice is necessary because of an unacceptably long waiting time for a heart by an HLA match-based allocation system, and is justified by the observed results. HLA-A, HLA-B, and HLA-DR matching is performed retrospectively.

There are four different surgical approaches that have been described for CHLT:

1. Transplantation of the heart but maintaining the patient on CBP during the liver transplantation was described in the first three cases of CHLT. Subsequent concerns about substantial coagulopathy and increased bleeding changed the strategy to performing liver implantation following separation from cardiopulmonary bypass [46, 47, 51, 53, 61]. However, improved surgical and anesthetic techniques during liver transplant and the potential benefits to the transplanted heart to remain on CPB during liver implantation led to revising this strategy for CHLT. Hennessey et al suggested that this technique provides a considerably shortened liver ischemia time and decreases blood transfusion compared with the sequential approach [68].
2. Transplantation of heart/lung /liver en block was described by Dennis et al [69]. This technique reduced the number of anastomoses but increases the warm ischemic time of the liver allograft.
3. Transplantation of the heart with discontinuation of CPB, leaving the chest opened. The liver transplantation was performed as a second step through a bilateral subcostal incision with extension in the midline to the sternotomy [70] and was accomplished by caval sparing hepatectomy with an anastomosis between the donor suprahepatic cava and the recipient left/middle hepatic vein trunk. Biliary tubes were inserted through the donor cystic duct stumps whenever possible, and the abdomen was closed over drains after achieving hemostasis [71]. One of the major advantages of this procedure is that CHLT can be performed with minimal deviation from the standard procedures of IHT and ILT.

4. Staged CHLT transplantation was first reported by Figuera et al [72] for patients who underwent IHT and were hemodynamically unstable after cardiac reperfusion. Subsequent liver transplantation was deferred, and the patients underwent deceased donor liver transplantation from a second donor. However, in the Mayo study simultaneous CHLT was feasible in 87% (13 of 15) of patients and appears favorable if cardiac function and hemodynamics are satisfactory [71].

As compared to IHT the mean ICU stay did not differ and the mean hospital stay was not significantly longer for CHLT [71].

In series of Mayo clinic there was no difference in immunosuppressive protocol between the CHLT and IHT group.[71] All patients received induction therapy with the monoclonal antibody OKT3 after transplantation for 5-14 days, which allowed for delayed introduction of calcineurin inhibitors following by triple-drug immunosuppression, including calcineurin inhibitor (cyclosporine or tacrolimus) as a primary immunosuppressant; azathioprine or MMF as a secondary immunosuppressant and prednisone. Cyclosporine target trough levels were: 300-400 ng/mL first 3 months, 150-200 ng/mL 4-12months, 100-150 ng/mL >12 months. A therapeutic tacrolimus level was 8-14 ng/ml. Azathioprine and MMF were dosed based on leukocyte counts.

Acute cellular rejection of the liver was infrequent. The more aggressive immunosuppressive regimen, including OKT3 induction employed for CHLT than used for isolated liver transplantation (ILT) may make rejection of liver allograft a relatively infrequent event. Interestingly, heart rejection was also less frequent in CHLT than in those receiving isolated heart transplantation (IHT). To explain the favorable low rejection rate an induction of partial tolerance has been proposed as a mechanism. The liver has been demonstrated to permit acceptance of other simultaneously transplanted organs operating via shedding soluble HLA antigens [73, 74]. It has been hypothesized that maintaining a proper concentration of soluble HLA in circulation would lead to tolerance to the allotype of the soluble HLA. This concept may help to explain the protection of a simultaneous heart transplant by a successful human liver transplant [75]. Therefore, less intensive immunosuppression therapy for these patients after CHLT than for IHT may be justified. Indeed, according to UNOS report 28.2% CHLT recipients were maintained on a single immunosuppressive agent. The most commonly used immunosuppressive agent was tacrolimus (91%) [48].

Based on the experience of several centers it seems that acute renal failure complicates the early postoperative course of many patients after CHLT [47, 76]. Therefore, renal function was significantly worse in the CHLT patients at the late follow-up as compared to IHT. It was previously demonstrated that the risk of chronic renal failure after transplantation of a non-renal organ depends on the type of organ transplanted and at 5 years cumulative incidence of chronic renal failure was lower after IHT (10.9±0.2) compared to ILT (18.1±0.20). [77, 78] CNI sparing (Sirolimus based) immunosuppression probably should be considered in CHLT group of patients to prevent progressive CNI-induced renal damage [76, 79].

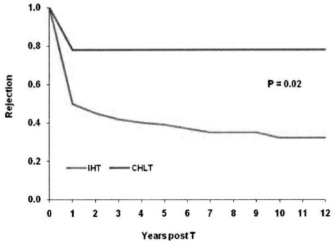

Freedom from cardiac allograft rejection (International Society for Heart and Lung Transplantation ≥Grade 2) for CHLT at 1 month was 83% and did not change further. For IHT freedom from rejection at 1 month, 1year, 3 years and 10 years was 80%, 48%, 42% and 32% respectively (p=0.02, Log-Rank test). Reproduced from [71] with permission.

IHT – isolated heart transplantation
CHLT – combined heart and liver transplantation
T–transplantation

Figure 1 *Freedom from* cardiac allograft rejection (International Society for Heart and Lung Transplantation ≥2) for CHLT (n=15) versus IHT (n=258).

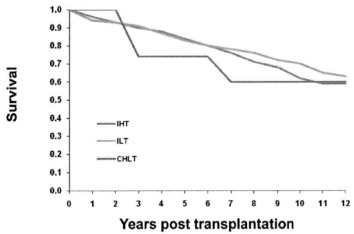

Survival rates at 1month, 1 year, 5 years and 10 years for the CHLT recipients were 100%, 100%, 75% and 60% respectively and was comparable with survival rate for IHT (97%, 93%, 83% and 65% respectively) and ILT (97%, 94%, 83% and 70% respectively, p=0.44, Log-Rank test).
IHT – isolated heart transplantation.
ILT – isolated liver transplantation.
CHLT – combined heart and liver transplantation.
Reproduced from [71] with permission.

Figure 2 Survival for CHLT (n=15) IHT (n=258) and ILT (n=1201).

Table 3. Comparative patient survival of CHLT with IHT and ILT

	OLT–OHT[a]	OLT[b]	OHT[b]
1 year	85%	88%	86%
3 years	77%	80%	79%
5 years	75%	74%	72%

[a] Based on OPTN data as of January 26, 2007.
[b] OPTN/SRTR data as of May 2004 —adjusted patient survival of cohorts are transplants performed 2001–2002 for 1 year, 1999–2000 for 3 years and 1997–1998 for 5 year.

OLT – orthotropic liver transplantation.
OHT – orthotropic heart transplantation.
Reproduced from [48] with permission.

Pulmonary embolism is a rare complication in early period post IHT [80]. However, the incidence of pulmonary embolism was higher in CHLT group as compared to IHT (13% vs. 1.7% respectively) probably reflecting prolongation of immobilization period and delayed recovery of anticoagulant proteins in this group of patients [81].

Overall, as reported by Mayo clinic, patient survival after CHLT did not differ from survival after IHT and ILT [79] (Figure 2). In the report of the Organ Procurement Transplant Network (OPTN) and Scientific Registry of Transplant Recipients (SRTR) the survival rate after CHLT was also comparable to IHT and ILT recipients [48] (Table3).

The most common indication for CHLT was familial amiloidosis (FA). FA is a multisystem disorder induced by deposition of abnormal serum TTR (prealbumin) protein, mainly produced in the liver, in several organs. Among the over 40 mutations described, the Portuguese variant (TTR Met30) is the most frequent and not associated with cardiomyopathy. Orthotopic liver transplantation is established as the treatment of choice for TTR Met30 FA with stabilization or remission of symptoms. In patients with a non-TTR Met30 mutation and cardiomyopathy, the amyloid fibrils deposition in the heart is increased after ILT suggesting that wild-type TTR constitutes amyloid in the hearts similar to the phenomenon observed in senile systemic amyloidosis [82-84]. This leads to progression of cardiomyopathy following ILT in patients carrying a non-TTR Met30 mutation and indicates CHLT as a procedure of choice [85]. Although cirrhotic patients theoretically present greater operative risks because of coagulopathy and portal hypertension, FA determines systemic involvement that, in advanced stages, can seriously affect the safety of the procedure with a negative impact on short- and long-term results. Indeed, ALA 60 has been reported as a mutation of particularly poor prognosis and five of eight patients with ALA60 mutation described in literature have died after isolated liver transplantation [86, 87]. Moreover, the Tyr 77 (German variant) mutation is also typically associated with prominent and progressive cardiac involvement after isolated liver transplantation [88]. Mayo clinic study suggests that specific FA mutations do not affect the therapeutic success of CHLT: during 4.4 years follow up, 3 of the 4 patients with ALA60 TTR mutation remain alive and one died of progressive renal failure. Three patients with the TYR77 TTR variant remain alive. No evidence of amyloid affecting cardiac grafts has been observed by endomyocardial biopsy. Autonomic disturbances, peripheral neuropathy, gastrointestinal and urinary tract dysfunction, however, remain the main signs of FA in most patients and optimizing the timing for CHLT appears to be crucial. Survival rate for patients with FA was comparable with survival rate for IHT [71] (Figure 3).

Since livers explanted from patients with FA contain only microscopic amyloid deposits and are otherwise essentially normal, and it typically takes approximately 50 years for TTR deposition to progress to clinically apparent disease, the FA liver can be used as a domino donor liver for selected older patients awaiting liver transplantation. CHLT does not preclude domino donation of FA recipients' liver. In contrast to caval sparing hepatectomy with an anastomosis between the donor suprahepatic cava and the recipient left/middle hepatic vein trunk caval excision with veno-venous and portal-venous bypass was employed for FA patients serving as domino liver donors. None of the domino donors experienced any technical problems related to donation or veno-venous and porto-venous bypass [71, 89].

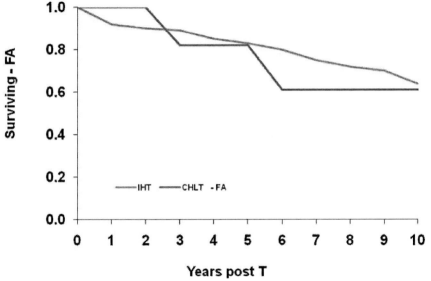

Survival rates for patients with FA patients at 1month, 1 year, 5 years and 10 years were 100%, 100%, 83%, and 63% and did not differ from IHT (p=0.91, Log-Rank test).
IHT – isolated heart transplantation.
CHLT – combined heart and liver transplantation.
T – transplantation.
FA-Familial amiloidosis.
Reproduced from [71] with permission.

Figure 3 Survival for FA patients, undergoing CHLT (n=11) and IHT (n=258).

Conclusion

Combined simultaneous cardiac surgery and liver transplantation is indicated for selected patients with advanced cardiac and liver disease. This is a feasible surgical option which can be performed safely and morbidity is not prohibitive for success.

References

[1] Keeffe EB. Liver transplantation at the millennium. Past, present, and future. *Clin. Liver Dis.* 2000; 4(1):241-55.

[2] Carey WD, Dumot JA, Pimentel RR, Barnes DS, Hobbs RE, Henderson JM, et al. The prevalence of coronary artery disease in liver transplant candidates over age 50. *Transplantation* 1995; 59(6):859-64.

[3] Johnston SD, Morris JK, Cramb R, Gunson BK, Neuberger J. Cardiovascular morbidity and mortality after orthotopic liver transplantation. *Transplantation 2002*; 73(6):901-6.

[4] Plevak DJ. Stress echocardiography identifies coronary artery disease in liver transplant candidates. *Liver Transpl. Surg.* 1998;4(4):337-9.

[5] Bizouarn P, Ausseur A, Desseigne P, Le Teurnier Y, Nougarede B, Train M, et al. Early and late outcome after elective cardiac surgery in patients with cirrhosis. *Ann. Thorac. Surg.* 1999; 67(5):1334-8.

[6] .Klemperer JD, Ko W, Krieger KH, Connolly M, Rosengart TK, Altorki NK, et al. Cardiac operations in patients with cirrhosis. *Ann Thorac Surg* 1998; 65(1):85-7.

[7] .Eagle KA, Guyton RA, Davidoff R, Ewy GA, Fonger J, Gardner TJ, et al. ACC/AHA Guidelines for Coronary Artery Bypass Graft Surgery: A Report of the American College of Cardiology/American Heart Association Task Force on Practice Guidelines (Committee to Revise the 1991 Guidelines for Coronary Artery Bypass Graft Surgery). American College of Cardiology/American Heart Association. *J. Am. Coll. Cardiol.* 1999; 34(4):1262-347.

[8] .Morris JJ, Hellman CL, Gawey BJ, Ramsay MA, Valek TR, Gunning TC, et al. Case 3-1995. Three patients requiring both coronary artery bypass surgery and orthotopic liver transplantation. *J. Cardiothorac. Vasc. Anesth.* 1995; 9(3):322-32.

[9] .Abramov D, Tamariz MG, Fremes SE, Guru V, Borger MA, Christakis GT, et al. Trends in coronary artery bypass surgery results: a recent, 9-year study. *Ann. Thorac. Surg.* 2000;70(1):84-90.

[10] .Csikesz NG, Nguyen LN, Tseng JF, Shah SA. Nationwide volume and mortality after elective surgery in cirrhotic patients. *J. Am. Coll. Surg.* 2009; 208(1):96-103.

[11] .Hayashida N, Shoujima T, Teshima H, Yokokura Y, Takagi K, Tomoeda H, et al. Clinical outcome after cardiac operations in patients with cirrhosis Does off-pump coronary artery bypass grafting really preserve renal function? *Ann. Thorac. Surg. 2004*; 77(2):500-5.

[12] .Plotkin JS, Johnson LB, Rustgi VK, Kuo PC, Liu AD. Dobutamine stress echocardiography for orthotopic liver transplant evaluation. *Transplantation* 2001; 71(6):818.

[13] .Kaplan M, Cimen S, Kut MS, Demirtas MM. Cardiac operations for patients with chronic liver disease. *Heart Surg. Forum* 2002; 5(1):60-5.

[14] .Suman A, Carey WD. Assessing the risk of surgery in patients with liver disease. *Cleve Clin. J. Med.* 2006; 73(4):398-404.

[15] .Hirata N, Sawa Y, Matsuda H. Predictive value of preoperative serum cholinesterase concentration in patients with liver dysfunction undergoing cardiac surgery. *J. Card Surg.* 1999; 14(3):172-7.

[16] .Downing SW, Edmunds LH, Jr. Release of vasoactive substances during cardiopulmonary bypass. Ann *Thorac. Surg.* 1992; 54(6):1236-43.

[17] .Hayashida N, Chihara S, Kashikie H, Tayama E, Yokose S, Akasu K, et al. Biological activity of endogenous atrial natriuretic peptide during cardiopulmonary bypass. *Artif. Organs.* 2000; 24(10):833-8.

[18] .Schrier RW, Gurevich AK, Cadnapaphornchai MA. Pathogenesis and management of sodium and water retention in cardiac failure and cirrhosis. *Semin. Nephrol.* 2001; 21(2):157-72.

[19] Okano N, Miyoshi S, Owada R, Fujita N, Kadoi Y, Saito S, et al. Impairment of hepatosplanchnic oxygenation and increase of serum hyaluronate during normothermic and mild hypothermic cardiopulmonary bypass. *Anesth. Analg.* 2002; 95(2):278-86.

[20] Chukwuemeka A, Weisel A, Maganti M, Nette AF, Wijeysundera DN, Beattie WS, et al. Renal dysfunction in high-risk patients after on-pump and off-pump coronary artery bypass surgery: a propensity score analysis. *Ann. Thorac. Surg.* 2005; 80(6):2148-53.

[21] Michalopoulos A, Alivizatos P, Geroulanos S. Hepatic dysfunction following cardiac surgery: determinants and consequences. *Hepatogastroenterology* 1997; 44(15):779-83.

[22] Della Rocca G, Costa MG, Pompei L, Chiarandini P. The liver transplant recipient with cardiac disease. *Transplant Proc.* 2008; 40(4):1172-4.

[23] Therapondos G, Flapan AD, Plevris JN, Hayes PC. Cardiac morbidity and mortality related to orthotopic liver transplantation. *Liver Transpl* 2004;10(12):1441-53.

[24] Kang YG, Freeman JA, Aggarwal S, DeWolf AM. Hemodynamic instability during liver transplantation. *Transplant. Proc.* 1989; 21(3):3489-92.

[25] Glauser FL. Systemic hemodynamic and cardiac function changes in patients undergoing orthotopic liver transplantation. *Chest* 1990; 98(5):1210-5.

[26] Stahl RL, Duncan A, Hooks MA, Henderson JM, Millikan WJ, Warren WD. A hypercoagulable state follows orthotopic liver transplantation. *Hepatology* 1990; 12(3 Pt 1):553-8.

[27] Plotkin JS, Johnson LB, Rustgi V, Kuo PC. Coronary artery disease and liver transplantation: the state of the art. *Liver Transpl.* 2000(4 Suppl 1):S53-6.

[28] Kniepeiss D, Iberer F, Grasser B, Schaffellner S, Stadlbauer V, Stauber R, et al. Simultaneous coronary artery bypass grafting and orthotopic liver transplantation. *Transpl. Int.* 2003; 16(3):207-9.

[29] Lebbinck H, Bouchez S, Vereecke H, Vanoverbeke H, Troisi R, Reyntjens K. Sequential off-pump coronary artery bypass and liver transplantation. *Transpl. Int.* 2006; 19(5):432-4.

[30] Axelrod D, Koffron A, Dewolf A, Baker A, Fryer J, Baker T, et al. Safety and efficacy of combined orthotopic liver transplantation and coronary artery bypass grafting. *Liver Transpl.* 2004; 10(11):1386-90.

[31] Manas DM, Roberts DR, Heaviside DW, Chaudhry S, Tocewicz K, Hudson M, et al. Sequential coronary artery bypass grafting and orthotopic liver transplantation: a case report. *Clin. Transplant.* 1996; 10(3):320-2.

[32] Massad MG, Benedetti E, Pollak R, Chami YG, Allen BS, DeCastro MA, et al. Combined coronary bypass and liver transplantation: technical considerations. *Ann. Thorac. Surg.*1998; 65(4):1130-2.

[33] Plotkin JS, Scott VL, Pinna A, Dobsch BP, De Wolf AM, Kang Y. Morbidity and mortality in patients with coronary artery disease undergoing orthotopic liver transplantation *Liver Transpl. Surg.*1996; 2(6):426-30.

[34] Benedetti E, Massad MG, Chami Y, Wiley T, Layden TJ. Is the presence of surgically treatable coronary artery disease a contraindication to liver transplantation? *Clin Transplant* 1999; 13(1 Pt 1):59-61.

[35] Wu YM, Voigt M, Rayhill S, Katz D, Chenhsu RY, Schmidt W, et al. Suprahepatic venacavaplasty (cavaplasty) with retrohepatic cava extension in liver transplantation: experience with first 115 cases. *Transplantation* 2001; 72(8):1389-94.

[36] Burtenshaw AJ, Isaac JL. The role of trans-esophageal echocardiography for perioperative cardiovascular monitoring during orthotopic liver transplantation. *Liver Transpl.* 2006; 12(11):1577-83.

[37] Destephano CC, Harrison BA, Mordecai M, Crawford CC, Shine TS, Hewitt WR, et al. Anesthesia for Combined Cardiac Surgery and Liver Transplant. *J. Cardiothorac. Vasc. Anesth.* 2009; 24:24.

[38] Ghobrial RM, Gornbein J, Steadman R, Danino N, Markmann JF, Holt C, et al. Pretransplant model to predict posttransplant survival in liver transplant patients. *Ann. Surg.* 2002; 236(3):315-22.

[39] Donovan CL, Marcovitz PA, Punch JD, Bach DS, Brown KA, Lucey MR, et al. Two-dimensional and dobutamine stress echocardiography in the preoperative assessment of patients with end-stage liver disease prior to orthotopic liver transplantation. *Transplantation* 1996; 61(8):1180-8.

[40] Mitruka SN, Griffith BP, Kormos RL, Hattler BG, Pigula FA, Shapiro R, et al. Cardiac operations in solid-organ transplant recipients. *Ann. Thorac. Surg.*1997; 64(5):1270-8.

[41] Eckhoff DE, Frenette L, Sellers MT, McGuire BM, Contreras JL, Bynon JS, et al. Combined cardiac surgery and liver transplantation. *Liver Transpl* 2001; 7(1):60-1.

[42] Pollard RJ, Sidi A, Gibby GL, Lobato EB, Gabrielli A. Aortic stenosis with end-stage liver disease: prioritizing surgical and anesthetic therapies. *J Clin Anesth* 1998;10(3):253-61.

[43] Fraccaro C, Napodano M, Tarantini G, Gasparetto V, Gerosa G, Bianco R, et al. Expanding the eligibility for transcatheter aortic valve implantation the trans-subclavian retrograde approach using: the III generation CoreValve revalving system. *JACC Cardiovasc. Interv.*2009; 2(9):828-33.

[44] Mack M. Percutaneous mitral valve therapy: when? Which patients? *Curr. Opin. Cardiol.*2009;24(2):125-9.

[45] Lutter G, Quaden R, Osaki S, Hu J, Renner J, Edwards NM, et al. Off-pump transapical mitral valve replacement. *Eur. J. Cardiothorac. Surg.* 2009; 36(1):124-8.

[46] Shaw BW, Jr., Bahnson HT, Hardesty RL, Griffith BP, Starzl TE. Combined transplantation of the heart and liver. *Ann. Surg.* 1985; 202(6):667-72.

[47] Befeler AS, Schiano TD, Lissoos TW, Conjeevaram HS, Anderson AS, Millis JM, et al. Successful combined liver-heart transplantation in adults: report of three patients and review of the literature. *Transplantation* 1999;68(9):1423-7.

[48] Te HS, Anderson AS, Millis JM, Jeevanandam V, Jensen DM. Current state of combined heart-liver transplantation in the United States. *J. Heart Lung Transplant.* 2008; 27(7):753-9.

[49] Alkofer BJ, Chiche L, Khayat A, Deshayes JP, Lepage A, Saloux E, et al. Liver transplant combined with heart transplant in severe heterozygous hypercholesterolemia: report of the first case and review of the literature. *Transplant. Proc.* 2005;37(5):2250-2.

[50] Arpesella G, Chiappini B, Marinelli G, Mikus PM, Dozza F, Pierangeli A, et al. Combined heart and liver transplantation for familial amyloidotic polyneuropathy. *J. Thorac. Cardiovasc. Surg.* 2003; 125(5):1165-6.

[51] Grazi GL, Cescon M, Salvi F, Ercolani G, Ravaioli M, Arpesella G, et al. Combined heart and liver transplantation for familial amyloidotic neuropathy: considerations from the hepatic point of view. *Liver Transpl.* 2003;9(9):986-92.

[52] Lauro A, Diago Uso T, Masetti M, Di Benedetto F, Cautero N, De Ruvo N, et al. Liver transplantation for familial amyloid polyneuropathy non-VAL30MET variants: are cardiac complications influenced by prophylactic pacing and immunosuppressive weaning? *Transplant. Proc* .2005;37(5):2214-20.

[53] Nardo B, Beltempo P, Bertelli R, Montalti R, Vivarelli M, Cescon M, et al. Combined heart and liver transplantation in four adults with familial amyloidosis: experience of a single center. *Transplant. Proc.* 2004; 36(3):645-7.

[54] Praseedom RK, McNeil KD, Watson CJ, Alexander GJ, Calne RY, Wallwork J, et al. Combined transplantation of the heart, lung, and liver. *Lancet* 2001; 358(9284):812-3.

[55] Ruygrok PN, Gane EJ, McCall JL, Chen XZ, Haydock DA, Munn SR. Combined heart and liver transplantation for familial amyloidosis. *Intern. Med. J.* 2001; 31(1):66-7.

[56] Stangou AJ, Hawkins PN. Liver transplantation in transthyretin-related familial amyloid polyneuropathy. *Curr. Opin. Neurol.* 2004;17(5):615-20.

[57] Surakomol S, Olson LJ, Rastogi A, Steers JL, Sterioff S, Daly RC, et al. Combined orthotopic heart and liver transplantation for genetic hemochromatosis. *J. Heart Lung. Transplant.* 1997 May; 16(5):573-5.

[58] Fricker FJ, Griffith BP, Hardesty RL, Trento A, Gold LM, Schmeltz K, et al. Experience with heart transplantation in children. *Pediatrics* 1987; 79(1):138-46.

[59] Gandhi SK, Reyes J, Webber SA, Siewers RD, Pigula FA. Case report of combined pediatric heart-lung-liver transplantation. *Transplantation* 2002; 73(12):1968-9.

[60] Olivieri NF, Liu PP, Sher GD, Daly PA, Greig PD, McCusker PJ, et al. Brief report: combined liver and heart transplantation for end-stage iron-induced organ failure in an adult with homozygous beta-thalassemia. *N.Engl. J. Med* .1994; 330(16):1125-7.

[61] Detry O, Honore P, Meurisse M, Defraigne JO, Defechereux T, Sakalihasan N, et al. Advantages of inferior vena caval flow preservation in combined transplantation of the liver and heart. *Transpl. Int* .1997; 10(2):150-1.

[62] Haynes H, Farroni J. Successful combined heart-liver transplantation in a patient with hemochromatosis. *Prog. Transplant* .2004; 14(1):39-40.

[63] Offstad J, Schrumpf E, Geiran O, Soreide O, Simonsen S. Plasma exchange and heart-liver transplantation in a patient with homozygous familial hypercholesterolemia. *Clin. Transplant* .2001; 15(6):432-6.

[64] Rela M, Muiesan P, Heaton ND, Corbally M, Hajj H, Mowat AP, et al. Orthotopic liver transplantation for hepatic-based metabolic disorders. *Transpl. Int* .1995; 8(1):41-4.

[65] Revell SP, Noble-Jamieson G, Johnston P, Rasmussen A, Jamieson N, Barnes ND. Liver transplantation for homozygous familial hypercholesterolaemia. *Arch. Dis. Child.* 1995; 73(5):456-8.

[66] Valdivielso P, Escolar JL, Cuervas-Mons V, Pulpon LA, Chaparro MA, Gonzalez-Santos P. Lipids and lipoprotein changes after heart and liver transplantation in a patient with homozygous familial hypercholesterolemia. *Ann. Intern. Med.* 1988; 108(2):204-6.

[67] Porrett PM, Desai SS, Timmins KJ, Twomey CR, Sonnad SS, Olthoff KM. Combined orthotopic heart and liver transplantation: the need for exception status listing. *Liver Transpl* .2004 ; 10(12):1539-44.

[68] Hennessey T, Backman SB, Cecere R, Lachapelle K, de Varennes B, Ergina P, et al. Combined heart and liver transplantation on cardiopulmonary bypass: report of four cases. *Can. J. Anaesth.* 2010; 57 (4):355-60.

[69] Dennis CM, McNeil KD, Dunning J, Stewart S, Friend PJ, Alexander G, et al. Heart-lung-liver transplantation. *J Heart Lung Transplant* 1996;15(5):536-8.

[70] Couetil JP, Houssin DP, Soubrane O, Chevalier PG, Dousset BE, Loulmet D, et al. Combined lung and liver transplantation in patients with cystic fibrosis. A 4 1/2-year experience. *J. Thorac. Cardiovasc. Surg* .1995; 110(5):1415-22; discussion 22-3.

[71] Raichlin E, Daly RC, Rosen CB, McGregor CG, Charlton MR, Frantz RP, et al. Combined heart and liver transplantation: a single-center experience. *Transplantation* 2009;88(2):219-25.

[72] Figuera D, Ardaiz J, Martin-Judez V, Pulpon LA, Pradas G, Cuervas-Mons V, et al. Combined transplantation of heart and liver from two different donors in a patient with familial type IIa hypercholesterolemia. *J. Heart Transplant* .1986; 5(4):327-9.

[73] Davies HS, Pollard SG, Calne RY. Soluble HLA antigens in the circulation of liver graft recipients. *Transplantation* 1989 Mar; 47(3):524-7.

[74] McMillan RW, Gelder FB, Zibari GB, Aultman DF, Adamashvili I, McDonald JC. Soluble fraction of class I human histocompatibility leukocyte antigens in the serum of liver transplant recipients. *Clin. Transplant* .1997 Apr;11(2):98-103.

[75] Vogel W, Steiner E, Kornberger R, Koller J, Spielberger M, Aulitzky W, et al. Preliminary results with combined hepatorenal allografting. *Transplantation* 1988 Feb; 45(2):491-3.

[76] Raichlin E, Khalpey Z, Kremers W, Frantz RP, Rodeheffer RJ, Clavell AL, et al. Replacement of calcineurin-inhibitors with sirolimus as primary immunosuppression in stable cardiac transplant recipients. *Transplantation* 2007; 84(4):467-74.

[77] Gonwa TA, Mai ML, Melton LB, Hays SR, Goldstein RM, Levy MF, et al. End-stage renal disease (ESRD) after orthotopic liver transplantation (OLT) using calcineurin-based immunotherapy: risk of development and treatment. *Transplantation* 2001 Dec 27; 72(12):1934-9.

[78] Ojo AO, Held PJ, Port FK, Wolfe RA, Leichtman AB, Young EW, et al. Chronic renal failure after transplantation of a non-renal organ. *N. Engl. J. Med* .2003 Sep 4; 349(10):931-40.

[79] Raichlin E, Bae JH, Khalpey Z, Edwards BS, Kremers WK, Clavell AL, et al. Conversion to sirolimus as primary immunosuppression attenuates the progression of allograft vasculopathy after cardiac transplantation. *Circulation* 2007; 116(23):2726-33.

[80] Berroeta C, Flament F, Lathyris D, Provenchere S, Paquin S, Desmonts JM, et al. Pulmonary embolism: an uncommon cause of dyspnea after heart transplantation. *J. Cardiothorac. Vasc. Anesth* .2006; 20(2):236-8.

[81] A hypercoagulable state follows orthotopic liver transplantation. *Hepatology* 1990 ; 12(3):553-8.

[82] Stangou AJ, Hawkins PN, Heaton ND, Rela M, Monaghan M, Nihoyannopoulos P, et al. Progressive cardiac amyloidosis following liver transplantation for familial amyloid polyneuropathy: implications for amyloid fibrillogenesis. *Transplantation* 1998 Jul 27; 66(2):229-33.

[83] Westermark P, Sletten K, Johansson B, Cornwell GG, 3rd. Fibril in senile systemic amyloidosis is derived from normal transthyretin. *Proc. Natl. Acad. Sci. U S A.* 1990 Apr; 87(7):2843-5.

[84] Yazaki M, Tokuda T, Nakamura A, Higashikata T, Koyama J, Higuchi K, et al. Cardiac amyloid in patients with familial amyloid polyneuropathy consists of abundant wild-type transthyretin. *Biochem. Biophys. Res. Commun.* 2000 Aug 11; 274(3):702-6.

[85] Pomfret EA, Lewis WD, Jenkins RL, Bergethon P, Dubrey SW, Reisinger J, et al. Effect of orthotopic liver transplantation on the progression of familial amyloidotic polyneuropathy. *Transplantation* 1998 Apr 15; 65(7):918-25.

[86] Kotani N, Hattori T, Yamagata S, Tokuda T, Shirasawa A, Yamaguchi S, et al. Transthyretin Thr60Ala Appalachian-type mutation in a Japanese family with familial amyloidotic polyneuropathy. *Amyloid.* 2002 Mar;9(1):31-4.

[87] Sharma P, Perri RE, Sirven JE, Zeldenrust SR, Brandhagen DJ, Rosen CB, et al. Outcome of liver transplantation for familial amyloidotic polyneuropathy. *Liver Transpl.* 2003 Dec;9(12):1273-80.

[88] Garcia-Herola A, Prieto M, Pascual S, Berenguer M, Lopez-Viedma B, Mir J, et al. Progression of cardiomyopathy and neuropathy after liver transplantation in a patient with familial amyloidotic polyneuropathy caused by tyrosine-77 transthyretin variant. *Liver Transpl. Surg.* 1999 May; 5(3):246-8.

[89] Azoulay D, Samuel D, Castaing D, Adam R, Adams D, Said G, et al. Domino liver transplants for metabolic disorders: experience with familial amyloidotic polyneuropathy. *J. Am. Coll. Surg* .1999; 189(6):584-93.

In: Cardiovascular Diseases and Liver Transplantation
Editor: Zoka Milan, pp. 157-167
ISBN: 978-1-61122-910-3
© 2011 Nova Science Publishers, Inc.

Chapter X

Previous Chemotherapy and Cardiac Function

Wafaa Abdel-Haidi[*]
Department of Clinical Oncology
Faculty of Medicine, Cairo, Egypt

Abstract

The past few years have seen remarkable progress in the development of anticancer treatment. Advances have led to better cure rates, median overall survival rates, and time to progression. New chemotherapeutic agents, targeted therapies, and even radioactively labeled molecules are being engineered to match the unique diagnosis and needs of each patient with as few side effects as possible. These measures often result in a better quality of life for patients. Each chemotherapeutic agent has a known spectrum of side effects affecting different parts of the body. One of the main side effects of chemotherapeutic agents is cardiotoxicity. It can occur either acutely or during or long after the course of treatment with certain drugs. Sometimes cardiotoxicity can be the limiting factor in giving the optimal chemotherapeutic dose and can act as an obstacle to a patient's hope for a cure. Chemotherapy-induced cardiotoxicity is extremely difficult both to treat and to manage; therefore, cardiac function should be given priority whenever a cardiotoxic agent is included in the course of treatment and should be monitored carefully with baseline, intercyclic, and post treatment assessments. Certain chemotherapeutic agents should be avoided in patients with a prior history of cardiac disease so as not to worsen the condition. If necessary, certain prophylactic measures and cardioprotective agents should be used with a very close follow-up of the cardiac functions.

Chemotherapy can be given prior to liver transplantation to control tumor growth and prevent progression, especially if the patient is expected to stay on the waiting list for surgery for more than six months. Some liver transplant patients have undergone chemotherapy before liver transplantation.

---

[*] Correspondence: Dr Wafaa Abdel-Haidi, MSc, Consultant Oncologist, Department of Clinical Oncology, Faculty of Medicine, Cairo, Egypt, E-mail: wafaa.abdelhaidi@gmail.com.

This chapter highlights the types of chemotherapeutic agents that affect the heart and discusses their mode of action and ways of minimizing their effects. There is a brief discussion of the proper methods of assessing cardiac function during and after the course of treatment. Various options are available for managing hepatocellular carcinoma, though the best approach is liver transplantation in early stages with curative intent.

Introduction

In recent years, remarkable progress has been made in the development of anticancer treatment. Advances have led to improvements not only in the cure rates of some early discovered types of tumors such as breast cancer, Hodgkin's lymphoma, testicular cancer, and some gynecological malignancies, but also in the overall survival rates and time to progression of other tumors, even in the metastatic settings [1]. However, this marked progress is dependent on rather intense chemotherapeutic protocols and their associated side effects. Some protocols can elicit nephrotoxicity, while others cause neurotoxicity. The specific side effects vary according to the type of chemotherapy administered, the number and type of drugs combined, their infusion rates, the dose schedule, the patient's age, and any underlying associated comorbidities. Certain types of chemotherapeutic agents can induce cardiac dysfunction in several ways. Cardiac effects can include simple hypotension, hypertension, arrhythmias, thromboembolism, ischemia, cardiomyopathy, and even congestive heart failure [2].

Cardiotoxicity can be divided into early acute events or late chronic events. The acute type can occur hours, a few days, or, subacutely, several weeks following the administration of chemotherapy. It is related to the acute insult of the drug on cardiac tissue, which makes quick recovery impossible. Hence, the time required to eliminate the toxic effect of the drug depends on the type of insult caused. Acute cardiotoxicity is not related to the cumulative total dose of the chemotherapy administered. Its manifestations can vary from arrhythmias, nonspecific ST-T wave changes in the electrocardiogram, pericardial effusion, and a clinically unapparent drop in the left ventricular ejection fraction (LVEF) with transient congestive heart failure. Acute cardiotoxicity rarely results in myocardial infarction and sudden death. On the other hand, chronic cardiotoxicity occurs months to years after finishing the course of treatment [3]. It is a consequence of the cumulative total dose of the chemotherapeutic agent used and leads to irreversible congestive heart failure—the heart becomes subsequently dilated over time as a result of muscle fiber degeneration and necrosis. These effects, evident in myocardial biopsy, are discussed later in this chapter [4,5].

Chemotherapeutic agents have different mechanisms of action. They are categorized according to the main mechanism of action, such that agents in the same category might share a pharmacological profile, a toxicity profile, or drug interactions. For example, chemotherapeutic agents can be classified as alkalizing agents, antimetabolites, antitumor antibiotics, mitotic spindle agents, topoisomerase inhibitors, tyrosine kinase inhibitors, monoclonal antibodies, or hormonal agents. As alkalizing agents, high-dose cyclophosphamide can cause acute myopericarditis and cardionecrosis, ifosfamide causes normal blood pressure disturbances such as hypotension or hypertension, and cisplatin can cause bradycardia, bundle branch block, and congestive heart failure. 5-Fluorouracil and its prodrug capecitabine (Xeloda), both antimetabolites, can induce myocardial ischemia, especially if given to a patient with a prior history of cardiac disease. Paclitaxel is classified as a mitotic spindle agent, with its side effects of atrioventricular conduction defects, ventricular tachycardia, and ischemia [6].

Trastuzumab (Herceptin), a humanized monoclonal antibody against the HER2/*neu* receptor, is an extracellular receptor tyrosine kinase in the human epidermal growth factor receptor (HER) family. The overexpression of the HER2 receptor at the cellular level or its amplification at the nuclear level leads to a large increase in the metastatic potential and aggression of certain tumors, especially breast cancer [9]. Trastuzumab is an FDA-approved monoclonal antibody against the HER2 receptor and has become crucial as a first-line treatment for breast cancer in the adjuvant and metastatic settings. It is also used in the neoadjuvant setting, where it is administered with the aim of cytoreduction, that is, of reducing the size of tumors and allowing them to be removed more easily with an acceptably safe negative surgical margin. However, the HER2 receptor (also known as ErbB-2) plays a crucial role in embryonic cardiogenesis and has also been found to be very important for normal adult cardiac function [7,8]. Hence, trastuzumab causes cardiotoxicity by blocking the HER2 receptors, where it blocks the growth factor signaling for both the cardiac muscles and the tumor cells [10]. Fortunately, trastuzumab-induced cardiotoxic events are reversible after stopping the treatment. Several studies have reviewed myocardial biopsies showing a predominant myocyte dysfunction with no typical morphological changes, unlike the changes seen with other cytotoxic drugs such as anthracyclines [11]. Trastuzumab-induced cardiotoxic events are not related to its cumulative dose. The drug potentates the cardiotoxic effect of anthracyclines; therefore, the two should never be given concurrently [12].

The list of cardiotoxic chemotherapeutic agents also includes other targeted therapies, for example, tyrosine kinase inhibitors such as nilotinib for the management of chronic, accelerated, or the blast phase of chronic myeloid leukemia; sunitinib for metastatic renal cell carcinoma; and sorafenib for renal cell and hepatocellular carcinoma. Bevacizumab (Avastin) is a humanized monoclonal antibody that blocks the receptors for vascular endothelial growth factor. It is used in the treatment of metastatic breast, colorectal, lung, and renal cancer. Of all cardiotoxic chemotherapeutic agents, anthracyclines are by far the most harmful. Classified as antitumor antibiotics, they are effective in a large variety of tumors and are included in most of the international cancer treatment protocols.

In 1970, anthracyclines were shown to elicit cumulative dose-related cardiotoxicity [13]. Agents include doxorubicin, daunorubicin, epirubicin, idarubicin, liposomal doxorubicin, and mitoxantrone—an anthracycline analog. Doxorubicin is a key in the treatment of a majority of solid tumors and some hematological ones. It has, by far, the most harmful effects on the myocardium; therefore, it is the most studied chemotherapeutic agent when it comes to drug-induced cardiotoxic effects. All the drugs classified as anthracyclines have a tolerance dose, after which their harmful effects on the myocardium become evident. For example, there is a 5% increased risk of cardiomyopathy at 450 mg/m^2 for doxorubicin, 900 mg/m^2 for daunorubicin, 935 mg/m^2 for epirubicin, and 223 mg/m^2 for idarubicin [14]. It is extremely important to monitor the cumulative total dose per body surface area, which is how most chemotherapy doses are calculated for patients. The term "anthracycline" is automatically associated with irreversible myocardial damage. Although the etiology of such damage is still under investigation, a well-known mechanism is the powerful ability of anthracyclines to generate reactive oxygen species and hydrogen peroxide, which form toxic free radicals that intercalate the DNA base pairs, leading to their breakdown and, ultimately, to cell death.

Toxic free radicals also alter the structure of the cell membrane and its function, leading to an increase in calcium influx. Anthracyclines induce this influx, resulting in intracellular calcium overload that might also lead to myocyte death. Free radicals can cause further damage at intracellular sites such as the nuclear envelope, mitochondria, and sarcoplasmic reticulum, through which doxorubicin activates the calcium-release channel [15]. Disturbances in calcium metabolism at the cellular level will lead to decreased contractility and the activation of proteases, causing myofibrillar damage [16,17]. Free radicals also induce topoisomerase II-dependent DNA damage and inhibit preribosomal DNA and RNA. The generation of hydrogen peroxide is responsible for the peroxidation of myocardial lipids, which contributes to myocardial damage, as proven by biopsy. The resultant formation of a ferric-doxorubicin complex also greatly increases the formation of free radicals. Ultimately, the major mechanism of chemotherapy-induced cardiotoxicity mainly depends on the harmful effect of toxic free radicals, which applies to both normal and tumor cells [18]. Other mechanisms include cytokine formation and chemotherapy-mediated apoptosis. Endomyocardial biopsy specimens are obtained from the right ventricle via a transjugular approach or using a long, flexible bioptome via the femoral vein. The procedure is the most sensitive but most invasive method of proving myocardial damage. Following a heavy course of treatment with a cardiotoxic chemotherapeutic agent, the biopsy might be characterized by predominantly multifocal areas of patchy and interstitial fibrosis known as "stellate scars" and may also show occasional vacuolated myocardial cells called "adria cells" [19,20].

It is of the utmost importance to investigate the cardiac history of a patient and perform a baseline echocardiography prior to starting treatment with any cardiotoxic chemotherapeutic agent, especially in anthracycline-based chemotherapy. Knowing that anthracycline-related cardiotoxic events are inevitable, oncologists should tailor the protocols to each patient in order to attain the best anticancer treatment while making the associated toxicity tolerable. Several important factors must be taken into consideration before prescribing an anthracycline-based chemotherapy regimen in order to prevent the development of dilated cardiomyopathy and other cardiac insults. For example, the method of anthracycline administration, whether by bolus, short, or long infusion rates, must be considered, as longer infusion rates have been shown to reduce the toxicity of the agent. The concurrent administration of other agents known to be cardiotoxic could lead to an interaction with the anthracycline and aggravate its toxic effect on the myocardium. For this reason, the sequential administration of such agents is preferable. Age should definitely be taken into account, especially in patients under the age of 15 years and over the age of 65 years. Thus, a child under the age of 15 years with a curable disease such as Hodgkin's lymphoma receiving a strong anthracycline-based regimen should be given the treatment cautiously, with the aim of preventing dilated cardiomyopathy from occurring later in life. Other factors to consider include dose modifications, better infusion rates, avoidance of concomitant chemoradiotherapy on the mediastinum, and the use of better follow-up imaging techniques like positron emission tomography-computed tomography. Such new imaging techniques have led to better-tailored protocols that offer patients the best management with the least side effects. In adults aged 65 years and over, special attention must be paid to their current cardiac status and close follow-up is mandatory, as any coexisting cardiac condition, or a previous one that has been proven to affect the LVEF, might lead to ischemic events and even sudden death [21]. Prescribing a chemotherapy protocol should be a careful balance between optimizing the clinical response and minimizing the side effects in the short and long term.

Thorough cardiac investigations should be requested for patients about to receive a cardiotoxic chemotherapy protocol, especially those with a prior history of cardiac disease. Most commonly, the LVEF is measured by using echocardiography. The value of the LVEF should not be less than 50%. For patients with a known cardiac disease, more sophisticated baseline cardiac tests should be conducted in addition to the echocardiography, including radionuclide angiography such as multiple-gated acquisition (MUGA) scintigraphy. The MUGA scan is a noninvasive nuclear imaging technique that uses a radioactive isotope such as technetium-99m to evaluate cardiac function, including the LVEF and other indices, and reflect the condition of the cardiac muscles and the blood flow within. Echocardiography uses ultrasound waves to create an image that reflects the cardiac status in terms of contractility and hence the strength of the cardiac muscles and the LVEF and also elicits any abnormalities in wall motion. It gives an idea about the shape and size of the cardiac chambers by testing the function of the valves and the direction of blood flow through them.

Echocardiography and the MUGA scan are the most commonly used imaging techniques used to investigate the cardiac condition prior to and after administration of a cardiotoxic chemotherapeutic agent [22]. However, the cardiac damage is sometimes not evident by either clinical evaluation or imaging techniques as a result of the myocardial compensatory reserve that allows adequate cardiac output despite the unapparent myocardial damage [23]. Therefore, serial echocardiography should be scheduled to monitor the cumulative chemotherapy-induced cardiotoxic effects that might be already present but are subclinical and need a time lag to become evident and considerable. For high-risk patients, close follow-up of cardiac function should be performed before, during, and at the end of the chemotherapy treatment course and then at 3, 6, 9 and 12 months after treatment [24]. In a prospective study, Nousiainen et al. [25] indicated the possibility of distinguishing the patients who are likely to develop cardiac dysfunction by measuring the LVEF at baseline and again at 200 mg/m^2 doxorubicin. A reported fall of 10% or more in the LVEF at this low cumulative dose had 72% specificity and 90% sensitivity at detecting late cardiac dysfunction. A low LVEF at baseline is a contraindication for anthracycline therapy [26]. Further, since serum cardiac troponin is a biological marker for myocardial damage, it can be used as a follow-up tool for monitoring patients on anthracyclines as well as a strong predictor for myocardial damage preceding a poor cardiac outcome, especially if there is a persistent increase in its levels [27]. Other biological markers under investigation include the B-type natriuretic peptide, which reflects ventricular dysfunction well, as this polypeptide is produced and secreted rapidly by the heart in response to ventricular wall stress and distension. In this case, chemotherapy-induced cardiomyopathy will elicit volume overload, which will result in distension of the ventricle walls and the consequent release of high levels of BNP in the serum [28,29].

With the great progress in cancer treatment development, researchers have been increasingly intrigued by the impact of chemotherapeutic agents on the heart, especially on the myocardium. Great efforts have been made to find a way to protect the heart during treatment with cardiotoxic agents so as not to deprive patients of their chance of being cured or having prolonged survival with a good quality of life. Some methods have evolved. For example, longer infusion rates have been shown to be less harmful than bolus or short infusions because the anthracyclines will have a low, sustained serum level rather than a peak. Adult cardiomyocytes are well-differentiated muscle cells that can no longer proliferate, similar to hepatocytes and nerve cells, but they retain the capability of regenerating, though on a small scale and only with the proper growth signals. A sudden high serum level of anthracyclines prevents cardiomyocytes from having sufficient time to switch on their regenerative capacity, leading to irreversible chemotherapy-induced cardiotoxicity [30].

Researchers have spent a lot of time trying to understand the mechanism of action of each chemotherapeutic agent and to match each agent with its pharmacokinetics. Their aim is to develop a counteraction against the pathophysiology of the underlying cardiac dysfunction caused by these agents and, most importantly, against the myocardial damage. One promising development is dexrazoxane (Cardioxane), a prodrug analog of the metal chelator EDTA. The concurrent administration of dexrazoxane with each dose of anthracyclines has been shown to significantly reduce chemotherapy-associated cardiotoxicity. The cardioprotective effect of dexrazoxane depends on iron chelation: It prevents the formation of doxorubicin-iron complexes, which are responsible for the formation of toxic free radicals that lead to oxidative stress on the cardiac muscles and subsequent cell death. Dexrazoxane is considered a free radical scavenger. Marty et al. [31], as part of the Dexrazoxane Study Group, noted the unique effect of dexrazoxane on reducing the impact and severity of anthracycline-induced cardiotoxicity in patients at increased risk of cardiac dysfunction as a result of previous anthracycline treatment. Dexrazoxane was also shown not to interfere with the antitumor efficacy of the chemotherapeutic regimen [32,33]. It should be prescribed to patients who are about to receive more than 300 mg/m^2 of doxorubicin, as recommended by Swain et al. [34]. It is infused intravenously over approximately 15 minutes at a fixed ratio according to the type of anthracycline used. There are also novel trials underway on the use of angiotensin-converting enzyme inhibitors, angiotensin II receptor blockers, and carvedilol (beta blocker). Cardinale et al. [35] showed some promising results in cancer patients on an anthracycline-based regimen. Patients experienced a complete LVEF recovery and a reduction in cardiac dysfunction, indicating that the use of an angiotensin-converting enzyme inhibitor in combination with a beta blocker can help improve cardiac dysfunction. Beta blockers such as carvedilol have been shown to have antioxidant and antiapoptotic properties, and some studies have already demonstrated the protective effects of beta blockers against anthracycline-induced cardiomyopathy, with more studies yet to come [36].

Other strategies for preserving myocardial damage include lowering the total cumulative dose of the anthracycline, substituting doxorubicin with less cardiotoxic analogs such as epirubicin or mitoxantrone, modifying the anthracycline treatment schedule to include longer infusion rates [37,38], and using lower doses on a weekly basis rather than high doses every three weeks [39]. It is also advisable to use other cardiotoxic agents in a sequential manner rather than concomitantly with an anthracycline so as not to aggravate its toxic effect on the cardiac muscles. Furthermore, the unique delivery system and small size (100 nm) of pegylated liposomal doxorubicin allow it to access small, tortuous tumor vasculature, concentrating the drug in the tumor while minimizing the systemic toxic effect and thereby reducing the cardiotoxic effect [40,41]. The advantage of pegylated liposomal doxorubicin is that it has comparable efficacy with conventional anthracyclines and can be given after prior anthracycline therapy as retreatment or rechallenge following a previous good response to anthracyclines. In this way, it liberates oncologists from the limiting factor of these cardiotoxic agents, namely, the total cumulative dose of anthracyclines that prevents them from offering the optimal treatment. Instead, oncologists can prescribe the liposomal form along with special monitoring of cardiac function [42].

Hepatocellular carcinoma is very difficult to treat and carries a poor prognosis. It is the fifth most common type of tumor and the third leading cause of cancer-related death worldwide, especially in patients with decompensated cirrhosis and few treatment options [43]. The proper staging of hepatocellular carcinoma is crucial to providing prognostic information that helps in choosing the most appropriate management for each patient. The Barcelona Clinic Liver Cancer staging system is the most commonly used classification and is recommended by the American Association for the Study of Liver Diseases [44]. It combines tumor burden with its consequent hepatic functions in addition to the performance status and an evidence-based treatment algorithm. Very early and early stages of hepatocellular carcinoma can be potentially curable by surgical resection, liver transplantation, and percutaneous therapy, whether radiofrequency ablation or ethanol injection [44,45]. Intermediate stages can be treated by trans catheter arterial chemoembolization (TACE), whereby a catheter is introduced using the Seldinger technique through the femoral artery to the aorta and into the liver, and the drug is directed into the tumor. The use of TACE reduces the hazards of systemic chemotherapy. Cisplatin, doxorubicin, mitomycin-C or 5-fluorouracil can be used in TACE, depending on the protocol followed by the particular cancer center. Transcatheter arterial chemoembolization causes tissue necrosis that can be used prior to liver transplantation to control tumor growth and prevent its progression, especially if the patient is expected to be on the waiting list for more than six months [46]. Drug-eluting beads are a novel addition to TACE. The drug is encapsulated in microspheres, allowing its sustained, slow release over time and leading to better distribution of the drug inside the tumor and decreased systemic side effects [47]. Other intra-arterial approaches include radioembolization with yttrium-90 radioactive microspheres. This method allows the internal delivery of high-dose radiation to the tumor capillary bed with limited radiation exposure to the surrounding normal tissues [48]. As for advanced stages and the metastatic setting, sorafenib has become the standard of care. An oral multikinase inhibitor, sorafenib suppresses tumor proliferation and angiogenesis and increases the rate of apoptosis. It blocks several molecular pathways that are responsible for hepatocarcinogenesis [49,50]. Furthermore, it has been shown statistically to improve the overall survival rate and median time to tumor progression in the SHARP trial [51]. Like all the other targeted therapies that block the receptors for vascular endothelial growth factor, sorafenib increases the risk of bleeding and arterial thromboembolic events [52,53]. Its use should be stopped prior to any surgical procedure and a thorough bleeding tendency profile is recommended preoperatively.

Conclusion

Chemotherapy-induced cardiotoxicity is one of the most disappointing drawbacks when it comes to offering the optimal management to cancer patients. Major advances have been made in anticancer treatment, but intensifying some chemotherapeutic protocols has led to expanding the toxicity profile and undesirable side effects. Modern clinical pharmacology has played a role in helping patients manage side effects, but the impairment of vital organs such as the heart poses a tremendous problem. Researchers have worked hard to identify the cardiotoxic chemotherapeutic agents, their mechanisms of action, factors increasing their toxicity, and how to diagnose, manage, and prevent their effects. Proper clinical examination of patients and thorough investigations should be conducted before administering a cardiotoxic agent, especially to those with a known cardiac condition or a previous one. Anthracyclines are the chemotherapeutic agents with the most harmful effects on the heart. They specifically affect the myocardium, causing dilated cardiomyopathy that results in congestive heart failure. Special attention should be paid to the total cumulative dose, infusion rate, dose schedule, and administration of other concurrent cardiotoxic agents. Monitoring the left ventricular ejection fraction by echocardiography and MUGA scan is crucial in this situation. Biological markers like troponin I and B-type natriuretic peptide are showing promise in eliciting ventricular injury before it is noticeable by modern imaging techniques. A low left ventricular ejection fraction is a contraindication for chemotherapeutic agents known to induce cardiotoxicity. Using anthracycline analogs or liposomal forms decreases the cardiotoxicity with comparable results. As trastuzumab potentiates the cardiotoxic effect of anthracyclines, it should not be given concurrently. However, it has the advantage of causing nonmorphological myocyte damage, such that its cardiotoxicity is reversible upon discontinuation of the drug. Dexrazoxane is a cardioprotective agent that has been shown to reduce the impact and severity of anthracycline-induced cardiotoxicity, but does not interfere with the antitumor efficacy of the chemotherapeutic agent. Angiotensin-converting enzyme inhibitors, angiotensin receptor blockers, and carvedilol are the subjects of ongoing investigations with promising results towards solving this problem.

A careful treatment algorithm for hepatocellular carcinoma should be derived to choose the most appropriate method of management. The Barcelona Clinic Liver Cancer staging system is used most commonly to determine the prognosis of the disease and the subsequent course of treatment. Liver resection, transplantation, and percutaneous ablation procedures are considered potentially curable therapeutic options in early stages. Transcatheter arterial chemoembolization is used in intermediate stages and as a bridge for liver transplantation, and sorafenib is the standard of care in advanced and metastatic hepatocellular carcinoma. Targeted therapy has shown great potential in treating such difficult tumors, with more advancements still to come in the near future.

References

[1] Verdecchia A, Francisci S, Brenner H, Gatta G, Micheli A, Mangone L et al. Recent cancer survival in Europe: a 2000–02 period analysis of EUROCARE-4 data. *Lancet Oncol* 2007; 8 (9): 784–96.

[2] Yeh ET. Cardiotoxicity induced by chemotherapy and antibody therapy. *Ann Rev Med* 2006; 57: 485-98.

[3] Pai VB, Nahata MC. Cardiotoxicity of chemotherapeutic agents. Incidence, treatment and prevention. *Drug Safety* 2000; 22: 263-302.

[4] Haq MM, Legha SS, Choksi J, Hortobagyi GN, Benjamin RS, Ewer M, Ali M. Doxorubicin-induced congestive heart failure in adults. *Cancer* 1985; 56: 1361-5.

[5] Steinherz LJ, Steinherz PG, Tan C. Cardiac failure and dysrhythmias 6-19 years after anthracycline therapy: a series of 15 patients. *Med. Pediar. Oncol* 1995; 24: 352-61.

[6] Yeh ET, Bickford CL. Cardiovascular complications of cancer therapy: incidence, pathogenesis, diagnosis, and management. *J Am Col Cardio* 2009; 53(24): 2231–47.

[7] Crone SA, Zhao YY, Fan L, et al. ErbB2 is essential in the prevention of dilated cardiomyopathy. *Nat Med* 2002; 8 (5): 459–65.

[8] Negro A, Brar BK, Lee KF: Essential roles of Her2/erbB2 in cardiac development and function. *Recent Prog Horm Res* 2004; 59:1-12.

[9] Chazin VR, Kaleko M, Miller AD and Slamon DJ. Transformation mediated by the human *HER-2* gene independent of epidermal growth factor receptor. *Oncogene* 1992:7: 1859–66.

[10] Suter TM, Cook-Bruns N, Barton C: Cardiotoxicity associated with trastuzumab (Herceptin) therapy in the treatment of metastatic breast cancer. *The Breast* 2004; 13:173-83.

[11] Ewer MS, Vooletich MT, Durand JB, Woods M, Davis JR, Valero V et al: Reversibility of trastuzumab-induced cardiotoxicity: new insight based on clinical course and response to medical treatment. *J Clinical Oncology* 2005; 23(31): 7820-6

[12] Minotti G, Menna P, Salvatorelli E, Cairo G, Gianni L. Anthracyclines: molecular advances and pharmacologic developments in antitumor activity and cardiotoxicity. *Pharmacol Rev* 2004 ; 56(2):185–229.

[13] Lefrak E, Pitha J, Rosenheim S et al: A clinicopathologic analysis of adriamycin cardiotoxicity. *Cancer* 1973; 32: 302-14.

[14] Keefe DL. Anthracycline-induced cardiomyopathy. *Semin Oncol* 2001;28 (12):2.

[15] Holmberg SR, Cumming DV, Kusama Y, Hearse DJ, Poole-Wilson PA, Shattock MJ et al. Reactive oxygen species modify the structure and function of the cardiac sarcoplasmic reticulum calcium-release channel. *Cardioscience* 1991; 2:19-25.

[16] Kusuoka H, Futaki S, Koretsune Y, Kitabatake A, Suga H, Kamada T et al. Alterations of intracellular calcium homeostasis and myocardial energetics in acute adriamycin-induced heart failure. *J Cardiovasc Pharmacol* 1991; 18: 437-44.

[17] Holmberg SR, Williams AJ. Patterns of interaction between anthraquinone drugs and the calcium-release channel from cardiac sarcoplasmic reticulum. *Circ Res* 1990; 67: 272-83.

[18] Gianni L, Myers CE: The role of free radical formation in the cardiotoxicity of anthracycline. In: Muggia FM, Green MD, Speyer JL, ed. Cancer Treatment and the Heart, Baltimore: Johns Hopkins University Press; 1992:9-46.

[19] Speyer J, Wasserheit C. Strategies for reduction of anthracycline cardiac toxicity. *Semin Oncol* 1998; 25(5):525.

[20] Ewer M, Carrasco C, et al: Cardiac biopsy procedures at a cancer center. *Proc Am Soc Clin Oncol* 1991; 10:336.

[21] Wojtacki J, Lewicka-Nowak E, Leśniewski-Kmak K. Anthracycline-induced cardiotoxicity: clinical course, risk factors, pathogenesis, detection and prevention--review of the literature. *Med Sc Monit* 2000; 6: 411-20.

[22] Jannazzo A, Hoff man J, Lutz M. Monitoring of anthracycline-induced cardiotoxicity. *Ann. Pharmacother* 2008; 42: 99–104.

[23] Ewer MS, Lenihan DJ. Left ventricular ejection fraction and cardiotoxicity: is our ear really to the ground? *J. Clin. Oncol* 2008; 26: 1201–03.

[24] Meinardi MT, van der Graaf WT, van Veldhuisen DJ, Gietema JA, de Vries EG, Sleijfer DT. Detection of anthracycline-induced cardiotoxicity. *Cancer Treat Rev* 1999; 25 (4):237-247.

[25] Nousiainen T, Jantunen E, Vanninen E, Hartikainen J. Early decline in left ventricular ejection fraction predicts doxorubicin cardiotoxicity in lymphoma patients. *Br J Cancer* 2002; 86:1697-70.

[26] Schwartz RG, McKenzie WB, Alexander J, et al. Congestive heart failure and left ventricular dysfunction complicating doxorubicin therapy: seven-year experience using serial radionuclide angiocardiography. *Am J Med* 1987; 82:1109-18.

[27] Cardinale D, Sandri MT, Martinoni A, Borghini E, Civelli M, Lamantia G et al. Myocardial injury revealed by plasma troponin I in breast cancer treated with high-dose chemotherapy. *Ann. Oncol* 2002; 13:710-15.

[28] Sparano JA, Brown DL, Wolff AC. Predicting cancer therapy–induced cardiotoxicity: the role of troponins and other markers. *Drug Saf* 2002; 25:301-11.

[29] Dolci A, Dominici R, Cardinale D, Sandri MT, Panteghini M. Biochemical markers for prediction of chemotherapy-induced cardiotoxicity: systematic review of the literature and recommendations for use. *Am J Clin Pathol* 2008; 130 (5): 688–95.

[30] Gewirtz DA. A critical evaluation of the mechanisms of action proposed for the antitumor effects of the anthracycline antibiotics adriamycin and daunorubicin. *Biochem. Pharmacol* 1999;57:727–41.

[31] Marty M, Espié M, Llombart A, Monnier A, Rapoport BL, Stahalova V; Dexrazoxane Study Group. Multicenter randomized phase III study of the cardioprotective effect of dexrazoxane (Cardioxane) in advanced/metastatic breast cancer patients treated with anthracycline-based chemotherapy. *Ann Oncol* 2006; 17: 614–22.

[32] Swain SM, Vici P. The current and future role of dexrazoxane as a cardioprotectant in anthracycline treatment: expert panel review. *J Cancer Res Clin Oncol* 2004; 130: 1–7.

[33] Lipshultz SE, Rifai N, Dalton VM, Levy DE, Silverman LB, Lipsitz SR et al. The effect of dexrazoxane on myocardial injury in doxorubicin-treated children with acute lymphoblastic leukemia. *N Eng J Med* 2004; 351: 145–53.

[34] Swain SM, Whaley FS, Gerber MC, Ewer MS, Bianchine JR, Gams RA. Delayed administration of dexrazoxane provides cardioprotection for patients with advanced breast cancer treated with doxorubicin-containing therapy. *J Clin Oncol* 1997; 15: 1333–40.

[35] Cardinale D, Colombo A, Lamantia G, Colombo N, Civelli M, De Giacomi G et al. Anthracycline-Induced cardiomyopathy: Clinical relevance and response to pharmacologic therapy. *J Am Coll Cardiol* 2010; 55;213-20.

[36] Kalay N, Basar E, Ozdogru I, Er O, Cetinkaya Y, Dogan A et al. Protective effects of carvedilol against anthracycline-induced cardiomyopathy. *J Am Coll Cardiol* 2006; 48:2258-62.

[37] Torti FM, Bristow MR, Howes AE, Aston D, Stockdale FE, Carter SK et al: Reduced cardiotoxicity of doxorubicin delivered on a weekly schedule: assessment by endomyocardial biopsy. *Ann Intern Med* 1983; 99:745-49.

[38] Legha SS, Benjamin RS, Mackay B, Ewer M, Wallace S, Valdivieso et al. Reduction of doxorubicin cardiotoxicity by prolonged continuous intravenous infusion. *Ann Intern Med* 1982; 96:133-9.

[39] Benjamin RS: The schedule dependency of the cardiotoxiciy of Adriamycin: its relevance to pharmacokinetic parameters. In: Muggia FM, Green MD, Speyer JL, ed. *Cancer Treatment and the Heart*, Baltimore: Johns Hopkins University Press; 1992:278-85.

[40] O'Brien ME, Wigler N, Inbar M, Rosso R, Grischke E, Santoro A et al. Reduced cardiotoxicity and comparable efficacy in a phase III trial of pegylated liposomal doxorubicin HCL (CAELYX/Doxil) versus conventional doxorubicin for first-line treatment of metastatic breast cancer. *Ann. Oncol* 2004; 15:440-449

[41] Ewer MS, Martin FJ, Henderson IC, Shapiro CL, Benjamin RS, Gabizon AA. Cardiac safety of liposomal anthracyclines. *Semin Oncol* 2004; 31 (Suppl 13) :161-81.

[42] Safra T, Muggia F, Jeffers S, Tsao-Wei DD, Groshen S, Lyass O et al. Pegylated liposomal doxorubicin (Doxil): reduced clinical cardiotoxicity in patients reaching or exceeding cumulative doses of 500 mg/m2. *Ann. Oncol* 2000; 11:1029-33.

[43] El-Serag HB, Rudolph KL. Hepatocellular carcinoma: epidemiology and molecular carcinogenesis. *Gastroenterology* 2007; 132:2557–76.

[44] Bruix J, Sherman M. Management of hepatocellular carcinoma. *Hepatology* 2005; 42:1208–1236.

[45] Llovet JM, Bruix J. Molecular targeted therapies in hepatocellular carcinoma. *Hepatology* 2008; 48(4): 1312-27.

[46] Alba E, Valls C, Dominguez J, Martinez L, Escalante E, Lladó L, Serrano T. Transcatheter arterial chemoembolization in patients with hepatocellular carcinoma on the waiting list for orthotopic liver transplantation. *Am J Roentgenol* 2008;190:1341-8.

[47] Varela M, Real MI, Burrel M, Forner A, Sala M, Brunet M et al. Chemoembolization of hepatocellular carcinoma with drug eluting beads: efficacy and doxorubicin pharmacokinetics. *J Hepatol* 2007; 46:474–81.

[48] Kulik LM, Carr BI, Mulcahy MF, Lavandowski RJ, Atassi B, Ryu RK et al. Safety and efficacy of 90Y radiotherapy for hepatocellular carcinoma with and without portal vein thrombosis. *Hepatology* 2008; 47:71-81.

[49] Chang YS, Adnane J, Trail PA, Levy J, Henderson A, Xue D et al. Sorafenib (BAY 43-9006) inhibits tumor growth and vascularization and induces tumor apoptosis and hypoxia in RCC xenograft models. *Cancer Chemother Pharmacol* 2007; 59:561-74.

[50] Roberts LR, Gores GJ. Hepatocellular carcinoma: molecular pathways and new therapeutic targets. *Semin. Liver Dis* 2005; 25:212-25.

[51] Llovet JM, Ricci S, Mazzaferro V, Hilgard I, Gane E, Blanc JF et al. Sorafenib in advanced hepatocellular carcinoma. *N Engl J Med* 2008;359:378-90.

[52] Je Y, Schutz FA, Choueiri TK. Risk of bleeding with vascular endothelial growth factor receptor tyrosine-kinase inhibitors sunitinib and sorafenib: a systematic review and meta-analysis of clinical trials. *Lancet Oncol* 2009;10(10):967-74

[53] Choueri TK, Schutz FA, Je Y, Rosenberg JE, Bellmunt J. Risk of arterial thromboembolic events with sunitinib and sorafenib: a systematic review and meta-analysis of clinical trials. *J Clin Oncol* 2010; 28(13):2280-5.

Chapter XI

Cardiopulmonary Consequences of Transjugular Intrahepatic Portosystemic Shunts

Florence Wong[*]
Department of Medicine, Toronto General Hospital
Toronto, Ontario, Canada

Abstract

A transjugular intrahepatic portosystemic stent shunt (TIPS) is a radiological procedure designed to reduce portal pressure. It has been used for the management of complications of portal hypertension. The creation of the shunt transfers a large volume of blood from the splanchnic circulation to the systemic circulation, and therefore significant hemodynamic changes occur with TIPS insertion. The pulmonary circulation responds to the insertion of TIPS with and increase in mean pulmonary arterial pressure, which persists for at least 1 month. This post-TIPS pulmonary hypertension is partly related to an increase in pulmonary circulatory volume, and partly related to pulmonary vasoconstriction, leading to an increase in pulmonary vascular resistance. The systemic circulation responds to the TIPS insertion with systemic vasodilatation, which persists for at least 1 year post-TIPS. Vasodilatation rather than vasoconstriction occurs in the systemic circulation, related to hypo-responsiveness of the systemic circulation to various vasoconstrictors that are being channeled from the splanchnic to the systemic circulation. The volume overload presented to the heart, together with the high circulating vasoconstrictor levels, can lead to an increased left ventricular mass, with consequent diastolic dysfunction. This diastolic dysfunction, if present pre-TIPS, is associated with a decreased survival and reduced clearance of ascites post-TIPS. Diastolic dysfunction that is still detected at 1 month post-TIPS is also associated with a poor patient outcome. Therefore, patients who receive TIPS should undergo careful cardiovascular

---

[*] Correspondence: Florence Wong, 9th floor, North Wing, Room 983, Toronto Hospital, 200 Elizabeth Street, Toronto M5G 2C4, Ontario, Canada, Tel: (416) 340-3834, Fax: (416) 340-5019, e-mail: florence.wong@utoronto.ca.

investigations prior to TIPS insertion. Patients who have received TIPS should also be followed carefully for the detection of cardiopulmonary complications.

The Use of Transjugular Intrahepatic Portosystemic Stent Shunt in Cirrhosis

The transjugular intrahepatic portosystemic stent shunt or TIPS is a prosthesis that is inserted into a channel that is created within the liver parenchyma, connecting a branch of the portal vein and a branch of the hepatic vein. As such, a TIPS effectively functions as a side-to-side portocaval shunt, and is very effective in reducing sinusoidal portal pressure. Therefore, it has been mainly used to treat complications of portal hypertension in cirrhosis, such as refractory variceal bleeds or refractory ascites [1]. By removing the obstruction to portal flow, the insertion of TIPS allows the transfer of a significant blood volume from the splanchnic circulation to the pulmonary circulation, and thence to the systemic circulation. The sudden "dumping" of a significant blood volume into pulmonary and systemic circulations is associated with significant hemodynamic changes. The usually high cardiac output has been reported to increase further by another 50%, and the systemic circulation undergoes further dilatation in order to accommodate the increased cardiac output [2], further exacerbating the already hyperdynamic circulation. TIPS also appears to have significant effects on cardiac function [3,4], as congestive heart failure, sudden cardiac death, and myocardial infarction have all been reported in the immediate post-TIPS period in cirrhotic patients without known pre-existing cardiovascular disease [5]. Various recent investigations into these post-TIPS complications have led to significant advances in our understanding of the cardiovascular effects of TIPS.

The Effects of TIPS on the Pulmonary Circulation

In an elegant study performed by van der Linden et al [6], the authors serially measured pulmonary hemodynamics from the time of sedation to the post-procedure period in a cohorts of cirrhotic patients who underwent TIPS placement for the indications of refractory variceal bleed or refractory ascites. The authors found that the mean pulmonary artery pressure (MPAP) increased significantly immediately upon opening of the TIPS shunt from a mean of 12.3±3.0mmHg to 20.3±5.3mmHg (Figure 1). Since 1 litre of cardiac output increase can only account for 2-3mmHg increase in MPAP [7], the authors concluded that factor(s) other than an acute shift of vascular volume from the splanchnic circulation to the central circulation would have contributed to the increase in MPAP. They confirmed their interpretation by blocking the TIPS shunt, and immediately observed a reduction in MPAP, but to a level higher than pre-TIPS value (Figure 1). Upon reopening of the TIPS, the MPAP returned to the high immediate post-TIPS level. The authors postulated that neurohormonal factors might also be involved in mediating the increase in MPAP in the post-TIPS period.

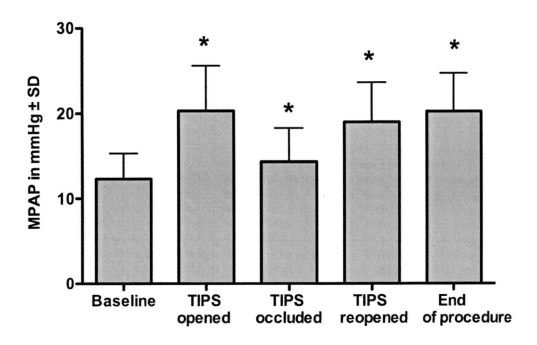

Figure 1. Changes in mean pulmonary artery pressure before and at various time points after TIPS insertion. * p<0.05 versus baseline. Adapted from reference [6] with permission.

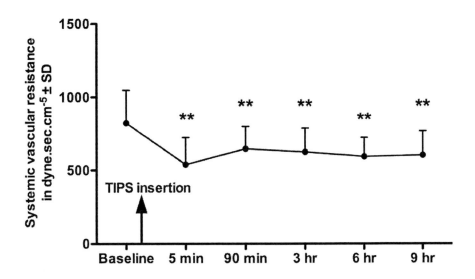

Figure 2. (Continued).

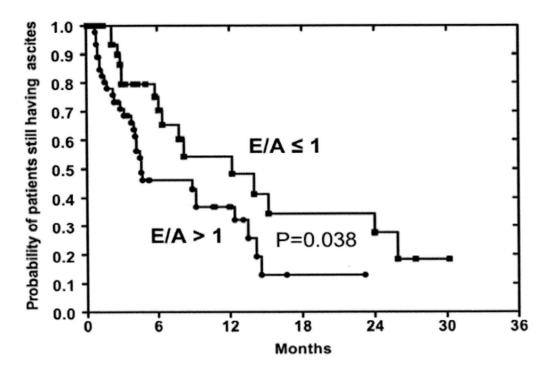

Figure 2. a) Cardiac output and b) systemic vascular resistance before and after TIPS insertion over a 9-hour period. **p<0.01 versus baseline, * p<0.05 versus baseline. Adapted from reference [3] with permission.

Similar findings have also been reported by Huonkers at al, who observed an immediate rise in the MPAP, and this increase persisted for 9 hours post-TIPS [3]. There was a concomitant but transient rise in pulmonary vascular resistance. We have also observed an increase of MPAP of similar magnitude at 30 minutes post-TIPS (personal unpublished data), associated with a parallel increase in pulmonary vascular resistance. This increase in MPAP persisted for at least 30 days after TIPS insertion [6]. Long-term follow-up reveals that the MPAP returns to baseline levels by 3 months, and remains stable for at least 12 months post-TIPS [8].

Collectively, these data suggest that acutely there is an inability of the right ventricle and the pulmonary circulation to dilate to accommodate the increased blood volume that is being shifted from the splanchnic to the pulmonary circulation following TIPS placement. The former may be related to some alterations in the intrinsic property of the myocardium, while the latter may be related to an enhanced response of the pulmonary vasculature to the presence of excess vasoconstrictors being delivered there. Patients with decompensated cirrhosis are known to have increased production of endothelins, a family of potent vasoconstrictors, from the liver, gut and the spleen [9,10]. To corroborate the notion that increased levels of vasoconstrictors such as endothelins are being delivered from the splanchnic to the pulmonary circulation following TIPS insertion, patients with cirrhosis and refractory ascites were found to have significantly elevated levels of endothelin I in the portal venous blood before TIPS insertion [11], and immediately after TIPS insertion, there was a significant rise in the arterial concentrations, suggesting a transfer of endothelin I from the portal to the systemic circulation via the pulmonary circulation [11]. Over the course of the following weeks to months, the increased volume in the pulmonary circulation would have been redistributed to other vascular beds. In addition, when endothelin levels were re-measured at 1-2 months post-TIPS insertion, there was a significant fall in the endothelin I levels in the systemic circulation [12]. Both these factors would have contributed to the fall in MPAP and pulmonary vascular resistance with time.

The Effects of TIPS on the Systemic Circulation

In contrast to the pulmonary circulation, the vascular resistance in the systemic circulation decreases and the cardiac output increases immediately post-TIPS [3, 8,13,14] (Figure 2), that is, the already hyperdynamic circulation becomes more hyperdynamic after TIPS insertion. These hemodynamic changes in the systemic circulation peak at about 1 month after TIPS insertion [14,15] and thereafter, slowly return towards their pre-TIPS levels over the course of the following 12 months [6,8], although the cardiac output may still be significant higher and the systemic vascular resistance significantly lower than the pre-TIPS levels at 12 months [8]. The rise in cardiac output is predominantly related to an increase in stroke volume rather than an increase in heart rate [3,8]. An increase in the left ventricular end-diastolic volume immediately post-TIPS, related to an acute transfer of the portal venous blood from the splanchnic circulation into the systemic circulation, appears to be responsible for the increased stroke volume [14]. It seems that the pulmonary and the systemic circulations deal with this sudden influx of volume differently; the pulmonary vasculature vasoconstricts to produce pulmonary hypertension, whereas the systemic circulation vasodilates and the mean arterial pressure either remains relatively unchanged or decreases [8]. Although it is possible that any vasoconstrictors being transferred from the splanchnic circulation following TIPS insertion would have been metabolized during their passage through the pulmonary circulation, a more plausible explanation would be hyporesponsiveness of the systemic circulation to the effects of vasoconstrictors [23-25], whereas the opposite is true of the pulmonary circulation [8,11]. There is evidence that the systemic circulation does not respond to vasoconstrictors post-TIPS, as high levels of endothelin I in the arterial circulation in the immediate post-TIPS period did not elicit any change in the mean arterial pressure or systemic vascular resistance [11]. In addition, differential responses of the pulmonary and systemic circulations to other stimuli, whether mechanical or humoral [26], may also be responsible for the opposite hemodynamic changes observed in these 2 circulations following TIPS insertion.

The Effects of TIPS on Cardiac Structure and Function

Patients with cirrhosis who receive a TIPS as a treatment for complications of portal hypertension usually undergo careful cardiovascular assessment prior to TIPS insertion, especially if the TIPS insertion is performed electively [21]. Despite this, there are cases of cardiac failure and unexplained sudden death following TIPS insertion [22,23], suggesting that the procedure itself does have a significant effect on cardiac function in cirrhosis. In a cohort of 34 patients who underwent TIPS insertion for either uncontrolled variceal bleed or refractory ascites, Salerno et al reported no significant systolic dysfunction after TIPS [24]. In fact, ejection fraction remained high and relatively unchanged. In contrast, the diastolic function has been reported as either unchanged [5,24] or worsened after TIPS [24]. Using the plasma renin activity (PRA) as a marker of the fullness of the effective arterial blood volume, the same authors were able to identify the patients who were likely to develop cardiac dysfunction post TIPS [25]. Those patients who had a PRA of >4ng/ml/hr, and hence a smaller effective arterial blood volume were the ones who could not increase their cardiac output post-TIPS. The same patients also displayed evidence of diastolic dysfunction as indicated by an E (early diastolic filling)/A (late or atrial contribution of diastolic filling) ratio of ≤ 1 [25]. Most of these patients continued to show evidence of diastolic dysfunction post-TIPS [24]. In some cases, diastolic dysfunction developed de novo after TIPS insertion.

Hitherto not yet described is the effect of TIPS on cardiac structure. In a cohort of 18 cirrhotic patients carefully followed for at least 12 months by the author, and who underwent TIPS insertion for the treatment of refractory ascites, there was an increase in left ventricular mass which peaked at 6 months (personal unpublished data). This left ventricular hypertrophy has been postulated as the result of increased volume load on the left ventricle [26] as well as the direct growth stimulation from the various vasoconstrictor hormones [27,28], which levels remain high for several months post-TIPS. Parallel with this increase in left ventricular mass, there is increase in left ventricular stiffness, which is the most likely explanation for the impediment to ventricular filling or diastolic dysfunction post-TIPS.

Clinical Significance of Cardiac Dysfunction Post-TIPS

The diastolic dysfunction post-TIPS is not simply an academic curiosity, but rather, this has been shown to have a negative impact on the prognosis on these patients. In the same cohort of 34 patients described earlier by Salerno et al, those patients who continued to show diastolic dysfunction at 1 month post TIPS had a decreased survival [24]. Most of the patients with diastolic dysfunction who died post-TIPS had hepatorenal syndrome as the cause of death [24], and poor cardiac function has been implicated in cirrhotic patients who developed hepatorenal syndrome in the setting of spontaneous bacterial peritonitis [29]. In a larger cohort of 101 cirrhotic patients who underwent elective TIPS insertion mostly for the indication of refractory ascites, Rabie et al reported that an E/A ratio of ≤ 1 pre-TIPS was also predictive of bad outcome post TIPS. These patients were more likely to have a decreased survival for up to 12 months post-TIPS (Figure 3), and the only cardiac deaths were noted in the patients who had a pre-TIPS E/A ratio of ≤ 1 [30]. In addition, there were proportionally more liver related deaths or death from renal failure in the same subgroup of patients. It has been suggested that the persistence of diastolic dysfunction post-TIPS identifies those patients who are not able to refill their central blood volume with the insertion of TIPS.

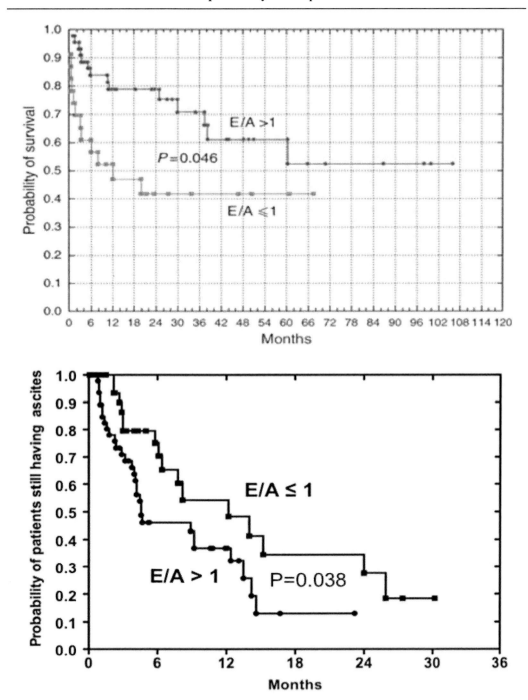

Figure 3. Probably of a) survival and b) ascites clearance in patients with or without pre-TIPS diastolic dysfunction as indicated by E/A ratio of ≤1. Reprinted from reference [30] with permission.

E/A, early maximal ventricular filling velocity/atrial maximal filling velocity.

This, in the presence of increased vasodilatation in the post-TIPS period may actually worsen the circulatory dysfunction that is already present in these patients, thereby predisposing them to other complications such as the development of hepatorenal syndrome.

It is interesting to note that the same subgroup of patients were less likely to clear their ascites post-TIPS insertion [30] (Figure 3). The corollary from this observation is that careful consideration should be given in assessing cirrhotic patients with evidence of diastolic dysfunction for TIPS placement, to determine whether the benefits outweigh the risks for the TIPS procedure.

Conclusion

The insertion of TIPS represents a significant advance in the management of complication of portal hypertension in cirrhosis. This initial enthusiasm in the 1990's of inserting a TIPS for every complication of portal hypertension has been dampened because of the appearance of many unexpected post-procedure cardiopulmonary events, many leading to the demise of the patient. Many physiological studies that followed in the next decade have provided us with valuable information on the cardiac and hemodynamic changes that accompany TIPS insertion. This has led many centres to lay down strict guidelines on patient selection for TIPS insertion, especially if this is done as an elective procedure. The advent of the knowledge on cirrhotic cardiomyopathy has helped to further fine tune patient selection for the procedure, as the presence of diastolic dysfunction, part of cirrhotic cardiomyopathy, may have a negative impact on patient outcome. All patients who undergo TIPS insertion should have careful follow-up for further complications, and timely liver transplant should be advised should these complications occur.

References

[1] Boyer TD. Transjugular intrahepatic portosystemic shunt in the management of complications of portal hypertension. *Curr. Gastroenterol. Rep.* 2008; 10: 30-35.

[2] Wong F, Sniderman K, Liu P, Allidina Y, Sherman M, Blendis LM. The effects of transjugular intrahepatic portasystemic shunt on systemic and renal hemodynamics and sodium homeostasis in cirrhotic patients with refractory ascites. *Ann. Int. Med.* 1995; 122: 816-22.

[3] Huonker M, Schumacher YO, Ochs A, Sorichter S, Keul J, Rossle M. Cardiac function and haemodynamics in alcoholic cirrhosis and effects of the transjugular intrahepatic portosystemic stent shunt. *Gut* 1999; 44: 743-8.

[4] Braverman AC, Steiner MA, Picus D, White H. High-output congestive heart failure following transjugular intrahepatic portal-systemic shunting. *Chest* 1995; 107: 1467-9.

[5] Merli M, Valeriano V, Funaro S, Attili AF, Masini A, Efrati C et al. Modifications of cardiac function in cirrhotic patients treated with transjugular intrahepatic portosystemic shunt (TIPS). *Am. J. Gastroenterol.* 2002; 97: 142-8.

[6] Van der Linden P, Le Moine O, Ghysels M, Ortinez M, Devière J. Pulmonary hypertension after transjugular intrahepatic portosystemic shunt: effects on right ventricular function. *Hepatology* 1996; 23: 982-7.

[7] Mélot C, Delcroix M, Closset J, Vanderhoeft P, Lejeune P, Leeman M, Naeije R. Starling resistor versus distensible vessel models for embolic pulmonary hypertension. *Am. J. Physiol.* 1995; 267: H817-H827.

[8] Lotterer E, Wengert A, Fleig WE. Transjugular intrahepatic portosystemic shunt: Short-term and long-term effects on hepatic and systemic hemodynamics in patients with cirrhosis. *Hepatology* 1999; 29: 632-9.

[9] Benjaminov FS, Prentice M, Sniderman KW, Siu S, Liu P, Wong F. Portopulmonary hypertension in decompensated cirrhosis with refractory ascites. *Gut* 2003; 52: 1355-62.

[10] Alam I, Bass NM, Bacchetti P, Gee L, Rockey DC. Hepatic tissue endothelin-1 levels in chronic liver disease correlate with disease severity and ascites. *Am. J. Gastroenterol.* 2000; 95: 199-203.

[11] Nolte W, Ehrenreich H, Wiltfang J, Pahl K, Unterberg K, Kamrowski-Kruck H et al. Systemic and splanchnic endothelin-1 plasma levels in liver cirrhosis before and after transjugular intrahepatic portosystemic shunt (TIPS). *Liver* 2000; 20:60-5.

[12] Martinet JP, Legault L, Cernacek P, Roy L, Dufresne MP, Spahr L, Fenyves D, et al. Changes in plasma endothelin-1 and big endothelin 1 induced by transjugular intrahepatic portosystemic shunts in patients with cirrhosis and refractory ascites. *J. Hepatol.* 1996; 25: 700-6.

[13] Wong F, Sniderman K, Liu P, Allidina Y, Sherman M, Blendis L. Transjugular intrahepatic portosystemic stent shunt: effects on hemodynamics and sodium homeostasis in cirrhosis and refractory ascites. *Ann Intern Med* 1995; 122: 816-22.

[14] Azoulay D, Castaing D, Dennison A, Martino W, Eyraud D, Bismuth H. Transjugular intrahepatic portosystemic shunt worsens the hyperdynamic circulatory state of the cirrhotic patient: preliminary report of a prospective study. Hepatology 1994; 19: 129-32.

[15] Colombato LA, Spahr L, Martinet JP, Dufresne MP, Lafortune M, Fenyves D, Pomier-Layrargues G. Haemodynamic adaptation two months after transjugular intrahepatic portosystemic shunt (TIPS) in cirrhotic patients. *Gut* 1996; 39: 600-4

[16] Umgelter A, Reindl W, Geisler F, Saugel B, Huber W, Berger H, Schmid RM. Effects of TIPS on global end-diastolic volume and cardiac output and renal resistive index in ICU patients with advanced alcoholic cirrhosis. *Ann. Hepatol.* 2010; 9: 40-5.

[17] Jimenez W, Rodes J. Impaired responsiveness to endogenous vasoconstrictors and endothelium-derived vasoactive factors in cirrhosis. *Gastroenterology* 1994; 107: 1201-3.

[18] Sieber CC. Endothelin and vascular reactivity in cirrhosis. *Hepatology* 1995; 22: 1609-11.

[19] Hartleb M, Moreau R, Cailmail S, Gaudin C, Lebrec D. Vascular hyporesponsiveness to endothelin 1 in rats with cirrhosis. *Gastroenterology* 1994; 107: 1085-93.

[20] Cahill PA, Redmond EM, Sitzmann JV. Endothelial dysfunction in cirrhosis and portal hypertension. *Pharmacol. Ther* .2001; 89: 273-93.

[21] Wong F. The use of TIPS in chronic liver disease. *Annals of Hepatology* 2006; 5: 5-15.

[22] Braverman AC, Steiner MA, Picus D, White H. High-output congestive heart failure following transjugular intrahepatic portal-systemic shunting. *Chest* 1995; 107: 1467-9.

[23] Pozzi M, Ratti L, Redaelli E, Guidi C, Mancia G. Cardiovascular abnormalities in special conditions of advanced cirrhosis. The circulatory adaptive changes to specific

therapeutic procedures for the management of refractory ascites. *Gastroenterol. Hepatol.* 2006; 29: 263-72.

[24] Cazzaniga M, Salerno F, Pagnozzi G, Dionigi E, Visentin S, Cirello I, Meregaglia D, et al. Diastolic dysfunction is associated with poor survival in patients with cirrhosis with transjugular intrahepatic portosystemic shunt. *Gut* 2007; 56: 869-75.

[25] Salerno F, Cazzaniga M, Pagnozzi G, Cirello I, Nicolini A, Meregaglia D, Burdick L. Humoral and cardiac effects of TIPS in cirrhotic patients with different "effective" blood volume. *Hepatology* 2003; 38: 1370-7.

[26] Ruzicka M, Skarda V, Leenen FHH. Effects of ACE inhibitors on circulating versus cardiac angiotensin II in volume overload-induced cardiac hypertrophy in rats. *Circulation* 1995; 92: 921-30.

[27] Wilke A, Funck R, Rupp H, Brilla CG. Effects of the renin-angiotensin-aldosterone system on the cardiac interstitium in heart failure. *Basic Res. Cardiol.* 1996; 91 (suppl 2) 79-84.

[28] Mancia G, Grassi G, Giannattasio C, Seravalle G. Sympathetic activation in the pathogenesis of hypertension and progression of organ damage. *Hypertension.* 1999; 34: 724-8.

[29] Ruiz del Arbol L, Urman J, Gonzales M, et al. Systemic, renal, and hepatic hemodynamic derangement in cirrhotic patients with spontaneous bacterial peritonitis. *Hepatology* 2003; 38: 1210-18.

[30] Rabie R, Cazzaniga M, Salerno M, Wong F. The use of E/A to predict the outcome of patients with cirrhosis treated with TIPS for complications of portal hypertension. *Am. J. Gastroenterology* 2009; 104: 2458-66.

Chapter XII

Hepatopulmonary Syndrome

*Pascal Fauconnet[1], Vincent Ho[2], Catherine Pastor[1]
and Eduardo Schiffer[1]**

[1]Hopitaux Universitaires de Geneve, 1205 Geneve, Switzerland
[2]School of Medicine, James Cook University Hospital, Department of Gastroenterology,
Townsville Hospital, Douglas Queensland 4810, Australia

Summary

Hepatopulmonary syndrome (HPS) is a pulmonary complication observed in patients with chronic liver disease and/or portal hypertension. HPS is attributable to an intrapulmonary vascular dilatation that induces severe hypoxemia. Considering the favorable long-term survival of HPS patients as well as the reversal of the syndrome with a functional liver graft, HPS is now an indication for liver transplantation (LT).

Both patients with mild cirrhosis who present with shortness of breath and all patients with end stage liver disease who are candidates for liver transplantation should undergo screening for HPS. Blood gas analysis and contrast-enhanced echocardiography are two main screening tools, together with lung function tests that can also detect additional pulmonary diseases that can contribute to impaired oxygenation.

If the partial pressure of oxygen in arterial blood (PaO_2) is > 80 mmHg, HPS can be excluded and no other investigation is needed. However, when PaO_2 is ≤ 80 mmHg, contrast-enhanced echocardiography should be performed to obtain evidence of or to exclude pulmonary vascular dilatation.

When the contrast-enhanced echocardiography is negative, HPS is excluded and no follow-up is needed. When the contrast-enhanced echocardiography is positive and PaO_2 < 60 mmHg, patients should obtain a severity score that provides them with a reasonable probability of being transplanted within 3 months. In mild-to-moderate HPS (60 mm Hg ≤ PaO_2 < 80 mmHg), periodic follow-up is recommended every 3 months to detect deterioration of PaO_2.

---

* Correspondence: Dr Eduardo Schiffer MD, Service of Anaesthesiology, Department APSI, Hospitaux Universitaires Geneve, Rue Gabrielle-Perret-Gentil 4, 1211 Geneve 14, Switzerland, Tel: +41 22 372 9366, Fax: +41 22 372 9366, E-mail: Eduardo.schiffer@hcuge.ch.

Although no intra-operative death has been directly attributed to HPS, the immediate post-LT oxygenation worsens in relation to the volume overload, and infections are commonly observed after LT surgery. Mechanical ventilation is often prolonged and the stay in the Intensive Care Unit is extended. A high postoperative mortality (mostly within 6 months) is observed in this group of patients in comparison with non-HPS patients. However, the recovery of an adequate PaO_2 within 12 months after LT explains the similar outcomes of HPS and non-HPS patients following LT.

Introduction

Because access to orthotopic liver transplantation (LT) has improved, an increasing number of candidates with impaired oxygenation that is attributable to hepatopulmonary syndrome (HPS)—which is a vascular pulmonary complication of liver disease—are included in the transplant waiting list. LT in patients with HPS was initially complicated by such high mortality that HPS was an absolute contraindication to LT twenty years ago. However, subsequent reports of better survival rates and the discovery that HPS disappears after graft replacement led to increased indications for LT in this group of patients. The aim of this review is to provide information on the management of HPS in LT candidates.

Diagnosis of Hepatopulmonary Syndrome

The diagnostic criteria of HPS associate impaired arterial oxygenation and intrapulmonary vascular dilatation in patients with chronic liver disease and/or portal hypertension (Table 1) [1]. Shortness of breath that may worsen on standing (platypnea) is a characteristic of HPS and likely reflects decreased oxygenation in patients moving from a supine to an upright position (orthodeoxia). When the patient is standing, the pulmonary blood flow is redistributed to the lower lung regions, thereby worsening pulmonary shunt and ventilation/perfusion mismatch [1]. Oxygen (O_2) diffusion impairment has also been described. Impaired arterial oxygenation is defined by a partial pressure of oxygen in arterial blood (PaO_2) ≤ 70 mmHg [1] or ≤ 80 mmHg [3]. Orthodeoxia is diagnosed when the decrease in PaO_2 is $\geq 5\%$ or ≥ 4 mmHg when the patient moves from a supine to an upright position [4]. Besides a $PaO_2 \leq 70$ or 80 mmHg, the definition of HPS and its severity score (Table 2) include an alveolar (A)-arterial (a) pressure gradient for O_2 ($AaPO_2$) ≥ 15 mmHg [3], ≥ 20 mmHg [2], or $\geq$ to the age-adjusted value [0.26 (age) - 0.43] [5]. $AaPO_2$ is calculated using atmospheric pressure (PB) at sea level, water vapor pressure at 37°C (47 mmHg), FIO_2 at room air (0.21). Assuming a ventilation/perfusion ratio of 0.8,

$P_AO_2 = [0.21 \times (PB - 47)] - (PaCO_2/0.8)$

$AaPO_2$ (mmHg) = $P_AO_2 - PaO_2$.

In HPS patients, low $PaCO_2$ results from an increase in alveolar ventilation. In the absence of pulmonary comorbidities, pulmonary function tests are within normal limits [4, 6].

Table 1. Diagnostic criteria of hepatopulmonary syndrome

Criteria 1: Chronic liver disease
Criteria 2: AaPO$_2$ ≥ 15 mmHg [3], or ≥ 20 mmHg [2], or ≥ to the age-adjusted value[a] [5] PaO$_2$ ≤ 80 mmHg [3] or ≤ 70 mmHg [2]
Criteria 3: Pulmonary vascular dilatation at contrast-enhanced echocardiography or ^{99m}TcMAA [3]

AaPO$_2$, alveolar-arterial pressure gradient for O$_2$.
[a] age-adjusted value: (0.26 x age) - 0.43
^{99m}TcMAA, perfusion body scan with Technetium-labeled macroaggregated albumin

Table 2. Severity score of hepatopulmonary syndrome

Stages	PaO$_2$ (mmHg)[a]
Mild	≥ 80
Moderate	60-80
Severe	50-60
Very severe	< 50

All stages also include an AaPO2 ≥ 15 mmHg.

A decrease in the single-breath diffusing capacity for carbon monoxide is the only routine pulmonary-function test that is consistently abnormal in patients with HPS [7]. However, the low diffusing capacity is not specific [8] and may not normalize (as do other gas exchange indexes) after liver transplantation.

Two techniques are used to confirm intrapulmonary vascular dilatation: contrast-enhanced echocardiography and perfusion lung scanning with ^{99m}technetium-labelled macroaggregated albumin (^{99m}Tc MAA). During transthoracic two-dimensional echocardiography, an intravenous injection of microbubbles is used to visualize the intrapulmonary shunt, which is defined by the appearance of microbubbles in the left heart 4-6 beats after the first appearance in the right heart (Figure 1). The timing of appearance in the left heart creates the distinction between the intrapulmonary and intracardiac shunt. In intracardiac shunts, microbubbles appear within 3 heartbeats in the left heart after the initial appearance in the right heart.

In normal subjects, perfusion lung scanning with ^{99m}Tc MAA shows macroaggregates that are almost completely trapped in the pulmonary circulation. In the presence of cardiac right-to-left shunts or intrapulmonary vascular dilatation, the uptake of ^{99m}Tc MAA can be visualized in other organs such as the brain or the spleen. Contrast-enhanced echocardiography seems more appropriate than scintigraphic perfusion scanning because it can differentiate between pulmonary and intracardiac shunts [1, 9].

Quantification of pulmonary shunts can be performed by several techniques. The oxymetric shunt ratio is estimated when patients are breathing 100% O$_2$. During lung perfusion scanning, the amount of ^{99m}Tc MAA injected is measured over the lungs and brain and the extrapulmonary shunt fraction is calculated assuming that the cerebral circulation receives approximately 13% of cardiac output.

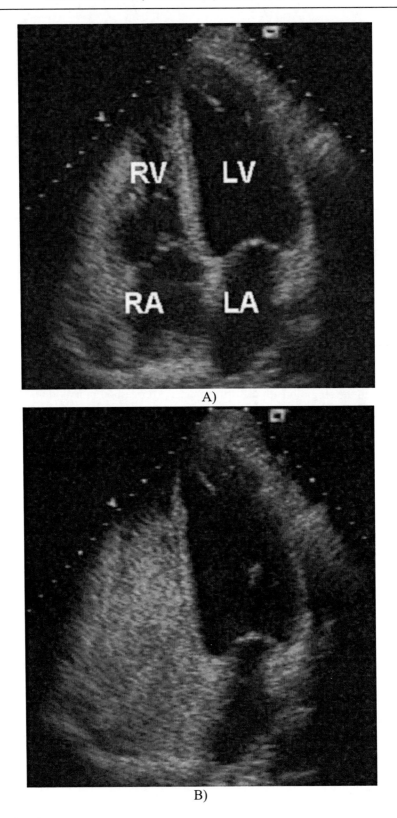

Figure 1 (Continued).

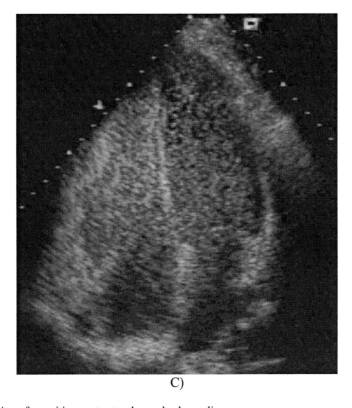

C)

Figure 1. Illustration of a positive contrast-enhanced echocardiogram.

A) A normal view of the four chambers of the heart in the absence of microbubbles. B) Four heartbeats after the injection of microbubbles, microbubbles are present in the right atrium (RA) and right ventricle (RV). C) Ten heartbeats after the injection of microbubbles, the left cardiac chambers (LA and LV) are filled with microbubbles. The timing of the appearance of microbubbles in the left heart distinguishes between an intrapulmonary shunt and an intracardiac shunt (with intracardiac shunts, microbubbles appear in the left heart within 3 heartbeats of their initial appearance in the right heart).

The pulmonary shunt fraction is increased if it is greater than 6%. Interestingly, an inverse relationship exists between the shunt fraction estimated by this technique and the arterial hypoxemia [9]. During contrast-enhanced echocardiography, the shunt can also be quantified according to the maximal echogenicity of the left atrium in comparison to that of the right atrium [10]: Grade 0, no microbubble; Grade 1, few bubbles without change in echogenicity; Grade 2, moderate microbubbles without complete filling; Grade 3, complete filling of the left atrium; Grade 4, same amount of bubbles in both atria. No correlation is shown between grades and arterial hypoxemia. Contrast injections provide a useful quantifiable indicator for detection of intrapulmonary shunts. Screening for HPS in patients with advanced cirrhosis should be done using contrast-enhanced echocardiography with patients in the upright position [11].

In patients with HPS, pulmonary angiography should be performed only when hypoxemia is severe (i.e., the partial pressure of oxygen is < 60 mmHg [8.0 kPa]), responds poorly to administration of 100% oxygen, and when there is a strong suspicion (on the basis of a chest computed tomography scan) of direct arterio-venous communication that would be amenable to embolization [12].

Pulse oximetry is a simple and widely available technique that reliably detects the presence and severity of hypoxemia in patients with HPS. With a threshold value of 96%, pulse oxymetry has a sensitivity and specificity of 100% and 88%, respectively, for detecting patients with a partial pressure of oxygen < 60 mmHg [13].

Pathogenesis of HPS

In patients with HPS, pulmonary vascular dilatation is attributed to a decreased vascular reactivity to constrictors, an increased response to vasodilators, and an impaired pulmonary hypoxic vasoconstriction. One of the mediators responsible for the vascular dilatation is nitric oxide (NO). Thus, an increased exhaled NO is measured in patients with HPS [14, 15]; exhaled NO decreases with the disappearance of HPS following LT [16, 17].

The pathogenesis of HPS has been more extensively studied in rats with biliary cirrhosis (Figure 2). Following ligation of the common bile duct, AaPO$_2$ increases concomitantly with the development of biliary cirrhosis and portal hypertension. In addition, pulmonary vascular dilatation is evidenced by an increased amount of microspheres injected in the femoral veins that pass through the pulmonary microcirculation [18-20]. High NO production in lungs is partly responsible for the vascular dilatation because chronic pharmacological inhibition of NO production prevents the occurrence of HPS [21]. NO originates from both endothelial constitutive and inducible forms of NO synthase (NOS); the inducible NOS is localized in pulmonary intravascular macrophages [21]. Following bile duct ligation in rats, the endothelial NOS expression in lungs increases over time and correlates with the onset of gas exchange abnormalities and pulmonary vascular dilatation [9, 22]. The pathophysiologic relationship between cirrhotic livers and pulmonary vascular dilatation may involve an overproduction of endothelin-1 by cirrhotic cholangiocytes and an increased expression of endothelin B receptors on pulmonary endothelial cells [23-25]. An excessive release of endothelin from the liver binds to endothelin B receptors on pulmonary endothelial cells releasing NO, which contributes to the pulmonary vascular dilatation. In contrast, the expression of endothelin A receptors on pulmonary vascular smooth muscle cells is not increased by the bile duct ligation, and the vascular contraction through endothelin is not enhanced [24].

In HPS rats, an increased expression of the inducible NOS in macrophages also contributes to the high pulmonary NO production [21]. Interestingly, prevention of bacterial translocation by norfloxacin (a quinolone predominantly active against Gram-negative bacteria) decreases the macrophage accumulation and the inducible NOS overexpression in lungs [26]. Because norfloxacin also reduces HPS severity, bacterial translocation is a key event in the pathophysiology of the disease. The tumor necrosis factor-α (TNF-α), which is a potent macrophage activator of iNOS, is increased in both cirrhotic patients and rats; however, interestingly, the TNF-α inhibitor pentoxifylline prevents HPS in rats [27].

Additionally, the high expression of heme oxygenase-1 in pulmonary macrophages participate in the pathogenesis of the pulmonary disease [25, 28]. Finally, Ca^{2+}-activated K^+ channels activation may be responsible for the blunted hypoxic pulmonary vasoconstriction that contributes to ventilation-perfusion mismatch and hypoxemia [28].

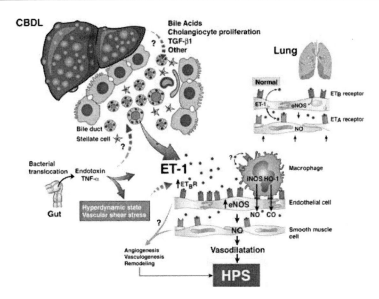

Figure 2. Hepatopulmonary syndrome: main findings in experimental and clinical studies.

Carbon monoxide (CO) and nitric oxide (NO) released by an increased expression of heme oxygenase 1 and inducible NO synthase (iNOS) pulmonary macrophages. Tumor-necrosis factor-α (TNF-α). Endothelial NO synthase (eNOS). Transforming growth factor-beta-1 (TGF-β1). Endothelin-1 (ET-1). See text for details. Reproduced from [38] with permission.

Treatment of HPS Patients who are on the Waiting List

Many pharmacological treatments have undergone clinical trials in the management of HPS. Small uncontrolled studies have reported a lack of efficacy with the use sympathomimethics, somatostatine, almitrine, indomethacin, and plasma exchange [29].

Consequently, oxygen administration is the only medical treatment used, and O$_2$ therapy should be considered at least during sleep and exercise for all HPS patients. Because no other medical treatment is available, eventually LT becomes a reasonable option for HPS patients.

However, pentoxifylline, a nonspecific phosphodiesterase-4 inhibitor, blocks TNF synthesis and TNF-induced macrophagic NO production. Pentoxifylline both attenuates and prevents the development of HPS in cirrhotic rats. Moreover, a recent pilot study shows improvement in clinical status after a 3 month period of treatment with pentoxifylline in cirrhotic adults with HPS [30].

Beneficial effects of inhaled prostaglandin including a decrease in respiratory symptoms and an improvement in oxygenation were recently described in patients with HPS [31].

An amplified production of pulmonary NO is thought to be important in development of this disorder in patients with liver cirrhosis. An inhibition of the effect of NO with methylene blue [32] or inhaled N(G)-nitro-L-arginine methyl ester [33] improves the hypoxemia or dyspnea associated with HPS.

In animal studies, administration of N-acetylcysteine showed an improvement in the liver enzymatic parameters and in arterial blood gases. This result suggests protective effects after treatment with N-acetylcysteine in cirrhotic rats with HPS [34].

Indications of LT and Liver Allocation in HPS Patients

All patients evaluated for LT must be screened for hypoxemia. When LT candidates have a $PaO_2 \leq 80$ mmHg and a $AaPO_2 \geq 15$ mmHg, contrast-enhanced echocardiography should be performed to evidence or exclude pulmonary vascular dilatation [1, 2]. When contrast-enhanced echocardiography is negative, HPS is excluded and no follow-up is necessary.

Because only a few patients with mild liver diseases may develop HPS over time, the pulmonary disease becomes the main problem [1]. Although LT can be performed to treat the pulmonary disease, no information is available on the number and outcomes of the patients with mild hepatic disease who benefit from LT because of the pulmonary complication.

LT for HPS is indicated only in severe hypoxemia ($PaO_2 < 60$ mmHg). Because HPS deteriorates over time, the severity of the syndrome should be regularly assessed while candidates are on the waiting list [2]. A 5 mmHg-decrease in PaO_2 each year has been documented in a small number of candidates., However, no prospective study determined the accuracy of pulse oximetry to detect deterioration of hypoxemia in patients who are on the waiting list. Moreover, because oxygen saturation by pulse oximetry overestimates PaO_2 [35], PaO_2 measurement should be regularly performed instead. A decrease in PaO_2 should also reflect an aggravation of pulmonary vascular dilatation and other causes of impaired oxygenation such as chronic obstructive pulmonary disease, bronchial asthma, and idiopathic pulmonary fibrosis should be excluded. Thus, 20-30% of patients with HPS have additional pulmonary abnormalities that impair oxygenation [36, 37].

Priorities for liver allocation are based on a severity score derived from total bilirubin and creatinine concentrations in serum as well as from the international normalized ratio, which is the Model for End-Stage Liver Disease (MELD) score. The United Network for Organ Sharing, the organization that controls organ allocation in the United States, applies a specific policy for LT candidates with HPS who benefit from a high priority to obtain a graft [38]. When contrast-enhanced echocardiography is positive and $PaO_2 < 60$ mmHg, patients obtain a MELD score that provides them a probability of being transplanted within 3 months [38, 39]. A similar policy has not been yet been defined in European countries.

Prevalence of HPS in LT Candidates

Before LT consideration, the prevalence of HPS among patients with liver diseases should vary from 4% to 24%, depending on the degree of hypoxemia chosen as the diagnostic criterion. New threshold values of impaired oxygenation were recently defined ($PaO_2 \leq 80$ mmHg and/or $AaPO_2 \geq 15$ mmHg) by the European Respiratory Society; these criteria should increase the homogeneity of future studies [1, 3]. In a recent study including 111 cirrhotic patients, 24 % had HPS [40].

The difficulty in assessing the prevalence of HPS in LT candidates is exacerbated because, as indicated in most previous studies, patients with severe hypoxemia were not included in the waiting list, or patients with minimal pulmonary vascular dilatation were not diagnosed as having HPS. In a recent prospective study from 2001 to 2004, there was a 10% prevalence of HPS among all candidates at the time of inclusion in the waiting list [6, 41].

Perioperative Management

Although no intraoperative death has been directly attributed to HPS (Table 3), there is evidence that immediate post-LT oxygenation worsens in relation to volume overload and infections commonly observed after major surgery. Mechanical ventilation is often prolonged and the stay in the Intensive Care Unit is extended [36]. Inhaled NO, intravenous methylene blue, and body positioning are used to improve peri-operative arterial oxygenation [36].

Mortality of HPS Patients

Before LT consideration, the 5-year survival rate is lower in patients with liver disease and HPS than in cirrhotic patients without pulmonary complication [2, 40]. Moreover, the survival rate is severely impaired when PaO2 is $\leq$ 60 mmHg. In contrast, the long term survival after LT is similar in patients with or without HPS [2]. Thus, LT is an indication in HPS patients because 1) they die earlier in the absence of LT and 2) HPS does not markedly impair the long-term survival rate of these patients after LT.

To determine the optimal time for LT in HPS patients, the survival after LT in HPS patients with preoperative PaO2 $\leq$ 60 mmHg was compared to that of HPS patients with preoperative PaO2 > 60 mmHg [2]. The long-term survival tends to be higher in patients who had a preoperative PaO2 > 60 mmHg in comparison with patients with a preoperative PaO2 $\leq$ 60 mmHg. Consequently, when contrast-enhanced echocardiography is positive and PaO2 < 60 mmHg, it seems reasonable to provide patients with the possibility of being transplanted within 3 months.

However, several studies found a high early postoperative mortality in HPS patients following LT: 9% within 3 months and 26 % within 12 months [42]; 16% [43] and 33% [6] within 6 months; 27% within 12 months [44]; and 9% within 20 months in a more recent study [45]. Causes of death were septic shock with multiple organ failure [6]; opportunistic pulmonary infection or abdominal sepsis [2]; abdominal sepsis or billiary duct leakage or hepatic vessel thrombosis [43]; multiple organ failure or ventilation-acquired pneumonia or cerebral hemorrhage or liver abscess [42]. A low preoperative PaO2 is either associated with an early postoperative mortality [2, 43, 44] or not [6, 42].

Thus, LT is an indication for HPS patients because they die earlier in the absence of LT and because the long-term survival is similar to that of non-HPS patients.

Table 3. Main studies on outcomes of HPS patients

Study characteristics	Main findings	References
HPS (33) LT performed (21) Two centers Retrospective study 2000-2008	Overall mortality 5%. Mortality in severe HPS (PaO$_2$ < 50 mmHg) 9%. Improved oxygenation in all 19 patients in whom PaO$_2$ were recorded (from 52.2±13.2 to 90.3±11.5 mmHg room air).	Gupta et al. [45]
HPS (31) Non-HPS (30) Single center Prospective study 2004-2006	26 of 31 HPS patients and all non-HPS patients underwent LT. Post operative survival rate 79% (immediate), 62% (1 year), 58% (4 years) in HPS patients. All HPS patients who did not receive LT died soon after evaluation (mean survival time was 34.4 days).	Yi et al. [47]
HPS (9)* Non-HPS (72) Single center Prospective study 2001-2004	No peroperative mortality. Postoperative mortality within 6 months: 33 % in HPS patients vs. 9% in non-HPS patients. All HPS patients had a 52 mmHg ≤ PaO$_2$ ≤ 70 mmHg. Improved postoperative PaO$_2$ in all patients who survived within 6 months	Schiffer et al. [6]
HPS (61) LT performed (24) LT denied (37) Non-HPS (77) LT performed (30) LT denied (47) Single center Retrospective study 1985 - 2002	LT increases the 5-year survival in HPS patients. Mean decline of PaO$_2$ awaiting LT is 5.2 ± 2.3 mmHg / year. No peroperative mortality. Long-term survival after LT is close in HPS and non-HPS patients. The long-term survival after LT of HPS patients tends to be higher when the preoperative PaO$_2$ > 60 mmHg. Resolution of the syndrome in all patients within 12 months.	Swanson et al. [2]
HPS = 40 Non-HPS (0) Multicenter Retrospective study Study period: 1996-2001	20 % HPS patients were denied LT (patients with the lower PaO$_2$). Early postoperative mortality in HPS patients: 16% (all patients who died had a low preoperative PaO$_2$).	Krowka et al. [43]
HPS (24) Non-HPS (0) Prospective study Two centers Study period: 1996-2001	27% of HPS patients died within 12 months. HPS more severe in patients who died. Resolution of the syndrome in all patients who survived.	Arguedas et al. [44]
HPS (6) Non-HPS (0) Single center Retrospective study Study period: 1993-1997	No postoperative mortality. Resolution of the syndrome in all patients.	Collisson et al. [46]
HPS (23) Non-HPS (0) Multicenter Retrospective study Study period: 1991-2000	9% postoperative mortality (within 3 months) and 26 % (within 12 months) No correlation between preoperative PaO$_2$ and death Resolution of the syndrome in most patients The lower the preoperative PaO$_2$, the longer the time of normal PaO$_2$ recovery	Taillé et al. [42]

(x) = number of patients included.

However, a high mortality within 6 months in HPS patients should be kept in mind. Future studies should confirm these findings as well as the UNOS policy suggesting providing HPS patients with the possibility of being transplanted within 3 months when the preoperative PaO2 is < 60 mmHg.

Evolution of HPS after LT

Besides the favorable long-term survival rate, another reason to perform LT in patients with HPS is the reversal of impaired oxygenation after LT [42, 45]. Correction of hypoxemia occurs as early as 6-10 months after LT [6, 46]. The time for reversibility may be longer with severe HPS. An increased recovery time is observed when PaO_2 is ≤ 52 mmHg, $AaPO_2$ is ≥ 66 mmHg, age is > 48 years, or if the liver disease is due to alcohol abuse [42]. No study investigated whether a delayed recovery might parallel graft dysfunction. Finally, a delayed resolution of HPS may explain the increased mortality observed within 6 months following LT.

Conclusion

Hepatopulmonary syndrome (HPS) is a pulmonary complication observed in patients with chronic liver disease and/or portal hypertension. HPS is attributable to an intrapulmonary vascular dilatation that induces severe hypoxemia. HPS is now an indication for liver transplantation (LT).

A high postoperative mortality (mostly within 6 months) is observed in this group of patients in comparison with non-HPS patients. However, the recovery of an adequate PaO_2 within 12 months after LT explains the similar outcomes of HPS and non-HPS patients following LT.

References

[1] Rodriguez-Roisin R, Krowka MJ, Herve P, Fallon MB: Highlights of the ERS Task Force on pulmonary-hepatic vascular disorders (PHD). *J Hepatol* 2005;42:924-7.

[2] Swanson KL, Wiesner RH, Krowka MJ: Natural history of hepatopulmonary syndrome: Impact of liver transplantation. *Hepatology* 2005;41:1122-9.

[3] Rodriguez-Roisin R, Krowka MJ, Herve P, Fallon MB: Pulmonary-hepatic vascular disorders (PHD). *Eur Resp. J* 2004; 24(5):861-80.

[4] Gomez FP, Martinez-Palli G, Barbera JA, Roca J, Navasa M, Rodriguez-Roisin R: Gas exchange mechanism of orthodeoxia in hepatopulmonary syndrome. *Hepatology* 2004;40:660-6.

[5] Gaines DI, Fallon MB: Hepatopulmonary syndrome. *Liver Int* 2004; 24: 397-401.

[6] Schiffer E, Majno P, Mentha G, Giostra E, Burri H, Klopfenstein CE, Beaussier M, Morel P, Hadengue A, Pastor CM: Hepatopulmonary syndrome increases the postoperative mortality rate following liver transplantation: a prospective study in 90 patients. *Am J Transpl* 2006;6:1430-7.

[7] Martinez GP, Barbera JA, Visa J, Rimola A, Pare JC, Roca J, Navasa M, Rodes J, Rodriguez-Roisin R: Hepatopulmonary syndrome in candidates for liver transplantation. *J Hepatol* 2001;34:651-7.

[8] Lima BL, Franca AV, Pazin-Filho A, Araujo WM, Martinez JA, Maciel BC, Simoes MV, Terra-Filho J, Martinelli AL: Frequency, clinical characteristics, and respiratory parameters of hepatopulmonary syndrome. *Mayo Clin Proc* 2004;79:42-8.

[9] Luo B, Abrams GA, Fallon MB: Endothelin-1 in the rat bile duct ligation model of hepatopulmonary syndrome: correlation with pulmonary dysfunction. *J Hepatol* 1998;29: 571-8.

[10] Kim BJ, Lee SC, Park SW, Choi MS, Koh KC, Paik SW, Lee SH, Hong KP, Park JE, Seo JD: Characteristics and prevalence of intrapulmonary shunt detected by contrast echocardiography with harmonic imaging in liver transplant candidates. *Am J Cardiol* 2004;94:525-8.

[11] Lenci I, Alvior A, Manzia TM, Toti L, Neuberger J, Steeds R: Saline contrast echocardiography in patients with hepatopulmonary syndrome awaiting liver transplantation. *J Am Soc Echocardiogr* 2009; 22: 89-94.

[12] Poterucha JJ, Krowka MJ, Dickson ER, Cortese DA, Stanson AW, Krom RA: Failure of hepatopulmonary syndrome to resolve after liver transplantation and successful treatment with embolotherapy. *Hepatology* 1995; 21: 96-100

[13] Arguedas MR, Singh H, Faulk DK, Fallon MB: Utility of pulse oximetry screening for hepatopulmonary syndrome. *Clin Gastroenterol Hepatol* 2007; 5: 749-54

[14] Cremona G, Higenbottam TW, Mayoral V, Alexander G, Demoncheaux E, Borland C, Roe P, Jones GJ: Elevated exhaled nitric oxide in patients with hepatopulmonary syndrome. *Eur Respir J* 1995; 8: 1883-5.

[15] Rolla G: Hepatopulmonary syndrome: role of nitric oxide and clinical aspects. *Dig Liver Dis* 2004; 36: 303-8.

[16] Rolla G, Brussino L, Colagrande P, Scappaticci E, Morello M, Bergerone S, Ottobrelli A, Cerutti E, Polizzi S, Bucca C: Exhaled nitric oxide and impaired oxygenation in cirrhotic patients before and after liver transplantation. *Ann Intern Med* 1998; 129: 375-8.

[17] Battaglia SE, Pretto JJ, Irving LB, Jones RM, Angus PW: Resolution of gas exchange abnormalities and intrapulmonary shunting following liver transplantation. *Hepatology* 1997; 25: 1228-32.

[18] Chang SW, Ohara N: Pulmonary circulatory dysfunction in rats with biliary cirrhosis. An animal model of the hepatopulmonary syndrome. *Am Rev Respir Dis* 1992; 145: 798-805

[19] Fallon MB, Abrams GA, McGrath JW, Hou Z, Luo B: Common bile duct ligation in the rat: a model of intrapulmonary vasodilation and hepatopulmonary syndrome. *Am J. Physiol* 1997; 272:G779-84.

[20] Schraufnagel DE, Malik R, Goel V, Ohara N, Chang SW: Lung capillary change in hepatic cirrhosis in rats. *Am J Physiol* 1997; 272:L139-47.

[21] Nunes H, Lebrec D, Mazmanian M, Capron F, Heller J, Tazi KA, Zerbib E, Dulmet E, Moreau R, Dinh-Xuan A, Simmoneau G, Hervé P: Role of nitric oxide in hepatopulmonary syndrome in cirrhotic rats. *Am. J. Respir. Crit Care Med* 2001;164:879-885.

[22] Fallon MB, Abrams GA, Luo B, Hou Z, Dai J, Ku DD: The role of endothelial nitric oxide in the pathogenesis of a rat model of hepatopulmonary syndrome. *Gastroenterology* 1997; 13: 606-14.

[23] Luo B, Tang L, Wang Z, Zhang J, Ling Y, Feng W, Sun JZ, Stockard CR, Frost AR, Chen YF, Grizzle WE, Fallon MB: Cholangiocyte endothelin 1 and transforming growth factor beta1 production in rat experimental hepatopulmonary syndrome. *Gastroenterology* 2005;129: 682-95

[24] Ling Y, Zhang J, Luo B, Song D, Liu L, Tang L, Stockard CR, Grizzle WE, Ku DD, Fallon MB: The role of endothelin-1 and the endothelin B receptor in the pathogenesis of hepatopulmonary syndrome in the rat. *Hepatology* 2004;39:1593-602.

[25] Luo B, Liu L, Tang L, Zhang J, Stockard CR, Grizzle WE, Fallon MB: Increased pulmonary vascular endothelin B receptor expression and responsiveness to endothelin-1 in cirrhotic and portal hypertensive rats: a potential mechanism in experimental hepatopulmonary syndrome. *J Hepatol* 2003;38:556-63.

[26] Rabiller A, Nunes N, Lebrec D, Tazi KA, Wartski M, Dulmet E, Libert JM, Mougeot C, Moreau R, Mazmanian M, Humbert M, Hervé P: Prevention of Gram-negative translocation reduces the severity of hepatopulmonary syndrome. *Am J Resp Crit Care Med* 2002;166:514-517

[27] Sztrymf B, Rabiller A, Nunes H, Savale L, Lebrec D, Le Pape A, de Montpreville V, Mazmanian M, Humbert M, Hervé P: Prevention of hepatopumonary syndrome and hyperdynamic state by pentoxifylline in cirrhotic rats. *Eur Resp J* 2004; 23: 752-8.

[28] Imamura M, Luo B, Limbird JN, Vitello AM, Oka M, Ivy DD, McMurtry IF, Garat CV, Fallon MB, Carter EP: Hypoxic Pulmonary Hypertension is Prevented in Rats with Common Bile Duct Ligation. *J Appl Physiol* 2004; 29:29

[29] Rodriquez-Roisin R, Krowka MJ, Herve P, Fallon MB: Highlights of the ERS Task Force on pulmonary-hepatic vascular disorders (PHD). *J Hepatol* 2005; 42: 924-7

[30] Gupta LB, Kumar A, Jaiswal AK, Yusuf J, Mehta V, Tyagi S, Tempe DK, Sharma BC, Sarin SK: Pentoxifylline therapy for hepatopulmonary syndrome: a pilot study. *Arch Intern Med* 2008;168:1820-3.

[31] Krug S, Seyfarth HJ, Hagendorff A, Wirtz H: Inhaled iloprost for hepatopulmonary syndrome: improvement of hypoxemia. *Eur J Gastroenterol Hepatol* 2007; 19:1140-3.

[32] Rolla G, Bucca C, Brussino L: Methylene blue in the hepatopulmonary syndrome. *N Engl J Med* 1994; 331:1098

[33] Brussino L, Bucca C, Morello M, Scappaticci E, Mauro M, Rolla G: Effect on dyspnoea and hypoxaemia of inhaled N(G)-nitro-L-arginine methyl ester in hepatopulmonary syndrome. *Lancet* 2003; 362: 43-4

[34] Vercelino R, Tieppo J, Dias AS, Marroni CA, Garcia E, Meurer L, Picada JN, Marroni NP: N-acetylcysteine effects on genotoxic and oxidative stress parameters in cirrhotic rats with hepatopulmonary syndrome. *Basic Clin Pharmacol Toxicol* 2008;102:370-6'

[35] Abrams GA, Sanders MK, Fallon MB: Utility of pulse oximetry in the detection of arterial hypoxemia in liver transplant candidates. *Liver Transpl* 2002; 8: 391-396

[36] Arguedas MR, Drake BB, Kapoor A, Fallon MB: Carboxyhemoglobin levels in cirrhotic patients with and without hepatopulmonary syndrome. *Gastroenterology* 2005;128: 328-33.

[37] Krowka MJ: Hepatopulmonary syndrome and portopulmonary hypertension: implications for liver transplantation. Clin. Chest Med. 2005; 26: 587-597

[38] Palma DT, Fallon MB: The hepatopulmonary syndrome. *J Hepatol* 2006; 45: 617-25.

[39] UNOS:www.unos.org/policiesandbylaws/policies.asp?ressources=true.Organ distribution: allocation of livers

[40] Schenk P, Schoniger-Hekele M, Fuhrmann V, Madl C, Silberhumer G, Muller C: Prognostic significance of the hepatopulmonary syndrome in patients with cirrhosis. *Gastroenterology* 2003;125:1042-52.

[41] Mohamed R, Freeman JW, Guest PJ, Davies MK, Neuberger JM: Pulmonary gas exchange abnormalities in liver transplant candidates. *Liver Transpl* 2002;8:802-8

[42] Taille C, Cadranel J, Bellocq A, Thabut G, Soubrane O, Durand F, Ichai P, Duvoux C, Belghiti J, Calmus Y, Mal H: Liver transplantation for hepatopulmonary syndrome: a ten-year experience in Paris, France. *Transplantation* 2003;75:1482-9.

[43] Krowka MJ, Mandell MS, Ramsay MA, Kawut SM, Fallon MB, Manzarbeitia C, Pardo M, Marotta P, Uemoto S, Stoffel MP, Benson JT: Hepatopulmonary syndrome and portopulmonary hypertension: a report of the multicenter liver transplant database. *Liver Transpl* 2004;10:174-182

[44] Arguedas MR, Abrams GA, Krowka MJ, Fallon MB: Prospective evaluation of outcomes and predictors of mortality in patients with hepatopulmonary syndrome undergoing liver transplantation. *Hepatology* 2003;37:192-7.

[45] Gupta S, Castel H, Rao RV, Picard M, Lilly L, Faughnan ME, Pomier-Layrargues G: Improved Survival After Liver Transplantation in Patients with Hepatopulmonary Syndrome. *Am J Transplant* 2010;10(2):354-63.

[46] Collisson EA, Nourmand H, Fraiman MH, Cooper CB, Bellamy PE, Farmer DG, Vierling JM, Ghobrial RM, Busuttil RW: Retrospective analysis of the results of liver transplantation for adults with severe hepatopulmonary syndrome. *Liver Transpl* 2002;8: 925-31.

[47] Yi HM, Wang GS, Yi SH, Yang Y, Cai CJ, Chen GH: Prospective evaluation of postoperative outcome after liver transplantation in hepatopulmonary syndrome patients. *Chin Med J* 2009;122: 2598-602.

Chapter XIII

Pre-Operative Assessment of Cardiovascular Function before Liver Transplantation: A Practical Approach

James Y. Findlay[*]
Department of Anesthesiology and Critical Care Medicine
Mayo Clinic, Rochester MN 55905, USA

Abstract

Liver transplantation surgery presents a considerable cardiovascular challenge, and cardiovascular complications are one of the most frequent causes of both early and late transplant-related morbidity and mortality. Coronary artery disease is common; the identification of this and specific cirrhosis-related entities such as cirrhotic cardiomyopathy, portopulmonary hypertension and hepatopulmonary syndrome can result in significant alterations in management. Thus, cardiovascular assessment should be part of the routine evaluation of liver transplant candidates. All patients should have an appropriate history and physical examination, a 12-lead electrocardiogram and a resting echocardiogram. Evaluation for coronary artery disease should be in a protocolized, step-wise manner with non-invasive testing for selected at-risk patients and angiographic confirmation of positive studies. Currently, there is controversy between different published guidelines regarding which patients should undergo non-invasive testing; until further research clarifies the optimum strategy, transplant teams should make reasoned decisions regarding their own practice.

---

[*] Correspondence: James Y. Findlay, Consultant, Department of Anesthesiology and Critical Care Medicine, Mayo Clinic, First St S.W. Rochester MN 55905, USA, E-mail: Findlay.James@mayo.edu.

Introduction

Cardiovascular morbidity and mortality are frequent among patients who have undergone liver transplant, in both the early post-operative period [1] and the long term [2,3]. Patients with end-stage liver disease (ESLD) presenting for pre-liver transplantation evaluation have a significant prevalence of coronary artery disease (CAD) [4] as well as potential limitations in cardiovascular reserve secondary to cirrhotic cardiomyopathy [5]. Thus, liver transplantation surgery represents a considerable cardiovascular challenge. In an uncomplicated procedure there are significant changes in cardiac pre-load associated with the clamping and unclamping of the inferior vena cava, in addition to the potential for arrhythmia, myocardial stunning and hypotension following recirculation of the transplanted organ [6,7]. In the complicated case significant haemorrhage, sometimes sudden and substantial, can occur, necessitating massive transfusion; the surgical approach may necessitate aortic clamping (and subsequent unclamping), further increasing the potential cardiovascular stress.

For these reasons, for many years there has been interest in pre-transplant cardiovascular screening of liver transplant candidates. The first widely disseminated schema for screening [8] closely followed the first report of worrisome mortality and morbidity in patients with CAD undergoing liver transplantation [9]. Since then there have been considerable advances in the understanding of cardiovascular diseases in the ESLD and liver transplant populations, as well as considerable controversy about the appropriate means to investigate liver transplant candidates for cardiovascular comorbidities and to manage those who present with these conditions. These issues are dealt with in detail in Chapter 2-6; the aim of this chapter is to outline a practical approach for the pre-operative cardiovascular assessment of liver transplant candidates.

The most widely used guidelines for the cardiovascular assessment of patients undergoing non-cardiac surgery are those produced by the American College of Cardiology and the American Heart Association (ACC/AHA). These are regularly updated, most recently in 2007 [10,11]. In addition to revisions of the full document, focused updates are issued whenever there are significant developments in one of the areas covered (e.g. perioperative beta-blockade in 2009 [12]). A review of the pertinent literature is produced and the guidelines are evidence-based as far as is feasible; beyond that point the recommendations are a combination of expert opinion and consensus. While not specific to liver transplantation, the ACC/AHA guidelines provide a useful framework with which to approach the pre-operative cardiovascular evaluation of any patient and are also an excellent resource regarding the various topics to which the interested reader is referred. Similar information, with comparable though not identical conclusions, can be found in the latest European Society of Cardiology (ESC) and European Society of Anesthesiology (ESA) guidelines for peri-operative cardiac risk assessment and management in non-cardiac surgery [13].

Pre-Liver Transplant Assessment

ESLD and, to a greater or lesser extent, the expected cardiovascular and other pathophysiological changes seen with this condition (see Chapter 1). There are also patients without liver failure, most of whom will be undergoing transplantation for tumour; these patients will have a more normal baseline cardiovascular profile. A suggested schema for cardiovascular evaluation for liver transplantation is outlined in Table 1. Whatever the details of cardiovascular assessment undertaken in any single institution, a clinical protocol should be used for every patient evaluated. A consistent approach avoids the confusion of variable approaches to evaluation and also allows a clearer comparison of outcomes.

Table 1. Suggested cardiovascular evaluation schema for liver transplant candidates

All patients	History and physical
	12-lead ECG
	Chest X-ray
	Echocardiogram
Selected "CAD risk" patients	Non-invasive stress testing (DSE preferred)
If non-invasive test positive	Coronary angiography

CAD: coronary artery disease; DSE: dobutamine stress echo.

History and Physical Examination

As with any patient evaluation, the first stage is to take a relevant history and perform a physical examination. It should be noted whether there is any history of prior ischaemic heart disease, whether the patient has had a myocardial infarction and what treatment (medical or surgical, operative or percutaneous intervention) has been undertaken. If the patient has coronary artery stents it should be ascertained whether these are bare metal or drug-eluting and when they were placed. Current symptoms concerning for a cardiac cause should be sought in all patients. Other major clinical risk factors for peri-operative cardiovascular morbidity should be noted: in addition to ischaemic heart disease, these include compensated or prior heart failure, diabetes mellitus, renal insufficiency and cerebrovascular disease [14] (Table 2). Other cardiac risk factors should also be noted, including a family history of early cardiac disease, current or past tobacco smoking, and a history of hyperlipidaemia or hypertension. For the latter it should be noted that the haemodynamic changes associated with ESLD may result in a hypertensive patient no longer requiring antihypertensive management at the time of transplant evaluation.

An assessment of the patient's exercise capacity should be made. Reported exercise capacity is linked to peri-operative cardiovascular risk [15], with a capacity of more than 4 metabolic equivalents (METs) being associated with low risk. Four METs is approximated by the ability to climb a flight of stairs or walk at a brisk pace. Fatigue and shortness of breath are commonly seen secondary to liver disease, so exercise tolerance may be limited in ESLD patients for reasons unrelated to cardiovascular ones.

The physical examination should include measurement of vital signs, assessment of cardiac rhythm, cardiac and pulmonary auscultation, and evaluation for peripheral oedema. Aortic ejection murmurs are common in ESLD as a result of the high flow state.

Table 2. Major risk factors for peri-operative cardiovascular complications

History of ischemic heart disease
Compensated or prior heart failure
Diabetes mellitus
Renal insufficiency
Cerebrovascular disease

Modified from Lee [14], Fleisher [10], and Poldermans [13])

Investigations

All patients should have a 12-lead electrocardiogram performed and a chest X-ray obtained. All patients should have a resting echocardiogram. This allows assessment of baseline left ventricular function and an estimate of cardiac output, as well as evaluation for regional wall motion abnormalities suggestive of any previous infarction. Any valvular abnormalities can be identified and quantified. In addition, evaluation of right ventricular systolic pressure (and hence pulmonary artery systolic pressure) using Doppler estimation of tricuspid regurgitant flow allows initial screening for portopulmonary hypertension; a value >50 mmHg should instigate further investigation [16]. An echo-contrast injection using agitated saline can also be performed; delayed opacification of the left cardiac chambers suggests hepatopulmonary syndrome. Again, patients suspected of this should undergo further specialized evaluation.

Further Testing

It is in the area of further testing for CAD that the current practice for liver transplant candidates differs most from the ACC/AHA guidelines. The ACC/AHA step-wise approach to cardiac evaluation in patients over 50 years of age is shown in Figure 1. A considerable number of liver transplant candidates will reach step 5 (functional capacity less than 4 METs). Liver transplantation is regarded as 'intermediate-risk surgery', hence those with 1–3 major risk factors (ischaemic heart disease, compensated or prior heart failure, diabetes mellitus, renal insufficiency and cerebrovascular disease) are recommended either to proceed to surgery with no further testing or to undergo further evaluation if management would be changed.

The ESC/ESA guidelines give similar recommendations, again suggesting that non-invasive testing may be appropriate if peri-operative management may be altered by the results [13]. Many in the field would argue that the potential to exclude or discover CAD in liver transplant candidates would alter pre-operative and peri-operative management. In contrast to the ACC/AHA guidelines, the most recent American Association for the Study of Liver Diseases (AASLD) practice guidelines state that 'chronic smokers, patients over the age of 50 and those with a clinical or family history of heart disease or diabetes' should undergo further evaluation for CAD [17] (Table 3). Clearly, use of the AASLD guidelines will result in more patients undergoing further testing than would do were ACC/AHA or ESC/ESA recommendations followed. As the proportion of patients undergoing further testing increases, the likelihood of missing a true case of CAD decreases, but at the expense of an increasing false positive rate. This issue is discussed further in the Chapter 2.

Table 3. AASLD recommendations for non-invasive testing. Adapted from [17]

Age >50 years
Chronic smokers
Diabetes mellitus
Clinical or family history of heart disease

AASLD: American Association for the Study of Liver Diseases.

Currently, the practice in most liver transplant programmes (at least in the United States) is to use a protocol similar to the AASLD guidelines. The favoured strategy is to proceed to non-invasive testing, with dobutamine stress echocardiography (DSE) currently being the most frequently used and recommended test [17]. Pharmacological testing with radionucleotide myocardial perfusion imaging is an alternative, but the proficiency of the local stress-testing laboratory should be considered in choosing which method to employ. There is further discussion of non-invasive testing in Chapter 14. Given the uncertainty of the clinical evidence and the lack of consensus in expert opinion on proceeding to further cardiac evaluation in liver transplant candidates, each centre should consider and establish what criteria it will use. These should be re-evaluated at regular intervals based on both new evidence and the experience of the programme. Patients who have a non-invasive test result consistent with CAD should then go on to coronary angiography to confirm or refute the presence of CAD and to determine the extent and significance of the coronary artery lesions.

An alternative approach that is currently used in some programmes is to identify candidates considered to be at high risk of CAD and send them for coronary angiography without prior non-invasive testing. The logic of this approach is the avoidance of the high false-positive rate of non-invasive testing; however, depending on what criteria are used to select patients for coronary angiography, this may result in an increased number of coronary angiograms being performed. Currently the available evidence is inadequate to evaluate this strategy.

Management and Disposition

The patient who is cleared from a cardiovascular standpoint can go ahead to transplantation with the expectation of a low (but not zero) risk for peri-operative cardiovascular risk. The patient identified as having CAD requires both appropriate management for this and consideration of liver transplant candidacy given the increased risk of cardiovascular events. Unfortunately there is little good-quality evidence to guide the clinician toward the best approach to such patients. Until such evidence is available, each case should be evaluated by both the liver transplant team and a consulting cardiologist familiar with peri-operative and post-operative issues in liver transplantation to arrive at an appropriate management strategy that is in the best interests of each individual patient. Management strategies for the patient identified as having CAD are discussed in the Chapter 2.

The Patient with Known CAD

The presence of CAD is only one of the major risk factors used for cardiovascular risk stratification in current general pre-operative guidelines (see Table 2) [10,13] and has no special weighting. The liver transplant candidate with known CAD should have a functional assessment; if exercise capacity is poor or difficult to evaluate then a non-invasive test is indicated unless a recently performed adequate study is available. The need for coronary angiography should be evaluated on an individualized basis depending on the patient's symptomatology, results of non-invasive testing (if performed) and prior cardiac interventions and imaging. The appropriateness of the patient's current CAD management should be reviewed with a cardiologist, preferably one aware of the particular issues involved in liver transplantation and the post-operative period. Once this information is obtained the clinician is in the same position as that noted above for the patient identified as having CAD during the evaluation process and individualized patient decisions have to be reached regarding the appropriate management strategy.

Conclusion

Every patient being considered for liver transplantation merits a cardiovascular assessment. This should be carried out in a protocolized, step-wise approach with each patient undergoing basic clinical evaluation and testing, with further specialized evaluation and testing if indicated. Current practice favours the use of non-invasive screening tests in patients considered at higher risk of CAD, with confirmatory coronary angiography in those who test positive, although there are several controversies in this area. Each transplant programme should examine the available evidence and decide upon their own protocol, performing reviews at regular intervals.

References

[1] Fouad TR, Abdel-Razek WM, Burak KW, Bain VG, Lee SS. Prediction of cardiac complications after liver transplantation. *Transplantation* 2009;87(5):763–70.
[2] Johnston SD, Morris JK, Cramb R, Gunson BK, Neuberger J. Cardiovascular morbidity and mortality after orthotopic liver transplantation. *Transplantation* 2002;73(6):901–6.

[3] Pruthi J, Medkiff KA, Esrason KT, Donovan JA, Yoshida EM, Erb SR, et al. Analysis of causes of death in liver transplant recipients who survived more than 3 years. *Liver Transpl.* 2001;7(9):811–15.

[4] Carey WD, Dumot JA, Pimentel RR, Barnes DS, Hobbs RE, Henderson JM, et al. The prevalence of coronary artery disease in liver transplant candidates over age 50. *Transplantation* 1995;59(6):859–64.

[5] Henriksen JH, Moller S. Cardiac and systemic haemodynamic complications of liver cirrhosis. *Scand. Cardiovasc J.* 2009;43(4):218–25.

[6] Paugam-Burtz C, Kavafyan J, Merckx P, Dahmani S, Sommacale D, Ramsay M, et al. Postreperfusion syndrome during liver transplantation for cirrhosis: outcome and predictors. *Liver Transpl.* 2009;15(5):522–9.

[7] Hilmi I, Horton CN, Planinsic RM, Sakai T, Nicolau-Raducu R, Damian D, et al. The impact of postreperfusion syndrome on short-term patient and liver allograft outcome in patients undergoing orthotopic liver transplantation. *Liver Transpl* 2008;14(4):504–8.

[8] Plevak DJ. Stress echocardiography identifies coronary artery disease in liver transplant candidates. *Liver Transpl. Surg.* 1998;4(4):337–9.

[9] Plotkin JS, Scott VL, Pinna A, Dobsch BP, De Wolf AM, Kang Y. Morbidity and mortality in patients with coronary artery disease undergoing orthotopic liver transplantation. *Liver Transpl. Surg.* 1996;2(6):426–30.

[10] Fleisher LA, Beckman JA, Brown KA, Calkins H, Chaikof EL, Fleischmann KE, et al. ACC/AHA 2007 Guidelines on Perioperative Cardiovascular Evaluation and Care for Noncardiac Surgery: Executive Summary: a report of the American College of Cardiology/American Heart Association Task Force on Practice Guidelines (Writing Committee to revise the 2002 Guidelines on Perioperative Cardiovascular Evaluation for Noncardiac Surgery) developed in collaboration with the American Society of Echocardiography, American Society of Nuclear Cardiology, Heart Rhythm Society, Society of Cardiovascular Anesthesiologists, Society for Cardiovascular Angiography and Interventions, Society for Vascular Medicine and Biology, and Society for Vascular Surgery. *J. Am. Coll. Cardiol.* 2007;50(17):1707–32.

[11] Fleisher LA, Beckman JA, Brown KA, Calkins H, Chaikof EL, Fleischmann KE, et al. ACC/AHA 2007 Guidelines on Perioperative Cardiovascular Evaluation and Care for Noncardiac Surgery: a report of the American College of Cardiology/American Heart Association Task Force on Practice Guidelines (Writing Committee to revise the 2002 Guidelines on Perioperative Cardiovascular Evaluation for Noncardiac Surgery) developed in collaboration with the American Society of Echocardiography, American Society of Nuclear Cardiology, Heart Rhythm Society, Society of Cardiovascular Anesthesiologists, Society for Cardiovascular Angiography and Interventions, Society for Vascular Medicine and Biology, and Society for Vascular Surgery. *J. Am. Coll. Cardiol.* 2007;50(17):e159–241.

[12] Fleischmann KE, Beckman JA, Buller CE, Calkins H, Fleisher LA, Freeman WK, et al. 2009 ACCF/AHA Focused Update on Perioperative Beta Blockade: a report of the American College of Cardiology Foundation/American Heart Association Task Force on Practice Guidelines. *Circulation* 2009;120(21):2123–51.

[13] Poldermans D, Bax JJ, Boersma E, De Hert S, Eeckhout E, Fowkes G, et al. Guidelines for Pre-Operative Cardiac Risk Assessment and Perioperative Cardiac Management in Non-Cardiac Surgery: the Task Force for Preoperative Cardiac Risk Assessment and

Perioperative Cardiac Management in Non-cardiac Surgery of the European Society of Cardiology (ESC) and endorsed by the European Society of Anaesthesiology (ESA). *Eur. Heart J.* 2009;30(22):2769–812.

[14] Lee TH, Marcantonio ER, Mangione CM, Thomas EJ, Polanczyk CA, Cook EF, et al. Derivation and prospective validation of a simple index for prediction of cardiac risk of major noncardiac surgery. *Circulation* 1999;100(10):1043–9.

[15] Reilly DF, McNeely MJ, Doerner D, Greenberg DL, Staiger TO, Geist MJ, et al. Self-reported exercise tolerance and the risk of serious perioperative complications. *Arch. Intern. Med.* 1999;159(18):2185–92.

[16] Krowka MJ, Swanson KL, Frantz RP, McGoon MD, Wiesner RH. Portopulmonary hypertension: results from a 10-year screening algorithm. *Hepatology* 2006;44(6):1502–10.

[17] Murray KF, Carithers RL, Jr. AASLD practice guidelines: evaluation of the patient for liver transplantation. *Hepatology* 2005;41(6):1407–32.

In: Cardiovascular Diseases and Liver Transplantation
Editor: Zoka Milan, pp. 201-215

ISBN: 978-1-61122-910-3
© 2011 Nova Science Publishers, Inc.

Chapter XIV

A Role of Cardiopulmonary Exercise Testing (CPET) in Defining Cardiopulmonary Function before Liver Transplantation

James Prentis and Chris Snowden*

Department of Anaesthesia, Freeman Hospital, Newcastle Upon Tyne, UK

Abstract

Cardiorespiratory assessment is an important component of overall risk assessment in liver transplant candidates, especially in asymptomatic patients. Current investigative methods, often lack specificity and isolate cardiac and respiratory function rather than applying an integrative approach to assessment. Cardiopulmonary exercise testing gives an indication of the combined reserve of the cardiorespiratory system when under stress. In the peri-operative period, similar demands are placed on these organ systems to support an increase in metabolic rate. In this chapter, we review the evidence for the use of cardiopulmonary exercise testing in the assessment of patients planned to undergo liver transplantation.

Introduction

Elective liver transplantation is associated with significant mortality and morbidity in the immediate post transplantation period. Improvements in both surgical technique and donor organ management have emphasised the importance of cardiorespiratory dysfunction in the

---

[*] Correspondence: James Prentis MRCP FRCA, Consultant Anaesthetist, Department of Anaesthesia, Freeman Hospital, Newcastle Upon Tyne, NE7 7DN, Tel: +44 191 233 6161, E-mail: jamesprentis@btinternet.com.

development of early postoperative complications. As a consequence, the recognition and preoperative assessment of coexisting cardiorespiratory disease and abnormal function forms an integral component of overall risk assessment. In this chapter, we discuss current methods of preoperative risk assessment for early liver transplantation outcome, primarily focusing on Cardiopulmonary exercise testing (CPET) for cardiorespiratory functional assessment.

Multifactorial Models of Risk

Whilst the severity of liver disease as defined by the Model for End-Stage Liver Disease (MELD) score [1,2] is a preoperative predictor of mortality prior to liver transplantation, it does not predict post transplantation survival. Instead, a number of multi-variable prognostic models have been developed in an attempt to estimate the risk of post transplantation mortality. However, a systematic review of established models of outcome prediction found that none were able to accurately discriminate between survivors and non-survivors [3] . A recent model, based on data from the European Liver Transplant Registry [4] included operative variables, thereby limiting its usefulness in the pre-operative setting. Volk *et al.* have defined the Charlson Comorbidity Index [5] which considers the impact of multiple medical co-morbidities in predicting risk of longer term mortality. Unfortunately, this model proved no better in predicting mortality than the other published models mentioned previously.

Cardiorespiratory Assessment

The relative inability of multifactorial models to predict early outcome following liver transplantation has focused preoperative investigation on specific areas of co-morbidity. Wherever significant overt disease such as myocardial ischaemia, cirrhotic cardiomyopathy, hepatopulmonary syndrome and porto-pulmonary hypertension are present, there are well defined protocols to direct further evaluation. Even so, there is often limited consensus as to what constitutes effective intervention and optimisation for these patients as presented in details in chapters 2 and 13.

It remains the most important challenge in cardiorespiratory risk assessment of liver transplant candidates is not only the initial screening of asymptomatic patients for covert cardiorespiratory disease but also the need for justification of a multiple preoperative investigative approach in terms of outcome benefit.

As presented in details in Chapter 13, most cardiorespiratory screening protocols rely on the use of clinical history, electrocardiogram and non-invasive investigative tests including trans thoracic echocardiography, arterial blood gas analysis and static pulmonary function tests In addition some form of cardiac stress testing procedure is often introduced to identify coronary artery disease.

The success of any screening process is ultimately dependent on the sensitivity and specificity of the testing procedures. A high proportion of false positive results will trigger more complex, time consuming and expensive tests where they are neither required nor likely to give additional useful information. For example, dobutamine stress echocardiography

(DSE) in the preoperative setting is used to detect areas of myocardium which in a situation where oxygen requirements are increased peri-operatively, may put the patients at risk of cardiac related complications. However, given issues regarding sensitivity, the additive value of DSE over simple clinical examination has been questioned in a general surgical population [6], as has its value as a predictive tool for non-cardiac postoperative complications [7]. More specifically, in liver transplant candidates, both dobutamine stress echocardiography and stress myocardial perfusion scanning have an extremely low sensitivity (13-61%) for diagnosing severe CAD when compared to more invasive coronary angiography [8]. Furthermore, up to 25% of liver transplant candidates fail to reach their target heart rate during the test, making the interpretation questionable [9]. Despite this, patients with definitive reversible changes on stress echocardiography, even with normal coronary angiography, do have increased mortality rates from cardiovascular complications, sepsis and donor graft failure [10].

A further fundamental issue with this simplified multiple investigative screening process, not only when used in a general surgical population undergoing major surgery, but especially in the investigation of the potential transplant recipient, is that many tests are performed in isolation of other system responses and under resting conditions. Where multiple comorbidities exist, isolated testing is less able to elicit which of the existing cardiac, respiratory, liver disease (which may improve with transplantation) or a combination have the most relevance in a given individual. Furthermore, isolated testing is unlikely to give a true representation of the complex integrated response of the cardiorespiratory system in patients with severe liver disease about to undergo the profound physiological stress of transplantation. As a corollary, the results of these investigations are unlikely to be related to perioperative outcome. For example, a study investigating the role of echocardiography in liver transplant recipients demonstrated no significant difference in the pre-operative left ventricular ejection fraction between survivors and non-survivors [11].

In summary, in major surgery, including liver transplantation, there is a primary requirement for an integrated test of overall cardiopulmonary function, which would be efficient at screening for generalised cardiorespiratory impairment and which also has relevance to perioperative outcome. In addition, the ability to define the importance of specific cardiorespiratory disease, in patients with multiple comorbidities (i.e. liver transplant candidates), may inform a more targeted approach to further investigation.

The recent introduction of cardiopulmonary exercise testing (CPET) into the preoperative setting, may provide an opportunity to develop this as a screening test in liver transplantation recipients. Furthermore, an understanding of the general status of the recipient regarding comorbid disease may also benefit the appropriate allocation of donor organs, leading to an improvement in life years gained for the transplant population as a whole [12].

Cardiopulmonary Exercise Testing

Cardiopulmonary exercise testing (CPET) is a non-invasive, reproducible investigation that allows the clinician to gain an understanding of an individual's cardio-respiratory function. Specifically it gives an indication of the combined reserve of the cardiovascular and respiratory systems when under stress. Exercise requires the coordinated function of the heart, lungs, peripheral vasculature and pulmonary circulation to meet the increase in cellular energy demand. In the peri-operative period, similar demands are placed on these organ systems to support an increase in metabolic rate. Although direct extrapolation is not entirely proven, it is likely that a patient's capacity to increase oxygen delivery (DO_2) and consumption (CO_2) during exercise correlates with their ability to maintain organ function in the peri-operative period, thereby preventing complications [13] . Unlike other diagnostic tests previously mentioned which evaluate the function of isolated organ systems, CPET simultaneously evaluates every organ essential for exercise.

Performing the Test

The body's metabolic response to a known exercise stress is measured through the accurate measurement of gas exchange at the airway. All variables are recorded on a breath by breath basis then averaged over a short time period (typically 15-45 sec) and the integration of a 12 lead electrocardiography (ECG) also allows detection of myocardial ischaemia.

The aim of the test is to record multiple measures of the patients cardiopulmonary reserve including the anaerobic threshold, peak oxygen consumption, ventilatory equivalents (measures of pulmonary ventilation perfusion mismatch) and respiratory limitation whilst simultaneously assessing for the occurrence of myocardial ischaemia.

There are a number of different protocols for performing CPET. The majority of centers performing peri-operative testing primarily use cycle ergometers. They have the advantage of offsetting the work of walking in patients who have difficulty ambulating and have fewer problems with ECG and airflow measurement artifact.

Although each protocol may vary slightly, most protocols consist of four main phases:

1. Rest

2-5 minutes of resting data (breath by breath gas analysis, 12 lead ECG, oxygen saturation and blood pressure) should be recorded to ensure the patient is comfortable and the equipment is functioning correctly.

2. Unloaded cycling

The rest period should then be followed by a period of 1-3 minutes of unloaded cycling. This is a period of further stabilisation which allows for the measurement of the oxygen cost of turning the legs, with minimum resistance for the particularly detrained or functionally limited patients.

3. Increasing resistance to pedalling

This component of the test that lasts usually 10 minutes, consist of increases the resistance to pedalling. The gradient of the incremental resistance is predetermined depending upon age, sex, weight and patients reported fitness level. Although the constantly increasing resistance is the most commonly used protocol, a stepped increase by using one minute increments can also produce acceptable data. The patient should be given verbal encouragement throughout the test.

4. Recovery

The ECG should be monitored until heart rate is within 10 beat per minute of the pre – test level, or any dysrythmia or ST changes have reverted to pre-test levels. Blood pressure should be monitored until it returns to the pre-test level.

CPET Variables

The CPET results are presented on varying combination plots. This is commonly presented as a nine plot graphical representation. This facilitates the interpretation of the test and permits the diagnosis of an abnormal response to exercise.

The most important variables to assess overall integrated cardiopulmonary function are:

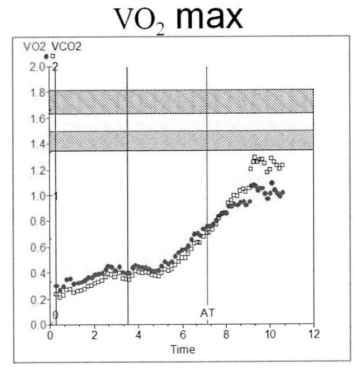

Figure 1. VO_2 max: Oxygen consumption (VO_2) max is the maximum rate of oxygen consumption during exercise and it cannot be exceeded despite increasing effort. In this plot of VO_2 vs time, it can be clearly seen that there is plateau in the VO_2. This could mean that the subject has reached their exercise capacity or there is underlying ischaemic changes occurring which would be revealed by ECG analysis. The latter is the most probably as the patient has not reached their predicted VO_2 (the hashed box).

Peak Exercise – Peak and Maximal Oxygen Consumption (VO_2) – Figure 1

VO_2 max is the maximum rate of oxygen uptake during exercise. It cannot be exceeded despite increasing effort – thus is an objective physiological endpoint. It is determined by the body's ability to transport and use oxygen. The strict definition is the plateau of oxygen consumption despite further increases in work rate. This should be determined by sequential, progressively increasing, constant work rate tests on different occasions. However, this is impractical in the majority of patients in the peri-operative period due to time constraints and access to testing. Therefore a surrogate is commonly used – VO_2 peak - the oxygen consumprion when the test is stopped. This variable is volitional, in that depends on the patient making maximal effort and is strongly linked to physiological factors. It is also more likely to be non-repeatable on different measurement occasions. Provided adequate effort is made, it has been related to clinical outcome in a number of studies particularly in the heart failure literature and is a useful easy to identify predictive parameter [14].

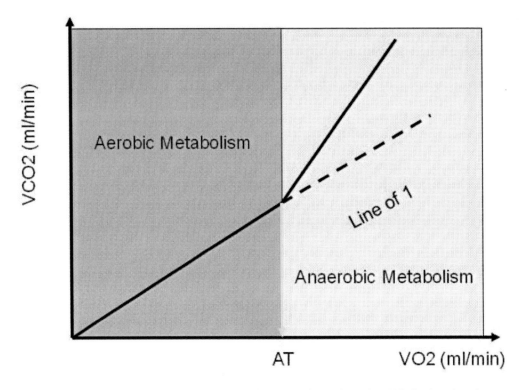

Figure 2. Anaerobic threshold determination : During incremental exercise, when VO_2 is plotted against VCO_2 there is a linear relationship during aerobic metabolism. As work rate increases, aerobic metabolism has to be supplemented by anaerobic metabolism. There is a resulting increase in the change of CO_2 production without a rise in the rate of change of oxygen consumption. This forms the basis of the V-Slope method of AT identification.

VO_2, oxygen consumption.

VCO_2, carbon dioxide production.

AT, anaerobic threshold.

Anaerobic Threshold (AT) Figure 2

The anaerobic threshold is a marker of the combined efficacy of the lungs, heart and circulation. During incremental exercise, there is a linear relationship between oxygen supply and demand. As work rate increases, there is point when oxygen demand will begin to exceed supply and aerobic metabolism has to be supplemented by anaerobic metabolism. Lactate levels start to rise and as it is a weak base it dissociates to release H^+ ions. These are buffered by the bicarbonate system leading to an increase in CO_2. Thus there is a resulting increase in the rate of CO_2 production without a rise in the rate of the oxygen consumption. The VO2 at the point at which this occur is called the AT. Graphically presented, the initial slope of the VCO_2/VO_2 line has a gradient of 1.0 or less, whereas the portion above the AT has a gradient of more than 1. The intersection of the linear regression lines of the two components identifies the AT.

The anaerobic threshold has some major theoretical advantages over the peak or maximal VO_2. It is a non-volitional, objective measure of exercise capacity and physiological reserve. The AT does not require the patient to achieve their maximal effort – occurring at approximately 47-64% of VO_2 max and has been shown to be highly reproducible [13] . This allows the patient to undergo sub-maximal testing and potentially improves the safety of the test. Concerns have been raised whether there is the potential for inter-observer variability in determining the AT. However, a recent study report has shown that there is a low error in the determination of the AT by experienced anaesthetic consultants [15] .

Ventilatory efficiency (V_E/VCO_2) Figure 3

Ventilation is more closely related to CO_2 output than O_2 uptake. Therefore, the ventilatory efficiency is defined by the relationship of the amount of ventilation required to eliminate 1 liter of CO_2. The efficiency of the elimination of CO_2 can be affected by many factors especially heart and lung pathology which alter the ventilation perfusion (VQ) mismatch. Ventilation of poorly perfused alveoli increases the alveolar dead space and thus the dead space:tidal volume ratio (V_D/V_T). This ratio is therefore a valuable measure to estimate the degree of VQ mismatching. V_D/V_T cannot accurately be measured without arterial blood gas analysis. However, it is proportional to the V_E/VCO_2 ratio which can be measured by gas analysis during CPET. V_E/VCO_2 is a stable, easily calculated parameter and in combination with AT has been found to be the best predictor of outcome in left ventricular failure [16] .

Cardiopulmonary Exercise Testing in Major Non-Cardiac Surgery

There is an increasing body of evidence that variables derived from CPET can predict patients at risk of increased rate of peri-operative mortality and morbidity. These studies vary in the type of surgery undertaken and the CPET variables used. However, the majority show that the use of CPET improves risk assessment for patients undergoing major surgery.

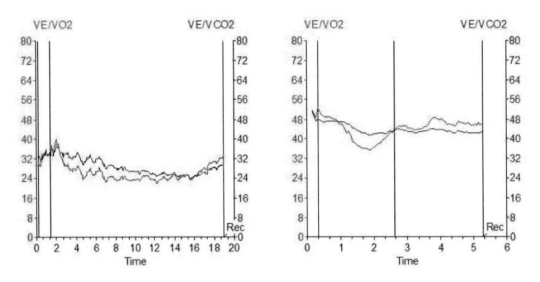

Figure 3. Normal and abnormal plots V_E/VCO_2 vs. time. Ventilatory efficiency in a normal patient compared to a patient with severe cirrhotic cardiomyopathy. During exercise the V_E/VCO_2 falls to a low level in the normal patient showing improved VQ due to the recruitment of the pulmonary capillary bed. This is in contrast to the patient with cirrhotic cardiomyopathy when the V_E/VCO_2 ratio remains elevated and does not fall with exercise. This is associated with a poor long term prognosis.

V_E/VCO_2, Ventilatory efficiency.

Open Abdominal Aortic Aneurysm Repair

Carlisle et al. measured a number of variables in 130 patients undergoing elective open abdominal aortic aneurysm repair [17]. All variables correlated with survival in univariate analysis. V_E/VCO_2 correlated best with 30 days and the total observational period survival [17]. AT was also associated with midterm survival but to a lesser degree [17]. In contrast, Nugent et al. investigated a small sample of 30 patients planned for abdominal aortic aneurysm surgery and followed outcome for 12 months, they found no significant difference in peak VO_2 in those who had postoperative complications compared to those who did not [18].

Upper Gastrointestinal (GI) surgery

There have been several studies investigating the use of CPET in upper GI surgery. Forshaw et al. [19] undertook CPET in 78 patients undergoing oesophagectomy. The patients that experienced postoperative cardiorespiratory complications had a significant lower peak VO_2. Analysis of receiver operator curve characteristics for the use of VO_2 and AT to predict complications was 0.63 (95% CI 0.50-0.76) and 0.62 (95% CI 0.49-0.75) respectively. Although the p values were significant the values are under 0.65 and therefore not related to strong prediction. However given the small population of "high risk" patients (defined as an AT <11ml/kg/min) it is unlikely that the current authors would be able to test the hypothesis that poor cardiorespiratory reserve is an important factor in determining postoperative complications after oesophagectomy. More importantly, Nagamatsu have shown that the maximum VO$_2$ correlates with the postoperative cardiopulmonary complication rate in patients undergoing surgery for upper GI malignancy [20,21]. A final study investigating CPET in bariatric patients demonstrated that peak VO$_2$ played a predictive role for postoperative complication rates in that population [22].

Intra-Abdominal Surgery

Older *et al.* [23] investigated 187 elderly patients undergoing intra-abdominal surgery. Patients with an anaerobic threshold (AT) <11ml/kg/min had a mortality rate of 18% compared to 0.8% in those with an AT>11ml/kg/min. Older produced a further follow on study showing that the risk stratification of these patients using anaerobic threshold, with admission of the high risk groups to the critical care unit postoperatively improved outcome [24].

Our recently published study further extends the supportive evidence for the use of CPET in preoperative risk assessment [25]. It demonstrated the relationship of submaximal cardiopulmonary parameters to postoperative morbidity in a group of surgical patients undergoing major intra-abdominal surgery (open aneurysm, pancreatic, liver resection and sarcoma surgery). 171 patients with a low subjective exercise tolerance underwent preoperative CPET. 116 patients underwent their planned operation. Those patients that had high rates of postoperative complications had reduced levels of preoperative anaerobic threshold when compared with those with fewer complications (AT 9.0 ml/min/kg vs. 12.1 ml/min/kg). Multivariate analysis demonstrated that a subjective measure of functional capacity, AT, peak VO$_2$, and early emergency surgical reintervention were all significant independent predictor variables for defining individuals at high- or low-risk of developing postoperative complications and prolonged hospital stay [25]. However, it was the variables derived from the CPET test that were more strongly associated with these complications and objective measurement of cardiorespiratory function significantly improved the predictive value of the model presented over subjective assessment alone.

Cardiopulmonary Exercise Testing and Outcome in Liver Transplantation

It has been increasingly recognised that patients with end stage liver disease have reduced exercise tolerance and aerobic capacity [26]. With the increasing body of evidence showing that reduced cardiorespiratory reserve can predict morbidity and mortality in major surgical patients there has been increasing interest in its use for assessment of the liver transplant candidate.

Epstein et al. [27] examined 100 day mortality after liver transplantation. 156 patients undertook CPET testing as part of their assessment prior to liver transplantation. Of 59 patients who underwent liver transplant, the 100-day mortality rate was 11.3% (6 out of 59).

There was no significant difference in baseline characteristics, resting echocardiography or cardiovascular function between survivors and non-survivors [27] . Non-survivors were more likely to have a peak VO2 < 60% or VO2–AT < 50% of predicted values . They were also more likely to have a combined peak VO2<60% and VO2 – AT < 50% predicted (p<0.001) [27]. Importantly, two deaths not predicted by a peak VO2 < 60%, occurred 1 and 4 days post transplantation were associated with technical difficulties at the time of operation thereby being unlikely to have been predicted by a pre-operative investigation.

A further study by Dharancy et al. has recently investigated the use of cardiopulmonary exercise testing in the assessment of liver transplantation candidates [11] . 149 patients were enrolled into the study. Analysis restricted to patients with a MELD higher than 17, showed that those patients with severe alterations of peak VO2 (peak VO2 <60% predicted) had lower 1 year survival with or without transplantation than the others (53.3+/-12% vs 87.5+/-11.6% p=0.05) whereas the overall MELD scores were not significantly different (22.7 vs 20.6). Of the 47 patients (34% of the study population) that were transplanted, six deaths occurred and those with a severe impairment of peak VO2 had a trend to increased mean length of hospital stay (22.8+/-5 days vs. 17.7 +/-2.2 days: p=0.06) and a significantly longer requirement for oxygen support to maintain SaO2 higher than 92% (3.3+/-1.1 days vs. 7.2+/-3.5 days, P=0.035).

Both these transplantation studies differ from the studies performed in high risk surgical populations in that they have used peak VO2<60% predicted as the main variable for predicting a high risk population. No discussion was made in either study as to why peak VO2<60% predicted was used. As discussed previously, peak VO2 is effort dependent and may vary from test to test. Therefore, peak VO2 is unlikely to be readily predicted from an equation using height, age and sex etc. This may lead to considerable variability in contrasting these studies.

Our own data aimed to assess the use of CPET as a preoperative predictor of 90 day survival in a consecutive group of patients undergoing liver transplantation [28] . 52 patients underwent submaximal cardiopulmonary exercise testing. 25 patients have subsequently undergone liver transplantation with a 90 day survival rate of 84% (21/25). Interestingly, age, body mass index (BMI), MELD, UKELD and time on waiting list were not statistically different between the survivors and non-survivors. In contrast, the mean AT in survivors was 12.1 (SD+/-2.2) ml/min/kg compared with 7.9 (SD+/-1.5) ml/min/kg in the non-survivors (p=0.003). Receiver operator curve analysis demonstrated an optimum AT value of >9.6 ml/min/kg demonstrated 100% positive predictive value for survival (Sensitivity 87%; Specificity 100%: AUC 0.95 (CI 0.74 -0.99); p=0.0001). (Figure 4)

Six patients had an anaerobic threshold < 9.6ml/min/kg. All 4 patient deaths occurred in this group, despite preoperative MELD, UKELD and donor risk index being comparable with the patient group with low risk of mortality. In the high risk group, both mean donor age and donor risk index were greater in the 4 non-surviving patients compared with the two survivors (mean DRI 1.51 vs 1.23; mean donor age 52.3 vs 20.0 respectively).

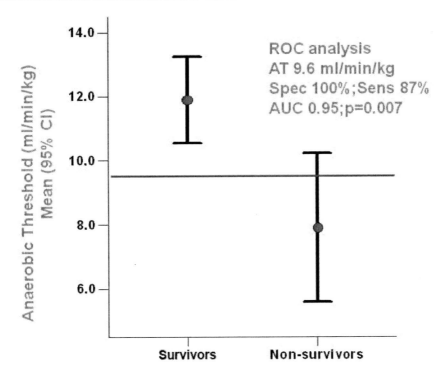

Figure 4. Mortality vs. Anaerobic threshold. ROC, Receiver Operating Characteristic curve, AUC, Area under the curve.

These suggest that in an unselected group of patients undergoing liver transplantation, a measure of cardiopulmonary reserve (AT), rather than standard scores of liver dysfunction, can predict those at risk of increased 90-day mortality rate. In this small study, we have found that the donor liver quality, as defined by the donor risk index, did not influence 90 day survival in those patients with an adequate cardiopulmonary reserve. However, in those patients with low cardiorespiratory reserve, the quality of the donor organ may impact upon survival (Figure 4).

CPET and Specific Disease Processes Related to Liver Transplant Recipients

Combinations of CPET variables can detect evidence of specific disease processes relating specifically to potential liver transplant recipients. These include ischaemic heart disease, diastolic dysfunction and pulmonary hypertension.

Ischaemic Heart Disease

Coronary artery disease is a common condition in potential liver transplant recipients. Studies have shown that at least one critical coronary artery lesion occurs in 5% to 26% of all liver transplant candidates who are asymptomatic [29] . Although, mild disease maybe difficult to diagnose, the simultaneous use of gas exchange may improve the sensitivity of the exercise test. When myocardial oxygen demand is not met during exercise, characteristic ST and T wave changes associated with ischaemia occur on the ECG. They are also distinctive gas exchange abnormalities. When deprived of oxygen, asynchronous contraction of the myocardium results in a reduction of stroke volume. This is illustrated by the consequent failure of VO_2 to increase in proportion to work rate.

Where VO_2 reaches a plateau despite increasing work it indicates that cardiac output has peaked. With further increases in heart rate, stroke volume must decrease reflecting the myocardial dyskinesia or ischaemia. If ECG changes occur without chest pain or gas exchange changes consistent with the diagnosis, functional myocardial ischaemia is unlikely.

Diastolic Dysfunction

Liver transplant candidates can overt cardiac dysfunction but the majority have more subtle defects that only become apparent under stress. Cardiac workload is often reduced due to the peripheral vasodilation caused by chronic liver failure, the high cardiac output demonstrated is often interpreted as normal cardiac function. Indices of left ventricular (LV) function (stroke index, LV stroke work and power) are also often greater than expected. Echocardiographic appearances of systolic function in the vast majority of patients are normal, even when cardiac mechanics are commonly disturbed. The early histological changes associated with "cirrhotic cardiomyopathy" commonly causes thickening of left ventricular wall. As wall thickening increases so does the degree of diastolic dysfunction. This leads to impairment of relaxation and impedance to left ventricular filling. If circulatory changes occur rapidly, such as during liver transplantation, this increase in filling pressure can result in congestive heart failure. CPET is especially suited for diagnosing diastolic dysfunction. The peak VO_2 and AT are commonly reduced reflecting reduced O_2 carriage to the tissues. There are associated increases in V_E/VCO_2 and V_D/V_T which reflect the decreased perfusion of ventilated lung units and are proportional to the underlying severity. The circulation of blood through the lung is slower than normal allowing time for diffusion of O_2 from the alveolus to the red cell. Thus, arterial oxygenation is normal in patients with chronic diastolic and systolic dysfunction [30].

Pulmonary Hypertension

Pulmonary vascular disease/hypertension causes a haemodynamic stenosis of the central circulation, making it difficult for the right ventricle to deliver blood to the left atrium at a sufficient rate to meet the increased cardiac output needed for exercise [14] . Therefore, a pattern similar to cardiac failure is seen with a decrease in AT and peak VO2 and increased V_E/VCO_2 and V_D/V_T. Pulmonary hypertension causes a decrease both in the functional pulmonary capillary bed and the availability of recruitable lung units reserved for exercise. Therefore, when the pulmonary blood flow increases during exercise, the red cell cannot remain in the pulmonary circulation long enough for the diffusion equilibrium of oxygen to occur. Arterial desaturation helps to distinguish between pulmonary vascular disease and cardiac failure. Another cause of hypoxaemia in pulmonary hypertension is the development of a right to left shunt resulting from a patent foramen ovale. This may cause marked exercise hypoxaemia which may be confirmed during CPET.

Conclusion

Liver transplant candidates commonly have normal resting cardiac function but by stressing the patient underlying cardiorespiratory dysfunction becomes evident. Quantification of this dysfunction is important in determining the postoperative risk for survival in the early post-transplant period. Cardiopulmonary exercise testing is a non-invasive test which objectively defines cardiorespiratory reserve. A limited number of studies have demonstrated that measures defined by preoperative CPET testing were able to predict a group of patients at high risk for mortality and morbidity post liver translpantation. These are being supported by our own observations. Furthermore, specific disease entities which are sometimes masked by liver disease may be uncovered by CPET which will more readily inform further investigative approaches. In summary, these findings need to be substantiated in a larger multi-centre study but if demonstrated to be consistent may have a profound effect on future risk assessment and donor – recipient organ allocation in liver transplantation.

References

[1] Kamath PS, Wiesner RH, Makinchoc M, Kremers W *et al*. A model to predict survival in patients with end-stage liver disease. *Hepatology* 2001;33:464-70.

[2] Meion RM. When is a patient too well and when is a patient too sick for a liver transplant. *Liver. Transpl.* 2004;10:S69-S73.

[3] Jacob M, Lewsey JD, Sharpin C *et al*. Systematic review and validation of prognostic models in liver transplantation. *Liver Transpl.* 2005;11(7):814-25.

[4] Burroughs A, Sabin C, Delvart V *et al*. 3-month and 12-month mortality after first liver transplant in adults in Europe: predicted models for outcome. *Lancet* 2006;367:225-32.

[5] Volk M, Hernandez J, Lok A, Marrero J. Modified Charlson comorbidity index for predicting survival after liver transplantation. *Liver Transplantation* 2007;13:1515-20.

[6] Mangano DT, London MJ, Tubau JF *et al*. Dipyridamole thallium-201 scintigraphy as a preoperative screening test. A re-examination of its predictive potential. Study of Perioperative Ischemia Research Group. *Circulation* 1991;84:493–502.

[7] Kertai MD, Boersma E, Bax JJ *et al*. A meta-analysis comparing the prognostic accuracy of six diagnostic tests for predicting perioperative cardiac risk in patients undergoing major vascular surgery. *Heart* 2003;89:1327–34.

[8] Aydinalp A, Bal U, Ertan C *et al*. Value of stress myocardial perfusion scanning in diagnosis of severe coronary artery disease in liver transplantation candidates. *Transplant Proc* .2009;41:3757-60.

[9] Harinstein ME, Flaherty JD, Ansari AH *et al*. Predictive value of dobutamine stress echocardiography for coronary artery disease detection in liver transplant candidates. *Am. J. Transplant.* 2008;8:1523-8.

[10] Guckelberger O, Byram A, Klupp J et al.Coronary event rates in liver transplant recipients reflect the increased prevalence of cardiovascular risk-factors. *Transpl. Int.* 2005; 18: 967-74.

[11] Dharancy S, Lemyze M, Boleslawski E et al. Impact of impaired aerobic capacity on liver transplant candidates. *Transplantation* 2008;86:1077-83.

[12] Brown RS Jr, Lake JR. The survival impact of liver transplantation in the MELD era, and the future for organ allocation and distribution. *Am J Transplant* 2005;5:203-4.

[13] Shoemaker WC, Wo CC, Thangathurai D et al. Hemodynamic patterns of survivors and nonsurvivors during high risk elective surgical operations. *World J. Surg.* 1999;23:1264-70.

[14] Wassermann K, Hansen JE, Sue DY, Stringer WW, Whipp BJ eds. Measurements during integrative cardiopulmonary exercise testing. In: *Principles of exercise testing and interpretation*. Lippincott, Williams and Wilkins: USA 2005

[15] Sinclair RCF, Danjoux GR, Goodridge V, Batterham AM. Determination of the anaerobic threshold in the per-operative assessment clinic:inter-observer measurement error. *Anaesthesia* 2009;64:1992-5.

[16] Gitt AK, Wasserman K, Kilkowski C et al. Exercise anaerobic threshold and ventilatory efficiency identify heart failure patients for high risk of early death. *Circulation* 2002;106:3079–84.

[17] Carlisle J, Myers M. Mid-term survival after abdominal aortic aneurysm surgery predicted by cardiopulmonary exercise testing. *Brit. J. Surg.* 2007;94(8):966-9.

[18] Nugent AM, Riley M, Megarry J et al. Cardiopulmonary exercise testing in the preoperative assessment of patients for repair of abdominal aortic aneurysm. *Irish Journal of Medical Science* 1998;167:238-41.

[19] Forshaw MJ, Strauss DC, Davies AR et al. Is cardiopulmonary exercise testing a useful test before oesophagectomy? *Annals of Thoracic Surgery* 2008;85:294-9.

[20] Nagamatsu Y, Yamana H, Fujita H et al. The simultaneous evaluation of preoperative cardiopulmonary functions of oesophageal cancer patients in the analysis of expired gas with exercise testing *Nippon Kyoba geka Gakkai Zasshi.* 1994;42:2037-40.

[21] Nagamatsu Y, Shima I, Yamana H et al. Preoperative evaluation of cardiopulmonary reserve with the use if expired gas analysis during exercise testing in patients with squamous cell carcinoma of the thoracic esophagus. *J. Thoracic. Cardiovasc. Surg.* 2001;121:1064-8.

[22] McCullough PA, Gallagher MJ, DeJong AT et al. Cardiorespiratory fitness and short-term complications in bariatric surgery. *Chest* 2006;130:517-25.

[23] Older P, Smith R, Courtney P, Hone R. Preoperative evaluation of cardiac failure and ischaemia in elderly patients by cardiopulmonary exercise testing *Chest* 1993;104:701-4.

[24] Older P, Hall A, Hader R. Cardiopulmonary exercise testing as a screening test for perioperative management of major surgery in the elderly. *Chest* 1999;116:355-62.

[25] Snowden CP, Prentis JM, Anderson HL. Submaximal cardiopulmonary exercise testing predicts complications and hospital length of stay in patients undergoing major elective surgery. *Ann. Surg.* 2010;251(3):535-41.

[26] [26] Epstein SK, Ciubotaru RL, Zilberberg MD et al. Analysis of impaired exercise capacity in patients with cirrhosis. *Dig. Dis. Sci.* 1998;43: 1701-7.

[27] Epstein SK, Freeman RB, Unterborn JN *et al.* Aerobic capacity is associated with 100-day outcome after hepatic transplantation. *Liver transplantation* 2004;10:418-24.

[28] Prentis J, Randles D, Snowden CP *et al.* Cardiopulmonary exercise testing predicts early postoperative survival following liver transplantation. Presented at The British Transplantation Society Feb 2009

[29] Plotkin JS, Scott VL, Pinna A *et al.* Morbidity and mortality in patients with coronary artery disease undergoing orthotopic liver transplantation. *Liver Transpl. Surg.* 1996;2:426-30.

[30] Guazzi M, Myers J, Arena R.Cardiopulmonary exercise testing in the clinical and prognostic assessment of diastolic heart failure. *J. Am. Coll. Cardiol.* 2005;46:1883-90.

In: Cardiovascular Diseases and Liver Transplantation
Editor: Zoka Milan, pp. 217-237
ISBN: 978-1-61122-910-3
© 2011 Nova Science Publishers, Inc.

Chapter XV

Pharmacotherapy of Cardiac Dysfunction in Liver Transplant Patients

Dina Jankovic[*]
Department of Pharmacy, Chelsea and Westminster Hospital, London, UK

Abstract

Liver transplant patients often present with cardiac dysfunction both independent and as a direct result of the liver disease, which can present a great challenge to anesthesiologists. Anesthesiologists need to be aware of the drug therapy available to treat cardiovascular complications that could arise during or shortly after surgery. Furthermore, they must be aware of the therapy for cardiovascular conditions initiated before surgery and how it could increase perioperative risk.

Cirrhotic cardiomyopathy is fairly common in patients with cirrhosis, but is usually latent unless the patient experiences significant physiological stress such as surgery. Heart failure is the third most common cause of death after liver transplant, following organ rejection and infection. Treatment for symptomatic cirrhotic cardiomyopathy involves the same therapy as treatment for noncirrhotic patients and includes diuretics, angiotensin-converting enzyme inhibitors, beta blockers, and aldosterone antagonists. Interactions between these and immunosuppressive agents must be taken into account. Portopulmonary hypertension can be treated with calcium channel blockers, prostanoids, endothelin receptor antagonists, and phosphodiesterase type 5 antagonists or combination therapy. The choice of therapy depends on the vasoreactivity of the patient and the severity of the disease. Oxygen, inhaled nitric oxide, diuretics, digoxin, and oral anticoagulants can be used as supportive therapy or in acute hypertensive episodes. Nitrates are not suitable vasodilators because of the risk of severe systemic hypotension. Surgery should be delayed in patients with cardiac stents who are taking dual antiplatelet therapy wherever possible until the dual therapy is completed. Where this is not possible,

---

[*] Correspondence: Dina Jankovic, Department of Pharmacy, Chelsea and Westminster Hospital, 369 Fulham Road, London SW10 9NH,Tel: +4420 8746 8000, E-mail: dina_jankovic_@hotmail.com.

a decision about whether to continue or to withdraw the antiplatelet agents should be made, taking into account the risk of bleeding and stent thrombosis.

Immunosuppressants used to prevent organ rejection can lead to or increase the risk of cardiovascular complications after surgery. Prednisolone, ciclosporin, tacrolimus, and mycophenolate mofetil have all been associated with hypertension in posttransplant patients. Calcium channel blockers are usually the agent of choice in the treatment of immunosuppressant-induced hypertension, along with beta blockers. Diuretics are not recommended. Tacrolimus has been known to cause cardiomyopathy in liver graft recipients, and where this occurs, the dose should be reduced, or the agent completely withdrawn. The risk of posttransplant heart failure does not appear to be greater when tacrolimus is the agent of choice. Increased incidence of hyperlipidemia has been reported in patients taking ciclosporin, tacrolimus, sirolimus, and azathioprine. This condition is treated with lipid-reducing agents as for nontransplant patients.

Introduction

Cardiac dysfunction in liver transplant patients can occur independently of or as a direct result of the liver disease. Examples of cardiovascular conditions associated with liver disease include cirrhotic cardiomyopathy, portopulmonary hypertension (POPH), hepatorenal syndrome, and hepatopulmonary syndrome. Anesthesiologists must be aware of issues that can arise from cardiac dysfunction during and after the liver transplantation, as these problems can affect the choice of anesthetic and monitoring during surgery. Furthermore, where treatment is initiated before the liver transplant, anesthesiologists need to be conscious of how to handle the different drugs in preparation for surgery, for example, when they should be discontinued and restarted to prevent complications. Some of the above-mentioned conditions resolve after liver function is restored, and therefore long-term treatment after surgery may not be necessary. However, immunosuppressive agents used to prevent organ rejection can lead to cardiomyopathy, hypertension, and hyperlipidemia, further increasing the risk of cardiovascular disease. Treatment of these conditions and prophylaxis of further complications may need to be initiated during the postoperative recovery period.

This chapter outlines the recommended treatment for cardiovascular dysfunction in patients with liver disease and addresses the issues anesthesiologists may face during liver transplant surgery. Conditions are organized into complications of the disease and those induced by immunosuppressants. Hepatorenal and hepatopulmonary syndrome, and portopulmonary hypertension are described in detail in chapters 5 and 12.

1. Disease Complications

1.1. Cirrhotic Cardiomyopathy

Cirrhotic cardiomyopathy refers to the occurrence of cardiac dysfunction in patients with cirrhosis, in the absence of any other associated cardiac disease. Portal hypertension is one of the main predisposing factors to circulatory abnormalities [1]. Cirrhotic cardiomyopathy is most commonly manifested as systolic dysfunction, diastolic dysfunction, and electrophysiological changes. It is usually clinically latent and only becomes apparent (manifested as heart failure or arrhythmias) during physiological stress, such as infection, hemorrhage, or liver transplantation [2,3].

In stable cirrhotic patients, cardiomyopathy is usually asymptomatic and overt ventricular failure is absent. Consequently, pharmacological therapy is not initiated [4]. Nevertheless, awareness of potential latent conditions is essential when patients are due to undergo liver transplant surgery, as the physical stress could precipitate symptomatic heart failure. Diagnostic tests can be carried out to predict the risk of cardiac complications during and after surgery. Treatment for these conditions involves the same therapy as for noncirrhotic patients, as few studies have been carried out to establish the optimal treatment specifically for cirrhotic cardiomyopathy [5]. Treatment for heart failure is outlined in section 1.2. Since hepatic hypertension is a predisposing factor, pharmacotherapy aimed at reducing the portal-collateral blood flow and the resistance opposing this flow can minimize the risk of cirrhotic cardiomyopathy [1].

1.2 Heart Failure

Heart failure is the third most common cause of mortality after liver transplantation, following infection and organ rejection. It can occur in patients with no previous structural heart disease [6] and therefore cannot always be predicted. Therapy for posttransplant heart failure is the same as that for nontransplant patients [2].

Diuretics are used for the relief of symptoms and fluid retention. [9] The use of angiotensin-converting enzyme (ACE) inhibitors should be considered for all patients with heart failure resulting from left ventricular systolic dysfunction, before beta blockers are initiated. Angiotensin-converting enzyme inhibitors are started at low doses and subsequently increased according to response and side effects [9]. Where ACE inhibitors are not tolerated because of persistent dry cough, angiotensin II receptor antagonists can be used as an alternative. Care should be taken when using ACE inhibitors, as hemodynamic disturbances specific to cirrhosis can lead to profound arterial hypotension in response to this therapy [5]. Beta blockers licensed for use in heart failure should be added after diuretics and ACE inhibitors in stable heart failure, regardless of whether symptoms persist. Although the effects of beta blockers on contractile dysfunction and electrophysiological abnormalities in cirrhotic patients have not yet been established [5], a single dose of propranolol has been associated with temporarily improved QT intervals [10].

In patients whose symptoms of heart failure resulting from left ventricular dysfunction remain moderate to severe despite therapy with diuretics, ACE inhibitor, and beta blockers, spironolactone should be considered (12.5–50 mg daily). Furthermore, there is some evidence that the aldosterone antagonist potassium canrenoate can improve left ventricular hypertrophy and wall thickness and, to some extent, left ventricular function indices in patients with overt congestive heart failure [11]. Digoxin is indicated in patients with worsening or severe heart failure caused by left ventricular systolic dysfunction despite treatment with ACE inhibitors, beta blockers, and diuretics, as well as in patients with atrial fibrillation and any degree of heart failure [7].

Table 1 Interactions between immunosuppressive agents used after liver transplant surgery and drugs used in the treatment of chronic cardiac failure [7,8]

Heart Failure Medication / Immuno-suppressant	ACE inhibitors	Diuretics	Beta blockers	Digoxin
Prednisolone	No known interaction	Prednisolone + loop or thiazide diuretics may lead to hypokalemia or precipitate potentially life-threatening torsade de pointes arrhythmias	No known interaction	Increased risk of digitalis toxicity when used with corticosteroids (as a result of potassium loss)
Azathioprine	Azathioprine + captopril or enalapril associated with anemia. Azathioprine + captopril can lead to leukopenia	No known interaction	No known interaction	No known interaction
Mycophenolate mofetil	No known interaction	No known interaction	No known interaction	No known interaction
Ciclosporin	Isolated cases of renal failure developed in kidney transplant patients taking ciclosporin when given enalapril. Ciclosporin + ACE inhibitors may lead to hyperkalemia.	Isolated cases of nephrotoxicity reported in patients taking ciclosporin + amiloride/hydrochlorothiazide/metolazone/mannitol. Frusemide can potentially protect the kidneys from ciclosporin-induced damage. Ciclosporin + potassium-sparing diuretics may exacerbate/increase the risk of hyperkalemia.	Carvedilol may modestly increase ciclosporin levels in some patients. Ciclosporin and beta blockers may exacerbate/increase the risk of hyperkalemia.	Ciclosporin causes a marked rise in digoxin levels in some patients.
Tacrolimus	Limited data, although concurrent use may increase the risk of hyperkalemia	Tacrolimus + potassium-sparing diuretics may exacerbate/increase the risk of hyperkalemia.	Tacrolimus + beta blockers may exacerbate/increase the risk of hyperkalemia.	No known interaction

When treating heart failure in patients who have undergone liver transplant, it is essential to take account of interactions between heart failure medicines and immunosuppressants. Table 1 shows the interactions between such agents.

1.3 Portopulmonary Hypertension

Portopulmonary hypertension (POPH) refers to pulmonary arterial hypertension (PAH) (mean pulmonary arterial pressure > 25 mmHg) [12] developed as a result of liver disease or portal hypertension. It has been suggested that mild to moderate POPH does not affect the outcome of liver transplant, with pulmonary arterial pressure falling after surgery. Severe pulmonary hypertension (systolic pulmonary arterial pressure > 60 mmHg) has been associated with an increased rate of perioperative mortality and an increased risk of right heart failure. Furthermore, pulmonary arterial pressure can remain high postoperatively in these patients [13].

The aims of pharmacological treatment for POPH are symptom control and pharmacodynamic improvement [14]. Response is considered satisfactory when

- The patient's symptoms are within WHO FC I or II (see below);
- Peak O_2 consumption is greater than 15 ml/min/kg;
- BNP/NT-proBNP plasma levels (parameters used to diagnose and grade the severity of heart failure) are normal or near normal;
- Echocardiography indicates no pericardial effusion;
- Right atrial pressure is below 8 mmHg; and
- Cardiac index (CI) is greater or equal to 2.5 l/min/m^2.

Pharmacotherapy for POPH is based on that for idiopathic pulmonary arterial hypertension (IPAH), but also considers common comorbidities in patients with POPH. Treatment depends on the predicted likely response to vasodilator agents and classification according to the World Health Organization's functional classes (WHO FCs) of the disease (classes are outlined in Table 2). Calcium channel blockers (CCBs) are indicated in vasoreactive patients, based on evidence mainly related to the use of nifedipine (120–240 mg), diltiazem (240–720 mg), and amlodipine (up to 20 mg) [15]. Doses of CCBs associated with satisfactory clinical response are relatively high; however, it is recommended to start with a low dose—nifedipine 30 mg slow release formulation twice daily, diltiazem 60 mg three times daily, or amlodipine 2.5 mg once daily—and slowly increase to the maximum tolerated dose. Patients should be monitored closely for side effects and efficacy for the first three to four months of therapy [14]. Patients who do not meet the criteria for a positive vasodilator response, and those not reaching a satisfactory response to CCBs, should be initiated on alternative PAH treatment.

Prostanoids. Prostacyclins are endogenous compounds produced predominantly by endothelial cells. They have vasodilatory, antiplatelet, cytoprotective, and antiproliferative properties [17]. It has been suggested that patients with PAH have dysregulated prostacyclin metabolic pathways [18].

Table 2 World Health Organisation (WHO) functional classes of pulmonary artery hypertension (PAH). Adapted from [16]

WHO functional class	Description
I	PAH with no effects on physical activity. Ordinary physical activity does not lead to dyspnea, fatigue, chest pain, or presyncope.
II	PAH with mild limitation of physical activity. No discomfort at rest, but normal physical activity causes increased dyspnea, fatigue, chest pain, or presyncope.
III	PAH with marked limitation of physical activity. No discomfort at rest, with less than ordinary activity causing increased dyspnea, fatigue, chest pain, or presyncope.
IV	PAH leading to an inability to perform any physical activity. Dyspnea and/or fatigue may be present at rest. Symptoms increased by almost any physical activity. Signs of right ventricular failure may be present.

Prostanoids are synthetic analogs of prostacyclins used in the treatment of PAH. Although prostanoids and prostacyclins have different pharmacokinetic properties, their pharmacodynamic actions are similar. The prostanoids used in the treatment of PAH are epoprostenol, iloprost, treprostinil, and beraprost.

Intravenous infusion of epoprostenol is recommended in the treatment of PAH in patients who fall under the categories of WHO FC III and IV. The initial recommended dose is 2–4 ng/kg/min, which is subsequently increased as permitted by side effects (flushing, headache, diarrhea, leg pain). The maintenance dose usually ranges from 20 to 40 ng/kg/min [19,20]. Epoprostenol is administered continuously via an infusion pump and a permanent tunneled catheter. Limitations of this treatment include the inconvenience of pumps, since pump malfunction, local infection, catheter obstruction, and sepsis have all been associated with their use. Abrupt discontinuation of epoprostenol infusion has been associated with rebound pulmonary hypertension with exacerbated symptoms and even death and thus should be avoided. Patients taking epoprostenol demonstrated improvement in their symptoms, exercise capacity, and hemodynamics in two randomized controlled trials in patients with IPAH [21,22] as well as in one retrospective study on patients with PAH associated with liver disease [23].

Iloprost is indicated for use in patients with PAH in WHO FC III. Although there is less evidence for its use, iloprost is available for intravenous infusion, as well as aerosol inhalation, making it an appealing choice of therapy. When administered intravenously, it has been suggested to be as effective as epoprostenol [24]. The effectiveness of inhalation therapy (6–9 times, 2.5–5 mg/inhalation, median 30 mg daily) has been shown to be beneficial compared with placebo [25]; however, no studies have been conducted comparing its efficacy with that of intravenous epoprostenol.

Treprostinil is recommended in the treatment of patients in WHO FC III and IV by the European Society of Cardiology [15], although it is currently not licensed for use in the United Kingdom. The main advantage of treprostinil is its chemical stability, which allows it to be administered via continuous subcutaneous infusion (using a microinfusion pump and a small subcutaneous catheter) at room temperature and changing reservoirs every 48 hours, compared with every 12 hours for epoprostenol. Subcutaneous treprostinil is initially given at a dose of 1–2 ng/kg/min. The dose is then increased gradually as permitted by side effects.

The maintenance dose varies between patients, usually ranging between 20 and 80 g/kg/min [14]. The main side effects include pain at the injection site (responsible for the discontinuation of treatment in 8% of patients), flushing, and headaches [26]. Subcutaneous treprostinil, like epoprostenol, has been shown to improve survival [27], exercise capacity, hemodynamics, and symptoms [28], with the greatest benefit seen in patients with more severe symptoms at baseline and in those able to tolerate higher doses (> 13.8 ng/kg/min). The effectiveness of intravenous treprostinil appears to be comparable to that of epoprostenol; however, higher doses of treprostinil are required [29,30]. The use of inhaled and oral treprostinil is still under investigation.

Beraprost is the only chemically stable prostacyclin analog that can be administered orally; however, its use is not recommended in PAH because it has a limited role in improving exercise capacity in treatment lasting longer than six months and little effect on hemodynamics [31].

Endothelin receptor antagonists. It has been suggested that the endothelin system plays a role in the pathogenesis of PAH because it is activated in both the plasma and the lung tissue of patients with PAH [32,33]. The binding of endothelin-1 to endothelin-A and endothelin-B receptors in pulmonary vascular smooth muscle cells results in vasoconstriction and mitogenesis. Furthermore, the activation of endothelin-B receptors in endothelial cells results in the release of vasodilators and antiproliferative substances such as nitric oxide and prostacyclins that may counteract the effects of endothelin-1. As a result, endothelin receptor antagonists have been incorporated in the treatment of PAH. There appears to be little difference between the clinical effects of blocking one particular isoform of the receptor (A or B) over the other.

Bosentan is an orally active endothelin (A and B) receptor antagonist that is recommended for use in patients in WHO FC II, III, and IV [14]. The initial recommended dose is 62.5 mg twice daily, which can be increased gradually to 125 mg twice daily after four weeks. In pediatric patients, doses are altered according to body weight. Several randomized controlled trials have shown that treatment with bosentan leads to improvements in exercise capacity functional class, echocardiographic variables, and time to clinical worsening in IPAH [34-38]. Furthermore, in patients with POPH, bosentan therapy led to improved symptoms and hemodynamics [39]. Bosentan has been associated with reversible, dose-dependent increases in hepatic aminotransferase levels as well as reductions in hemoglobin levels and impaired spermatogenesis [14].

Sitaxentan is an endothelin-A receptor antagonist. It is administered orally (100 mg daily). Sitaxentan therapy is recommended for patients in WHO FC II, III, and IV [14], although evidence for its use in patients in WHO FC II and IV is not as firm as that for bosentan. Two randomized controlled trials showed treatment with sitaxentan leads to improvements in exercise capacity and hemodynamics [40,41]. Its use has been associated with altered liver function tests and, consequently, requires monitoring of liver function.

Ambrisentan is a selective endothelin-A receptor inhibitor. The European Society of Cardiology recommends its use in patients in WHO FC II, III, and IV, with limited evidence for the latter classification [14]. Ambrisentan is started at 5 mg daily and, where tolerated, increased to 10 mg daily. Two randomized controlled trials have suggested ambrisentan therapy leads to improvements in symptoms, exercise capacity, hemodynamics, and time to clinical worsening in patients with PAH [42,43]. Like bosentan and sitaxentan, ambrisentan has been known to cause altered liver function tests and requires monthly monitoring of liver function. Ambrisentan has also been known to lead to peripheral edema, although it is generally well tolerated at a lower dose (5 mg) [44].

Phosphodiesterase type 5 inhibitors. Phosphodiesterase type 5 (PDE5) is an enzyme expressed in several sites in the body, including the pulmonary vasculature. Inhibition of PDE5 blocks the degradation of cyclic guanosine monophosphate (cGMP) and, consequently, leads to vasodilation through the nitric oxide/cGMP pathway. Phosphodiesterase type 5 inhibitors are primarily licensed for the treatment of erectile dysfunction; however, as a result of the considerable expression of the enzyme in the pulmonary vasculature, PDE5 inhibitors also cause pulmonary vasodilation. The three licensed agents are sildenafil, tadalafil, and vardenafil [14].

Sildenafil is an orally active, selective PDE5 inhibitor. It has been shown to increase exercise capacity, symptoms, and hemodynamics in patients with IPAH in one randomized controlled trial and several uncontrolled studies [45-48]. Furthermore, a case study on severe POPH in a patient with end-stage liver disease reported significant reduction in pulmonary arterial pressure with the use of sildenafil 50 mg twice daily and maintenance of satisfactory pulmonary arterial pressure with a maintenance dose of 50 mg once daily [49]. Sildenafil is fairly short acting and must be administered up to three times a day. The maximum effect is seen 60 minutes after administration [50]. The approved dose is 20 mg three times daily; however, in practice, the dose is often titrated to 40–80 mg three times daily [14]. Favorable effects of sildenafil on PAH in the long term are only seen with the dose of 80 mg three times daily. Side effects are mild to moderate and include headaches, flushing, and epistaxis [50].

Tadalafil is an oral PDE5 inhibitor administered once daily. The maximum effect is seen 75–90 minutes after administration [51]. The observed effective dose is 5, 10, 20 or 40 mg daily, although the evidence for its efficacy is not as strong as for sildenafil because of a lack of data on patients taking monotherapy tadalafil for PAH [52]. The side effects of tadalafil are similar to those of sildenafil in both their symptoms and frequency [14].

Nitrates (glyceryl trinitrate, isosorbide mononitrate), like PDE5 inhibitors, act on the cGMP pathway; however, they are contraindicated in PAH because there is a risk that they may precipitate severe systemic hypotension [53]. Agents used in the treatment of PAH in nonvasoreactive patients are summarized in Table 3, with their indications, side effects, advantages, and disadvantages.

Combination therapy. Combination therapy involves the use of more than one class of medicines. Although combination therapy is commonly used in the treatment of PAH, evidence for the long-term effectiveness and safety of most combinations is inconclusive [36]. . Several randomized controlled trials of combination therapies are discussed in this chapter.

As for the combined use of inhaled iloprost and bosentan, the evidence is inconclusive. One randomized controlled trial found a significant increase in exercise capacity (measured as six-minute walk distance) in patients using this combination therapy. Furthermore, although adding iloprost to their treatment did not significantly improve hemodynamics, it prolonged time to clinical worsening [54].

Table 3. Summary of drugs used in the treatment of PAH in non vasoreactive patients

Drug class	Agent	Side effects	Contraindications	Disadvantages of therapy
Prosta-cyclins	Epoprostenol Continuous IV infusion pump: initially 2–4 ng/kg/min, increased as permitted by side effects; maintenance dose usually 20–40 ng/kg/min	Pump malfunction, local infection at site of injection, catheter obstruction, sepsis	Severe left ventricular dysfunction	Inconvenience of using continuous IV infusion pump; reservoir changed every 12 hours; abrupt discontinuation can lead to rebound PAH with symptom exacerbation, possibly death.
	Iloprost Aerosol inhalation: 2.5–5 mg/inhalation, six to nine times daily	Hypotension, syncope, cough, headache, throat/jaw pain	Unstable angina within six months of myocardial infarction; decompensated cardiac failure, severe arrhythmias, congenital, or acquired heart valve defects within three months of cerebrovascular events; pulmonary veno-occlusive disease	Frequent administration; abrupt discontinuation can lead to rebound PAH with symptom exacerbation, possibly death.
	Treprostinil Continuous SC infusion: initially 1–2 ng/kg/min; increase gradually as permitted by side effects; maintenance dose 20–80 ng/kg/min; maximum daily dose 250 mg bd	Injection site pain, flushing, headaches, gastrointestinal disturbances, dry mouth, rectal hemorrhage, flushing, palpitations, edema, chest pain		Inconvenience of using continuous IV/SC pumps; reservoir changed every 48 hours; frequent irritation at injection site; abrupt discontinuation can lead to rebound PAH with symptom exacerbation, possibly death.
Endothelin receptor antagonists	Bosentan Oral: initially 62.5 mg bd; increase to 125 mg bd over four weeks.	Reversible, dose-dependent increase in hepatic aminotransferase; reduction in hemoglobin	Acute porphyria, pregnancy, breastfeeding	Potential hepatotoxicity
	Sitaxentan Oral: 100 mg od	Altered liver function tests, gastrointestinal disturbances, edema, flushing, headaches, insomnia, fatigue, dizziness	Breastfeeding	Evidence not as strong as for bosentan; potential hepatotoxicity
Endothelin receptor antagonists	Ambrisentan Oral: initially 5 mg od; increase to 10 mg od if tolerated	Altered liver function tests, abdominal pain, constipation, palpitations, flushing, peripheral edema, upper respiratory tract infections	Headache, anemia	Potential hepatotoxicity
Phospho-diesterase type 5 inhibitors	Sildenafil Oral: 20 mg tds; often titrated to 40–80 mg tds*; maximum effect after 60 min	Headaches, flushing, epistaxis	Recent history of stroke or myocardial infarction, history of nonarteritic anterior ischemia optic neuropathy, hereditary degenerative retinal disorders	Short half life; must be administered three times a day
	Tadalafil Oral: 5–40 mg od; effect observed after 75–90 min	Headaches, flushing, epistaxis	Moderate heart failure, uncontrolled arrhythmias, uncontrolled systemic hypertension	Less evidence than for sildenafil; longer acting than sildenafil
Oral anti-coagulant	Warfarin Varies according to INR; target INR range 2–3.	Hemorrhage	Peptic ulcers, severe hypertension, patients with increased risk of bleeding	Contraindicated in patients with esophageal varices because of the increased risk of bleeding
Oxygen therapy	Initially 28%, titrated towards a target oxygen saturation of 88%–92%			Long-term benefit not established
Nitric oxide	20–40 ppm			Used in acute PAH crisis only

Index: od = once daily, bd = twice a day, tds = three times daily, sc = subcutaneous, iv = intravenous.

Table 4. Stepwise therapy of PAH. Adapted from [14]

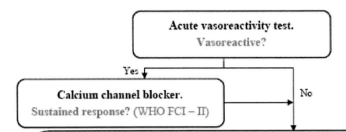

Single therapy

Recommendations summarised in table 4.

WHO FC	II	III	IV
First line	Ambisentan/ Bosentan/ Sildenafil	Ambisentan, bosentan, sitaxentan, sildenafil, epoprostenol (IV), iloprost (inhaled)	Epoprostenol (IV)
Second line	Tadalafil	Tadalafil, terliprostinil (subcutaneous or inhaled)	
Third line	Sitaxentan	Iloprost IV, terliprostinil IV (subcutaneous)	Ambisentan, bosentan, sitaxentan, sildenafil, tadalafil, iloprost (inhaled and IV), terliprostinil (subcutaneous)

Table 4 Recommendations for treatment of PAH. Adapted from (European society)

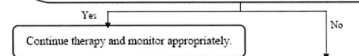

Combination therapy

No clear recommendations due to limited research. Trials carried out so far summarised in table 4.

Combination	Hæmodynamics	Exercise capacity	Time to clinical worsening	Additional comments
Bosentan + epoprostenol	↑			
Inhaled iloprost + bosentan	↔	↑	↑	Contrasting evidence. One RCT suggested no benefit in adding bosentan
Inhaled terliprostinil + bosentan		↑	↔	No effect on functional class
Sildenafil + epoprostenol		↑	↑	Compared to what??
Tadalafil + epoprostenol				WHO FC II study

Table 4. Combination therapy for PAH studied in RCTs and their findings.

However, another randomized controlled trial showed contrasting results, with the addition of iloprost showing no significant difference in hemodynamics, exercise capacity, or time to clinical worsening [55].

In one randomized controlled trial, adding inhaled treprostinil in patients already taking bosentan or sildenafil resulted in an improved six-minute walk distance; however, there was little effect on WHO functional class and time to clinical worsening [56]. By contrast, adding sildenafil to epoprostenol was shown to improve six-minute walk distance and prolong time to clinical worsening after 12 weeks [57].

The effects of adding sildenafil to bosentan therapy were studied in a randomized controlled trial of patients in WHO FC II, and a similar effect was achieved in both arms—with and without sildenafil [58]. Bosentan induces cytochrome P450 CYP3A4 and sildenafil inhibits it. When the two drugs are used concomitantly, plasma levels of bosentan rise, while levels of sildenafil decrease [59]. Although the interaction has not been shown to increase the toxicity of bosentan [60], its effects on the clinical efficacy of sildenafil have not yet been determined. Tadalafil and bosentan interact in a similar manner, and it has been suggested that their concurrent use can improve exercise capacity, though the increase is of borderline statistical significance [61].

The European Society of Cardiology emphasizes that research on combination therapy in PAH is insufficient for making clear recommendations with regard to which combinations are most beneficial or when to switch and when to combine agents. However, the society does recommend combined therapy in patients failing to produce a satisfactory response to monotherapy and optimizes background therapy [14].

In addition to PAH treatment aimed at reducing pulmonary arterial pressure, the following supportive therapies can be used [14]:

- Diuretics have been associated with symptomatic benefit in fluid-overloaded patients.
- Oral anticoagulants are recommended because of a high prevalence of vascular thrombotic lesions at postmortem in patients with PAH (target INR 2–3). The risks of starting oral anticoagulant therapy should be considered, as some patients may be at increased risk of bleeding (e.g., as a result of esophageal varices).
- Oxygen can reduce pulmonary vascular resistance (PVR) in patients with PAH. The long-term benefit of oxygen therapy has not been established. Guidance on the use of oxygen is based on that for patients with chronic obstructive pulmonary disease (COPD).
- Inhaled NO can be used to manage acute pulmonary hypertension. It causes vasodilation by stimulating an increase in cGMP levels. A dose of 20–40 ppm reduces arterial pressure and improves cardiac index without causing systemic vasodilation [61,62].
- Digoxin can be given to improve cardiac output acutely; the long-term benefits of its use are unknown [63].

Furthermore, it is important to consider comorbidities and weigh the risks and benefits of treating these conditions. For example, patients with chronic liver disease take adrenoceptor blockers to reduce the risk of variceal bleeding caused by portal hypertension; however, this medication can reduce exercise capacity and worsen hemodynamics in patients with pulmonary hypertension associated with liver disease [64].

For patients undergoing surgery assessment, the active management of PAH should be ensured. Respiratory function should be optimized and oxygen therapy given to achieve a blood oxygen saturation (by pulse oximetry) of more than 90% [65]. During surgery, anesthesiologists are required to minimize and manage rises in PVR as well as control systemic vascular resistance to ensure adequate cardiac perfusion. Most anesthetic drugs decrease this resistance; consequently, vasoconstrictors may need to be used. Finally, anesthesiologists must monitor for and treat right ventricular decompensation to prevent rapid deterioration and cardiac arrest [53].

1.4. Previous Myocardial Infarction—Patients with Coronary Stents

Percutaneous coronary intervention (PCI) is a common procedure used to treat infarcted myocardium resulting from an ST-segment elevation myocardial infarction (STEMI), as it has been shown to have better outcomes than fibrinolytic therapy [66-68]. Ninety percent of all patients undergoing PCI will have coronary stents inserted [69]. The coronary stent insertion is followed by dual antiplatelet therapy (clopidogrel 75 mg daily and aspirin 75 mg daily) to prevent stent thrombosis. The recommended dual antiplatelet therapy for bare metal stents (BMS) lasts four to six weeks. For drug-eluting stents (DES), therapy is recommended for 12 months, as the drugs used in DES inhibit endothelialization and, as a result, the stents remain thrombogenic for prolonged periods of time. After the stated dual therapy, low dose aspirin treatment is continued indefinitely [70].

Premature discontinuation of dual antiplatelet therapy in patients undergoing surgery significantly increases the risk of myocardial infarction and cardiac death compared with patients who continue taking dual therapy during surgery (30% and 0% incidence of major adverse cardiac events, respectively) [71]. As far as the effects of continuing dual therapy during noncardiac surgery on the risk of bleeding, findings are controversial, suggesting highly varied outcomes when antiplatelet therapy is continued [72-77]. In general, it has been suggested that aspirin therapy has a smaller effect on the risk of bleeding than dual antiplatelet therapy. Ultimately, patients with coronary stents represent a challenge for anesthesiologists because of the risk of bleeding associated with continuing antiplatelet therapy perioperatively and the risk of stent thrombosis when antiplatelet therapy is discontinued prematurely [78].

Several guidelines have been published on how to handle dual antiplatelet therapy during noncardiac surgery [70, 77, 79]. Usually vague, they tend to recommend individual assessments of all patients presenting for surgery while on dual antiplatelet therapy. Elective surgery should be postponed until dual therapy is completed—a minimum of 4–6 weeks and, wherever possible, 3 months after BMS-PCI and 12 months after DES-PCI [79,70].

In patients with DES where surgery is unavoidable, the risk of thrombosis and bleeding should be calculated [80]. Where the risk of thrombosis is higher than that of bleeding, dual antiplatelet therapy should be continued. When the risk of thrombosis is considered to be low and bleeding is likely, one or both antiplatelet agents may need to be discontinued. Aspirin should be continued wherever possible, whereas clopidogrel should be stopped seven days before surgery and restarted as soon as possible. Furthermore, patients with BMS should undergo noncardiac surgery 6 to 12 weeks after stent insertion, as the risk of restenosis after this period is relatively high [70]. Attempts have been made to use heparin (unfractioned or low molecular weight) as a "bridging" therapy to prevent stent thrombosis perioperatively while temporarily discontinuing the dual antiplatelet therapy. However, this treatment has been shown to be ineffective, possibly as a result of the lack of antiplatelet activity by heparins [81].

It is important to note that the above-mentioned recommendations are made for noncardiac surgery in general and do not consider individual types of surgery. Liver transplants are associated with a high risk of bleeding, and decisions on whether to perform surgery, continue dual antiplatelet therapy, or use a bridging therapy should only be made after discussion with the surgeon and a cardiologist.

2. Drug-Induced Cardiovascular Disease

Transplant patients are at a higher risk of developing metabolic cardiovascular complications, hypertension, and hyperlipidemia, all of which have been associated with an increased risk of major cardiovascular events [82]. Some of these conditions can be induced by immunosuppressants. This section discusses cardiovascular conditions associated with immunosuppressive agents and their treatment in posttransplant patients.

2.1. Immunosuppressant-Induced Hypertension

Prednisolone, ciclosporin, tacrolimus, and mycophenolate mofetil have all been associated with hypertension in posttransplant patients [83,84]. Hypertension is particularly common with the use of ciclosporin and tacrolimus [85, 86], possibly as a result of effects associated with decreased levels of calcineurin, [84] such as impaired sodium excretion [87], increased sympathetic nervous activity [88], and direct damage to endothelial cells followed by the release of the potent vasoconstrictor endothelin [89,90].

Hypertension that develops after transplantation can be difficult to treat with conventional antihypertensive agents, and interactions with immunosuppressive agents must be taken into account [91]. Calcium channel blockers are usually the first choice of therapy. Diltiazem increases the concentration of ciclosporin when given orally at doses of 80–160 mg daily, allowing ciclosporin doses to be reduced by one third on average and thus reducing the cost of therapy [92-94]. However, this effect does not occur in all patients and may depend on formulations. Consequently, patients taking ciclosporin and diltiazem concurrently should have their ciclosporin levels monitored [95,96]. Nifedipine and verapamil have been reported to play a role in protecting against ciclosporin-induced nephrotoxicity and may therefore be the drugs of choice [97-103]. Beta blockers can also be used in immunosuppressant-induced hypertension, whereas diuretics should be avoided [104].

2.2 Tacrolimus-Induced Cardiomyopathy

Tacrolimus has been associated with hypertrophic cardiomyopathy and heart failure in both pediatric and adult patients after liver grafting [105,106]. Echocardiographic monitoring has been recommended in patients receiving tacrolimus, and where hypertrophic changes develop, tacrolimus dose should be reduced or completely withdrawn [107]. However, two studies have suggested that the risk of cardiomyopathy in liver transplant patients is generally high and does not appear to increase with the use of tacrolimus [108, 109]. This topic is presented in more details in chapter 17.

2.3 Major Cardiovascular Events in Patients on Immunosuppressive Therapy

Aside from direct effects on the cardiovascular system, such as hypertension and cardiomyopathy, immunosuppressive agents have also been reported to contribute to the development of metabolic syndrome, with symptoms such as obesity, hypertension, hyperglycemia, and dyslipidemia [110]. Metabolic syndrome can then increase the risk of cardiovascular disease, including major cardiovascular events [111].

Hyperlipidemia is associated with the use of ciclosporin [112,113], tacrolimus [114], sirolimus, azathioprine [115], and corticosteroids [116-118]. Furthermore, corticosteroids and ciclosporin have an additive effect on blood lipids [119]. Drug-induced hyperlipidemia is treated with lipid-regulating agents, similar to those used in nontransplant patients, and drug-drug interactions are taken into account.

References

[1] Pozzi M, Ratti L, Guidi C, Milanese M, Mancia G. Potential therapeutic targets in cirrhotic cardiomyopathy. *Cardiovasc and Hematol Dis - Drug Targets* 2007; 7(1): 21-6.

[2] Sharma A, Fletcher A, Lipscomb GR. Pulmonary oedema after therapeutic ascitic paracentesis: a case report and literature review of the cardiac complications of cirrhosis. *Eur J Gastroenterol Hepatol* 2010; 22(2): 241–5.

[3] Moller S, Dumcke CW, Krag A. The heart and the liver. *Exp. Rev. of Gastroenterol. and Hepatol* .2009; 3(1): 51-64.

[4] Cohen-Solal A, Seghatol F, Durand F. Heart and liver cirrhosis. *Medecine Therapeutique – Cardio* 2007; 3(6): 448-52.

[5] Gaskari, SA, Honar H, Lee SS. Therapy insight: Cirrhotic cardiomyopathy. *Nat. Clin. Pract. Gastroenterol. Hepatol.* 2006; 3: 329-7.

[6] Myers RP, Lee SS. Cirrhotic cardiomyopathy and liver transplantation. *Liver Transpl.* 2000; 6: S44-52.

[7] Baxter K, et al. Stockley's Drug Interactions. The Pharmaceutical Press. London, 2009.

[8] Sweetman SC, et al. Martindale: the complete drug reference. The Pharmaceutical Press. London, March 2010.

[9] National Collaborating Centre for Chronic Conditions. Clinical guideline 5. Chronic heart failure: management of chronic heart failure in adults in primary and secondary care. *Nationl Institute for Clinical Excellence (NICE)*, July 2003.

[10] Henriksen JH, Bendtsen F, Hansen EF, Møller S. Acute non-selective beta-adrenergic blockade reduces prolonged frequency-adjusted Q-T interval (QTc) in patients with cirrhosis. *J. Hepatol.* 2004; 40: 239–46.

[11] Pozzi M, Grassi G, Ratti L, Favini G, Dell'Oro R, Redaelli E et al. Cardiac, neuroadrenergic, and portal hemodynamic effects of prolonged aldosterone blockade in postviral child A cirrhosis. *Am. J. Gastroenterol.* 2005; 100: 1110–6.

[12] Simonneau G, Gallen N, Rubin LJ, Langleben D, Seeger W, Domenighetti G et al. Clinical classification of pulmonary hypertension. *J. Am. Coll Cardiol* .2004; 43 (12 Suppl S):5S–12S.

[13] Ramsay MAE, Simpson BR, Nguyen A, Ramsay KJ, East C, Klintmalm GB. Severe Pulmonary Hypertension in Liver Transplant Candidates. *Liver Transpl* .1997; 3(5): 494-500.

[14] Galiè N, Hoeper MM, Humbert M, Torbicki A, Vachiery JL, Barbera JA et al. Guidelines for the diagnosis and treatment of pulmonary hypertension. *European Heart J* .2009: 30, 2493–537.

[15] Rich S, Kaufmann E, Levy PS. The effect of high doses of calcium-channel blockers on survival in primary pulmonary hypertension. *N. Engl. J. Med.* 1992; 327: 76-81.

[16] Barst RJ, McGoon M, Torbicki A, Sitbon O, Krowka MJ, Olschewski H, Gaine S. Diagnosis and differential assessment of the pulmonary arterial hypertension. *J. Am. Coll Cardiol* .2004; 43: S40-7.

[17] Jones DA, Benjamin CW, Linseman DA. Activation of thromboxane and prostacyclin receptors elicits opposing effects on vascular smooth muscle cell growth and mitogen-activated protein kinase signalling cascades. *Mol. Pharmacol* .1995; 48: 890-6.

[18] Galie N, Manes A, Branzi A. Prostanoids for pulmonary arterial hypertension. *Am. J. Respir. Med* .2003; 2: 123-37.

[19] Sitbon O, Humbert M, Nunes H, Parent F, Garcia G, Herve P et al. Long-term intravenous epoprostenol infusion in primary pulmonary hypertension: prognostic factors and survival. *J. Am. Coll Cardiol.* 2002; 40: 780- 8.

[20] McLaughlin W, Shillington A, Rich S, Survival in primary pulmonary hypertension: the impact of epoprostenol therapy. *Circulation* 2002; 106: 1477-82.

[21] Rubin LJ, Mendoza J, Hood M, McGoon M, Barst R, Williams WB et al. Treatment of primary pulmonary hypertension with continuous intravenous prostacyclin (epoprostenol). Results of a randomized trial. *Ann. Intern. Med* .1990; 112: 485–91.

[22] Barst RJ, Rubin LJ, Long WA, McGoon MD, Rich S, Badesch DB et al. A comparison of continuous intravenous epoprostenol (prostacyclin) with conventional therapy for primary pulmonary hypertension. The Primary Pulmonary Hypertension Study Group. *N. Engl. J. Med.* 1996; 334: 296–302.

[23] Kuo PC, Johnson LB, Plotkin JS, Howell CD, Bartlett ST, Rubin LJ. Continuous intravenous infusion of epoprostenol for the treatment of portopulmonary hypertension. *Transplantation* 1997; 63: 604–6.

[24] Hibenbottam T, Butt AY, McMahon A, Westerbeck R, Sharples L. Long-term intravenous prostaglandin (epoprostenol or iloprost) for treatment of severe pulmonary hypertension. *Heart* 1998; 80: 151-5.

[25] Olschewski H, Simonneau G, Galie N, Higenbottam T, Naeije R, Rubin LJ et al. Inhaled iloprost in severe pulmonary hypertension. *N. Engl. J. Med* .2002; 347: 322 – 9.

[26] Simonneau G, Barst RJ, Galie N, Naeije R, Rich S, Bourge RC et al. Continuous subcutaneous infusion of treprostinil, a prostacyclin analogue, in patients with pulmonary arterial hypertension. A double-blind, randomized, placebo-controlled trial. *Am. J. Respir. Crit. Care Med.* 2002; 165: 800– 4.

[27] Barst RJ, Galie N, Naeije R, Simonneau G, Jeffs R, Arneson C, Rubin LJ. Long term outcome in pulmonary arterial hypertension patients treated with subcutaneous treprostinil. *Eur. Respir. J.* 2006; 28: 1195–203.

[28] Lang I, Gomez-Sanchez M, Kneussl M, Naeije R, Escribano P, Skoro-Sajer N, Vachiery JL. Efficacy of long-term subcutaneous treprostinil sodium therapy in pulmonary hypertension. *Chest* 2006; 129: 1636–43.

[29] Tapson VF, Gomberg-Maitland M, McLaughlin VV, Benza RL, Widlitz AC, Krichman A, Barst RJ. Safety and fficacy of IV treprostinil for pulmonary arterial hypertension: a prospective, multicenter, open-label, 12-Week trial. *Chest* 2006; 129: 683–8.

[30] Sitbon O, Manes A, Jais X, Pallazini M, Humbert M, Presotto L et al. Rapid switch from intravenous epoprostenol to intravenous treprostinil in patients with pulmonary arterial hypertension. *J. Cardiovasc. Pharmacol*.2007; 49:1–5.

[31] Barst RJ, McGoon M, Mc Laughlin VV, Tapson V, Rich S, Rubin L et al. 2532 ESC Guidelines Beraprost therapy for pulmonary arterial hypertension. *J. Am .Coll Cardiol* .2003; 41: 2119- 25.

[32] Giaid A, Yanagisawa M, Langleben D, Michel RP, Levy R, Shennib H et al. Expression of endothelin-1 in the lungs of patients with pulmonary hypertension. *N Engl. J. Med.* 1993; 328: 1732–9.

[33] Galie N, Manes A, Branzi A. The endothelin system in pulmonary arterial hypertension. *Cardiovas.c Res* .2004; 61: 227–37.

[34] Channick RN, Simonneau G, Sitbon O, Robbins IM, Frost A, Tapson VF et al. Effects of the dual endothelin-receptor antagonist bosentan in patients with pulmonary hypertension: a randomised placebo-controlled study. *Lancet* 2001; 358: 1119- 23.

[35] Rubin LJ, Badesch DB, Barst RJ, Galie N, Black CM, Keogh A et al. Bosentan therapy for pulmonary arterial hypertension. *N. Engl. J. Med* .2002; 346: 896–903.

[36] Humbert M, Barst RJ, Robbins IM, Channick RN, Galie N, Boonstra A et al. Combination of bosentan with epoprostenol in pulmonary arterial hypertension: BREATHE-2. *Eur. Respir. J.* 2004; 24: 353–9.

[37] Galie N, Rubin LJ, Hoeper M, Jansa P, Al-Hiti H, Meyer GMB et al. Treatment of patients with mildly symptomatic pulmonary arterial hypertension with bosentan (EARLY study): a double-blind, randomised controlled trial. *Lancet* 2008; 371:2093–100.

[38] Galie N, Beghetti M, Gatzoulis MA, Granton J, Berger RMF, Lauer A et al. Bosentan therapy in patients with Eisenmenger syndrome: a multicenter, double-blind, randomized, placebo-controlled study. *Circulation* 2006;114: 48–54.

[39] Hoeper MM, Halank M, Marx C, Hoeffken G, Seyfarth HJ, Schauer J et al. Bosentan therapy for portopulmonary hypertension. *Eur. Respir. J.* 2005;25:502–8.

[40] Barst RJ, Langleben D, Frost A, Horn EM, Oudiz R, Shapiro S et al. Sitaxsentan therapy for pulmonary arterial hypertension. *Am. J. Respir. Crit. Care Med.* 2004;169:441–7.

[41] Barst RJ, Langleben D, Badesch D, Frost A, Lawrence EC, Shapiro S et al. Treatment of pulmonary arterial hypertension with the selective endothelin-A receptor antagonist sitaxsentan. *J. Am. Coll Cardiol.* 2006;47: 2049–56.

[42] Galie N, Badesch BD, Oudiz R, Simonneau G, McGoon M, Keogh A et al. Ambrisentan therapy for pulmonary arterial hypertension. *J. Am. Coll. Cardiol.* 2005;46:529–35.

[43] Galie N, Olschewski H, Oudiz RJ, Torres F, Frost A, Ghofrani HA et al. Ambrisentan for the treatment of pulmonary arterial hypertension. Results of the ambrisentan in pulmonary arterial hypertension, randomized, double-blind, placebo-controlled, multicenter, efficacy (ARIES) study 1 and 2. *Circulation* 2008;117:3010–9.

[44] McGoon M, Frost A, Oudiz R, Badesch BD, Galie` N, Olschewski H et al. Ambrisentan therapy in patients with pulmonary arterial hypertension who discontinued bosentan or sitaxsentan due to liver function test abnormalities. *Chest* 2009; 135:122–9.

[45] Bhatia S, Frantz RP, Severson CJ, Durst LA, McGoon MD. Immediate and long- term hemodynamic and clinical effects of sildenafil in patients with pulmonary arterial hypertension receiving vasodilator therapy. *Mayo Clin. Proc.* 2003;78: 1207 – 13.

[46] Michelakis ED, Tymchak W, Noga M, Webster L, Wu XC, Lien D et al. Long-term treatment with oral sildenafil is safe and improves functional capacity and hemodynamics in patients with pulmonary arterial hypertension. *Circulation* 2003; 108:2066 –9.

[47] Ghofrani HA, Schermuly RT, Rose F, Wiedemann R, Kohstall MG, Kreckel A et al. Sildenafil for long-term treatment of nonoperable chronic thromboembolic pulmonary hypertension. *Am. J. Respir. Crit. Care Med.* 2003;167:1139 – 41.

[48] Galie N, Ghofrani HA, Torbicki A, Barst RJ, Rubin LJ, Badesch D et al. The Sildenafil Use in Pulmonary Arterial Hypertension (SUPER) Study Group. Sildenafil citrate therapy for pulmonary arterial hypertension. *New. Engl. J. Med.* 2005;353:2148–57.

[49] Cadden IS. The use of sildenafil to treat portopulmonary hypertension prior to liver transplantation. *Ann. Hepatol* .2009: 8: 158-61.

[50] Sildenafil summary of product characteristics. Pfizer ltd. *Medicines compendium*. Available at www.emc.medicines.org.uk Last updated on the eMC: 23/02/2009.

[51] Tadalafil summary of product characteristics. Eli Lilly and Company ltd. *Medicines compendium*. Available at www.emc.medicines.org.uk Last updated on the eMC: 23/04/2010.

[52] Galie N, Brundage B, Ghofrani A, Oudiz R, Simonneau G, Safdar Z et al. Tadalafil therapy for pulmonary arterial hypertension. *Circulation* 2009;119:2894 – 903.

[53] Teo YW, Greenhalgh DL. Update on anaesthetic approach to pulmonary hypertension. *Eur. J. Anaesthesiol.* 2010; 27(4): 317-22.

[54] McLaughlin VV, Oudiz RJ, Frost A, Tapson VF, Murali S, Channick RN et al. Randomized study of adding inhaled iloprost to existing bosentan in pulmonary arterial hypertension. *Am. J. Respir. Crit. Care Med.* 2006;174:1257 – 63.

[55] Hoeper M, Leuchte H, Halank M, Wilkens H, Meyer FJ, Seyfarth HJ et al. Combining inhaled iloprost with bosentan in patients with idiopathic pulmonary arterial hypertension. *Eur. Respir. J* 2006;4:691–4.

[56] McLaughlin V, Rubin L, Benza RL, Channick R, Vosswinkel R, Tapson V et al. TRIUMPH I: efficacy and safety of inhaled treprostinil sodium in patients with pulmonary arterial hypertension. *Am. J. Respir. Crit. Care Med.* 2009;177: A965.

[57] Simonneau G, Rubin L, Galie N, Barst RJ, Fleming T, Frost A et al. Addition of sildenafil to long-term intravenous epoprostenol therapy in patients with pulmonary arterial hypertension. *Ann. Intern. Med.* 2008;149:521 – 30.

[58] Galie N, Rubin LJ, Hoeper M, Jansa P, Al-Hiti H, Meyer GMB et al. Treatment of patients with mildly symptomatic pulmonary arterial hypertension with bosentan (EARLY study): a double-blind, randomised controlled trial. *Lancet* 2008;371:2093 – 100.

[59] Paul GA, Gibbs JS, Boobis AR, Abbas A, Wilkins MR. Bosentan decreases the plasma concentration of sildenafil when coprescribed in pulmonary hypertension. *Br. J. Clin. Pharmacol* .2005;60:107 – 12.

[60] Humbert M, Segal ES, Kiely DG, Carlsen J, Schwierin B, Hoeper MM. Results of European post-marketing surveillance of bosentan in pulmonary hypertension. *Eur. Respir. J.* 2007; 30: 338 – 44.

[61] Beck JR, Mongero LB, Kroslowitz RM, Choudhri AF, Chen JM, DeRose JJ et al. Inhaled nitric oxide improves hemodynamics in patients with acute pulmonary hypertension after highrisk cardiac surgery. *Perfusion* 1999; 14:37–42.

[62] Pepke-Zaba J, Higenbottam TW, Dinh-Xuan AT, Stone D, Wallwork J. Inhaled nitric oxide as a cause of selective pulmonary vasodilatation in pulmonary hypertension. *Lancet* 1991; 338:1173–4.

[63] Rich S, Seidlitz M, Dodin E, Osimani D, Judd D, Genthner D et al. The short-term effects of digoxin in patients with right ventricular dysfunction from pulmonary hypertension. *Chest* 1998;114:787 – 92.

[64] Provencher S, Herve P, Jais X, Lebrec D, Humbert M, Simonneau G, Sitbon O. Deleterious effects of beta-blockers on exercise capacity and hemodynamics in patients with portopulmonary hypertension. *Gastroenterology* 2006;130: 120–6.

[65] Hoeper MM, Barbera JA, ChannickRN, Hussoun PM, Lang IM, Manes A. et al. Diagnosis, assessment, and treatment of nonpulmonary arterial hypertension pulmonary hypertension. *J. Am. Coll Cardiol.* 2009; 54(1Suppl):S85–S96.

[66] Keeley EC, Boura JA, Grines CL. Primary angioplasty versus intravenous thrombolytic therapy for acute myocardial infarction: A quantitative review of 23 randomised trials. *Lancet* 2003;361:13–20.

[67] Grines CL, Browne KF, Marco J, Rothbaum D, Stone GW, O'Keefe J et al. A comparison of immediate angioplasty with thrombolytic therapy for acute myocardial infarction. The Primary Angioplasty in Myocardial Infarction Study Group. *N. Engl. J. Med* .1993;328:673–9.

[68] Zijlstra F, Hoorntje JC, de Boer MJ, Reiffers S, Miedema K, Ottervanger JP et al. Long-term benefit of primary angioplasty as compared with thrombolytic therapy for acute myocardial infarction. *N. Eng. J. Med* .1999; 341:1413–9.

[69] Steinhul SR, Berger PB, Mann III JT, Fry ETA, DeLago A, Wilmer G, et al . Clopidogrel for the reduction of events during observation. Early and sustained dual oral antiplatelet therapy following percutaneous coronary intervention: a randomised controlled trial. *JAMA* 2002; 288: 2411–20.

[70] Grines CL, Bonow RO, Casey DE Jr, Gardner TJ, Lockhart PB, Moliterno DJ et al. Prevention of Premature Discontinuation of Dual Antiplatelet Therapy in Patients With Coronary Artery Stents. *Circulation* 2007;115:813-18.

[71] Schouten O, van Domburg RT, Bax JJ, de Jaegere PJ, Dunkelgrun M, Feringa HH. et al. Noncardiac surgery after coronary stenting: early surgery and interruption of antiplatelet therapy are associated with an increase in major adverse cardiac events. *J. Am. Coll Cardiol.* 2007; 49:122– 4.

[72] Kaluza GL, Joseph J, Lee JR, Raizner ME, Raizner AE. Catastrophic outcomes of noncardiac surgery soon after coronary stenting. *J. Am. Coll. Cardiol.* 2000; 35:1288– 94.

[73] Vicenzi MN, Meislitzer T, Heitzinger B, Halaj M, Fleisher LA, Matzier H. Coronary artery stenting and noncardiac surgery: a prospective outcome study. *Br. J. Anaesth.* 2006; 96:686–93.

[74] Rabbitts JA, Nuttall GA, Brown MJ, Hanson AC, Oliver WC, Holmes DR, Rihal CS. Cardiac risk of noncardiac surgery after percutaneous coronary intervention with drug-eluting stents. *Anesthesiology* 2008; 109:596–604.

[75] van Kuijk JP, Flu WJ, Schouten O, Hoeks SE, Schenkeveld L, de Jaegere PP et al. Timing of noncardiac surgery after coronary artery stenting with bare metal or drug-eluting stents. *Am. J. Cardiol* .2009; 104:1229-34.

[76] Burger W, Chemnitius JM, Kneissl GD, Rucker G. Low-dose aspirin for secondary cardiovascular prevention – cardiovascular risks after its perioperative withdrawal versus bleeding risks with its continuation – review and meta-analysis. *J. Intern. Med.* 2005; 257:399–414.

[77] Chassot PG, Delabays A, Spahn DR. Perioperative antiplatelet therapy: the case for continuing therapy in patients at risk of myocardial infarction. *Br. J. Anaesth* .2007; 99: 316–28.

[78] Iakovou I, Schmidt T, Bonizzoni E, Ge L, Snagiorgi G, Stankovic G. et al. Incidence, predictors, and outcomes of thrombosis after successful implantation of drug eluting stents. *JAMA* 2005;293: 2126–30.

[79] Poldermans D, Bax JJ, Boersma E, De Hert S, Eeckhout E, Fowkes G. et al. Guidelines for preoperative cardiac risk assessment and perioperative cardiac management in noncardiac surgery: the Task Force for Preoperative Cardiac Risk Assessment and Perioperative Cardiac Management in Noncardiac Surgery of the European Society of Cardiology (ESC) and endorsed by the European Society of Anaesthesiology (ESA). *Eur. Heart J.* 2009; 30:2769–812.

[80] Bornemann H, Pruller F Metzler H. The patient with coronary stents and antiplatelet agents: what to do and how to deal? *Eur. J. Anaesthesiol*.2010; 27(5): 406-10.

[81] Vicenzi MN, Meislitzer T, Heitzinger B, Halaj M, Fleisher LA, Metzler H. Coronary artery stenting and non-cardiac surgery-a prospective outcome study. *BJA* 2006; 96:686–93.

[82] Laryea M, Watt KD, Molinari M, Walsh MJ, McAlister VC, Marotta PJ et al. Metabolic Syndrome in Liver Transplant Recipients: Prevalence and Association With Major Vascular Events. *Liver Transpl.* 2007; 13:1109-14.

[83] Booth CJ. Intravenous tacrolimus may induce severe hypertension in renal transplant recipients. *Arch. Dis. Child.* 1999; 80 (suppl 1): A27.

[84] Koomans HA, Ligtenberg G. Mechanisms and consequences of arterial hypertension after renal transplantation. *Transplantation* 2001; 72 (suppl): S9–12.

[85] Textor SC, Canzanello VJ, Taler SJ, Wilson DJ, Schwartz LL, Augustine JE et al. Cyclosporine-induced hypertension after transplantation. *Mayo Clin. Proc.* 1994; 69: 1182–93.
[86] Porter GA, Bennett WM, Sheps SG. Cyclosporine-associated hypertension. *Arch. Intern. Med.* 1990; 150: 280–3.
[87] Weinman EJ. Cyclosporine-associated hypertension. *Am J Med* 1989; 86: 256–7.
[88] Mark AL. Cyclosporine, sympathetic activity, and hypertension. *N Engl J Med* 1990; 323: 748–50.
[89] Zaal MJW, De Vries J, Boen-Tan YN. Is cyclosporin toxic to endothelial cells? *Lancet* 1988; 332: 956–7.
[90] Deray G, Carayon A, Le Hoang P. Increased endothelin level after cyclosporine therapy. *Ann. Intern. Med.* 1991; 114: 809.
[91] Weinman EJ. Cyclosporine-associated hypertension. *Am. J .Med .*1989; 86: 256–7.
[92] Wagner K, Neumayer H-H. Prevention of delayed graft function in cadaver kidney transplants by diltiazem. *Lancet* 1985; ii: 1355–6.
[93] Neumayer H-H, Wagner K. Diltiazem and economic use of cyclosporin. *Lancet* 1986; ii: 523.
[94] Bourge RC, Kirkin JK, Naftel DC, White C, Mason DA, Epstein AE. Diltiazem-cyclosporine interaction in cardiac transplant recipients: impact on cyclosporine dose and medication costs. *Am. J. Med .*1991; 90: 402–4.
[95] Jones TE, Morris RG. Diltiazem does not always increase blood cyclosporin concentration. *Br. J. Clin. Pharmacol .*1996; 42: 642–4.
[96] Jones TE, Morris RG, Mathew TH. Formulation of diltiazem affects cyclosporin-sparing activity. *Eur. J. Clin. Pharmacol .*1997; 52: 55–8.
[97] Feehally J, Walls J, Mistry N, Horsburgh T, Taylor J, Veitch PS, Bell PR. Does nifedipine ameliorate cyclosporin A nephrotoxicity? *BMJ* 1987; 295: 310.
[98] Shin GT, Cheigh JS, Riggio RR, Suthanthiran M, Stubenbord WT, Serur D et al. Effect of nifedipine on renal allograft function and survival beyond one year. *Clin. Nephrol.* 1997; 47: 33–6.
[99] Weinrauch LA, D'Elia JA, Gleason RE, Shaffer D, Monaco AP. Role of calcium channel blockers in diabetic renal transplant patients: preliminary observations on protection from sepsis. *Clin. Nephrol.* 1995; 44: 185–92.
[100] Mehrens T, Thiele S, Suwelack B, Kempkes M, Hohage H. The beneficial effects of calcium channel blockers on long-term kidney transplant survival are independent of blood-pressure reduction. *Clin. Transplant.* 2000; 14: 257–61.
[101] Dawidson I, Rooth P. Improvement of cadaver renal transplantation outcomes with verapamil: a review. *Am. J. Med.* 1991; 90 (suppl 5A): 37S–41S.
[102] Dawidson I, Rooth P, Lu C, Sagalowsky A, Diller K, Palmer B et al. Verapamil improves the outcome after cadaver renal transplantation. *J. Am. Soc. Nephrol .*1991; 2: 983–90.
[103] Chan C, Maurer J, Cardella C, Cattrani D, Pei Y. A randomized controlled trial of verapamil on cyclosporine nephrotoxicity in heart and lung transplant recipients. *Transplantation* 1997; 63: 1435–40.
[104] Taler SJ, Textor SC, Canzanello VJ, Schwartz L. Cyclosporin-induced hypertension: incidence, pathogenesis and management. *Drug Safety* 1999; 20: 437–49.

[105] Atkison P, Joubert G, Barron A, Grant D, Paradis K, Seidman E et al. Hypertrophic cardiomyopathy associated with tacrolimus in paediatric transplant patients. *Lancet* 1995; 345: 894–6.

[106] Natazuka T, Ogawa R, Kizaki T, Ueno H, Shiotani H, Koizumi T et al. Immunosuppressive drugs and hypertrophic cardiomyopathy. *Lancet* 1995; 345: 1644.

[107] Committee on Safety of Medicines/Medicines Control Agency. Tacrolimus (Prograf) and hypertrophic cardiomyopathy in transplant patients. *Current Problems* 1995; 21: 6.

[108] Dollinger MM, Plevris JN, Chauhan A, MacGilchrist AJ, Finlayson ND, Hayes PC. Tacrolimus and cardiotoxicity in adult liver transplant recipients. *Lancet* 1995; 346: 507.

[109] Coley KC, Verrico MM, McNamara DM, Park SC, Cressman MD, Branch RA. Lack of tacrolimus-induced cardiomyopathy. *Ann. Pharmacother*. 2001; 35: 985–9.

[110] Perkins JD. Metabolic syndrome: a new view of some familiar transplant risks. *Liver Transpl.* 2006;12: 485-6.

[111] Lakka HM, Laaksonen DE, Lakka TA, Niskanen LK, Kumpusalo E, Tuomilehto J, Salonen JT. The metabolic syndrome and total and cardiovascular disease mortality in middle-aged men. *JAMA* 2002; 288: 2709-16.

[112] Luke DR, Beck JE, Vadiei K, Yousefpour M, LeMaistre CF, Yau JC. Longitudinal study of cyclosporine and lipids in patients undergoing bone marrow transplantation. *J. Clin. Pharmacol*. 1990; 30: 163–9.

[113] Ballantyne CM, Podet EJ, Patsch WP, Harati Y, Appel V, Gotto AM Jr, Young JB. Effects of cyclosporine therapy on plasma lipoprotein levels. *JAMA* 1989; 262: 53–6.

[114] Taylor DO, Barr ML, Radovancevic B, Renlund DG, Mentzer RM Jr, Smart FW et al. A randomized, multicenter comparison of tacrolimus and cyclosporine immunosuppressive regimens in cardiac transplantation: decreased hyperlipidemia and hypertension with tacrolimus. *J. Heart Lung Transplant.* 1999; 18: 336–45.

[115] van den Dorpel MA, Ghanem H, Rischen-Vos J, Man in't Veld AJ, Jansen H, Weimar W. Conversion from cyclosporine A to azathioprine treatment improves LDL oxidation in kidney transplant recipients. *Kidney Int*. 1997; 51: 1608–12.

[116] Ng MKC, Celermajer DS. Glucocorticoid treatment and cardiovascular disease. *Heart* 2004; 90: 829–30.

[117] Souverein PC, Berard A, Van Staa TP, Cooper C, Egberts AC, Leufkens HG, Walker BR. Use of oral glucocorticoids and risk of cardiovascular and cerebrovascular disease in a population based case-control study. *Heart* 2004; 90: 859–65.

[118] Wei L, MacDonald T, Walkeet BR.. Taking glucocorticoids by prescription is associated with subsequent cardiovascular disease. *Ann. Intern. Med.* 2004; 141: 764–70.

[119] Moore R, Hernandez D, Valantine H. Calcineurin inhibitors and post-transplant hyperlipidaemias. *Drug Safety* 2001; 24: 755–66.

In: Cardiovascular Diseases and Liver Transplantation
Editor: Zoka Milan, pp. 239-258
ISBN: 978-1-61122-910-3
© 2011 Nova Science Publishers, Inc.

Chapter XVI

Cardiovascular Monitoring During Liver Transplantation

Giorgio Della Rocca[*1], *Maria Gabriella Costa*[1] *and Zoka Milan*[2]

[1]Department of Anesthesia and Intensive Care Medicine
Medical School of the University of Udine
Piazzale S. Maria della Misericordia 15, 33100 Udine, Italy
[2]Department of Anaesthesia and Intensive Care Medicine
St James's University Hospital, Leeds LS9 7TF, UK

Abstract

Our understanding of the cardiovascular changes in end stage liver disease is increasing. Accurate presentation of the changes that occur during liver transplantation (LT) is vital to good anaesthetic management, and the speed at which they take place makes effective monitoring essential. To date perioperative haemodynamic monitoring has been largely based on thermodilution techniques. New developments in this field offer opportunities to monitor preload using variables such as right ventricular ejection fraction (RVEF) and right ventricular end diastolic volume (RVEDV) that seem preferable to those derived from pressures. Trans-oesophageal echocardiography (TEE) is receiving more attention because it is non invasive and can visualise heart structures, filling and dynamic function, but results are operator dependent and prolonged training is needed. Currently other less invasive techniques that provide continuous cardiac output monitoring are being evaluated but different levels of accuracy have been reported in LT recipients. The trend in intraoperative haemodynamic monitoring, a key feature of anaesthetic practice in LT, is towards systems that provide continuous information and are less invasive. A balance is needed between the hazards of an invasive approach and the desire for a continuous stream of accurate information that is robust enough to withstand the surgical and physiological challenges of LT. Despite its importance for

---

[*] Correspondence: Prof. Giorgio Della Roca, Department of Anesthesia and Intensive Care Medicine, Medical School of the University of Udine, Piazzale S. Maria della Misericordia 15, 33100 Udine , Italy, Tel: +39 0432 559900-1, Fax: +39 0432 559512, E-mail: giorgio.dellarocca@uniud.it

anaesthetists, there is no consensus as to which system is best. In this chapter we shall examine recent developments in haemodynamic monitoring during LT.

Introduction

End-stage liver disease is characterised by a hyperdynamic, hyporeactive circulation with reduced effective circulating volume [1, 2, 3]. Amongst the many factors that contribute to intra-operative haemodynamic instability during liver transplantation (LT) are associated cardiovascular disease (presented in detail in preceding chapters), anaesthetic agents, mechanical ventilation, hypothermia, surgical stress and manipulation, rapid fluid shift, bleeding, clamping of the inferior vena cava and portal vein, absence of liver function in the anhepatic phase, reperfusion syndrome, renal failure, and marginal grafts.[4,5,6]. Tissue hypoperfusion during surgery is associated with poor outcome following liver transplantation (LT) and consequently a cornerstone of management is maintenance of adequate volume. To achieve this during LT effective and detailed haemodynamic monitoring is necessary to provide the anaesthetist with a continuous overview of cardiovascular status. This in turn, allows rapid identification of problems with accurate direction of treatment strategies, and subsequent reduction in ICU stay and improved outcome [7,8,9,10,11]. There is no consensus amongst anaesthetists as to the best form of haemodynamic monitoring during LT despite its importance for intraoperative management. The forms of monitoring currently available are considered below.

Arterial Pressure Monitoring

During LT haemodynamic and metabolic changes are both rapid and frequent, and consequently direct arterial pressure monitoring is essential [12]. The accuracy of radial arterial blood pressure monitoring (RAP) during LT has been questioned since several studies have shown that during vasopressor therapy in critically ill patients or during LT, systolic RAP may underestimate central aortic pressure [13,14]. Two practical solutions are to use the femoral artery (FAP) rather than the radial, but should that prove unsuitable, the mean rather than systolic RAP has been suggested [15]. A recent study conducted on 36 patients found that RAP together with non invasive blood pressure monitoring, was a reliable alternative to FAP even during the most unstable phases of LT [15].

Central Venous Pressure

The use of central venous pressure monitoring (CVP) is traditional during LT despite evidence that it is not an accurate marker of right ventricular end-diastolic volumes, cannot define the degree of ventricular filling, nor the potential response to fluid challenge. Nevertheless some centres still use it as the only invasive form of haemodynamic monitoring during LT [16,17,18].

Pulmonary Artery Catheter

Since the first liver transplant procedure, the flow-directed balloon-tipped pulmonary artery catheter (PAC) has been used as a "gold standard" to guide fluid management and vasoactive/inotropic therapy [5,19]. Relevant haemodynamic variables measured by the PAC are pulmonary artery pressures (PAP), mixed venous oxygen saturation (SvO_2) and cardiac output (CO). The latter two are the main determinants of oxygen delivery. CO measurement with the intermittent thermodilution technique requires injection of a known quantity of cold indicator through the proximal lumen of the PAC into the right atrium. The indicator mixes with the surrounding circulation in the right ventricle (RV) and enters the PA where the change in temperature is detected by a thermistor located near the catheter tip, to produce a thermodilution curve. From this the CO is calculated by an equation shown in Figure 1[20].

PA catheterisation during LT is used less frequently today because its shortcomings are better appreciated, the procedure is better understood, and monitoring technology has seen new developments [21-25] The current generation of modified PAC, introduced in the late 1990s [26-28], allows continuous monitoring of CO (CCO), right ventricular ejection fraction (RVEF) and right ventricular end diastolic volume (RVEDV). CCO monitoring is based on the same intermittent thermodilution principle Instead of applying cool saline in a bolus fashion, blood flowing through the superior vena cava is heated intermittently by an electric filament attached to the PAC some 15 to 25 cm before its tip. The resulting heat signals from the thermistor on the tip of the PAC are analysed stochastically to determine a single thermodilution curve [20]. A proprietary averaging algorithm is applied to reduce the influence of thermal noise. The monitoring system automatically repeats measurements at regular intervals and displays the current CO with trends.

Currently there are two continuous cardiac output (CCO) monitors available: the "Vigilance II System" (Edwards, Lifesciences, Irvine, CA, USA) and the "OptiQ" System (Abbott Laboratories, North Chicago, IL, USA) [22-25]. They have different signal generation and signal processing technologies. Both systems have a response time of 3-6 minutes. Their advantage is the elimination of technical error associated with bolus measurement, but delays in the response of CCO measurement (semi-continuous CO) limit its clinical application during acute haemodynamic instability [26-27]. Significant infused volumes of cold fluids, and sudden changes in temperature, for example during graft reperfusion, can influence the accuracy and reliability of this method.

The relationships between stroke volume index (SVI), right ventricular end diastolic volume index (RVEDVI) and filling pressures have been analysed in a multicentre prospective study in 244 LT recipients [29]. Based on the stronger correlation between SVI and RVEDVI rather than between filling pressures and SVI, the results indicate that RVEDVI is a better reflection of preload than CVP and pulmonary artery occlusion pressure (PAOP) (Table 1). RVEDVI is a promising tool in intraoperative fluid management but several problems with the clinical applicability of RVEDV and RVEF have yet to be resolved. The advanced PAC catheter shows delayed reactivity to rapid changes of intravascular volume and accuracy of data is dependent on catheter position with respect to the tricuspid valve, and the proximity of the thermistor to the pulmonary valve. Right ventricular (RV) monitoring using RV volumetric catheters may be unreliable with irregular or high heart rates (HR) (HR>130-150 beats/min), because the R-R interval becomes too short to identify the ejection fraction. Finally the RVEDV is calculated from stroke volume, which in turn is derived from cardiac output measurements, raising concerns about mathematical coupling as a potential limitation to its use as a preload index. In response, Chang and Nelson have shown that concerns over mathematical coupling do not justify limiting the use of these variables in clinical practice [30,31].

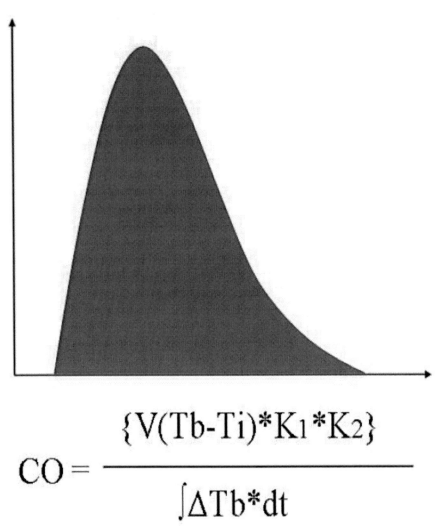

$$CO = \frac{\{V(T_b - T_i) * K_1 * K_2\}}{\int \Delta T_b * dt}$$

Legend: CO=cardiac output, V=volume of injectate, Tb=blood temperature, Ti=injectate temperature, K1=catheter constant, K2=apparatus constant, $\int \Delta T_b * dt$ = change in blood temperature over a given time.

Figure 1. Intermittent thermodilution: the Stewart Hamilton principle.

Table 1. Cardiac output agreement and precision (obtained from different devices vs gold standard)

Author	Year	Pts	Device	Data	Bias	LOA	PE
Greim [23]	1997	14	PAC	ICO-CCO*	-0.8 to 1.6	0.6 to 1.9	//
Bottiger [24]	1997	12	PAC	ICO-CCO	-0.24	±1.789	//
Bao [25]	2008	13	PAC	ICO-CCO	-0.18±1.91	//	//
Lazor [26]	1997	10	PAC	STATCCO-ICO CCO-ICO	0.06 0.06	-0.08 to 0.18 -0.04 to 0.16	// //
Della Rocca [59]	2002	62	PiCCO	COart-ICO PCCO-CCO PCCO-ICO	0.15 -0.03 0.04	±1.74 ±1.75 ±1.69	// // //
Tzenkov [60]	2003	35	PiCCO	PCCO-ICO	0.18	±4.27	//
Costa [75]	2008	23	LiDCO	COLi-ICO PulseCO_ICO	0.11 0.29	-1.8 to 2.1 -1.9 to 2.5	16% 17%
Biasis [91]	2008	20	Vigileo	APCO-ICO	0.80	-1.8 to 3.5	43%
Della Rocca [90]	2008	18	Vigileo	APCO-ICO APCO-CCO	0.95 1.29	±1.41 ±1.28	26% 29%
Biancofiore [92]	2009	29	Vigileo	APCI-ICI	1.3	-1.5 to 4.1	54%
Costa [93]	2009	10	LiDCORapid	PulseCOLiR-ICO PulseCOLiR-CCO			30% 26%

Legend: PAC, pulmonary artery catheter; ICO, intermittent cardiac output (from PAC); CCO, continuous cardiac output (from PAC); STATCCO, Steady State CCO (from PAC); PCCO, pulse contour cardiac output (from PiCCO); COart, intermittent cardiac output (from PiCCO); APCO, continuous cardiac output (from Vigileo/FloTrac); COLi, intermittent cardiac output (from LiDCOplus); PulseCO, continuous cardiac output (from LiDCOplus). APCI, continuous cardiac index (from Vigileo/FloTrac); ICI intermittent cardiac index (from PAC); PulseCOLiR, uncalibrated continuous cardiac output (from LiDCORapid). * mean bias during all the study period (from-to).

Using the PAC and SvO_2 for continuous monitoring of oxygen supply and demand might be another useful haemodynamic tool during LT. The main problems when promoting SvO_2 measurement are difficulties in interpreting whether changes result from variations in cardiac output, oxygen supply or demand, or carrying capacity variations, which are important when the graft is re-establishing metabolic function [32]. For example, immediately after graft reperfusion, when sudden hypotension can occur, a sharp decrease in SvO_2 is expected due to the return of pooled venous blood to the circulation, but recovery should be rapid if cardiac output is well maintained. If a prolonged reduction in SvO_2 is seen, then a low cardiac output should be suspected, assessed and aggressively treated. The introduction of central venous oxygen saturation ($ScvO_2$) in LT as a surrogate for SvO_2, as in critically ill patients, is even more questionable, as the over-representation of the oxygen consumption of the upper half of the body complicates interpretation [33].

Pulmonary artery catheterisation and its clinical value in terms of outcome benefit have been under debate now for more than a decade [34]. Minor and major complications associated with PAC use have been reported to occur in 23% and 4.4% of insertions, respectively [35]. Ventricular arrhythmias during catheterisation in LT patients have occurred [36]. Among fatal complications related to the PAC use, rupture of the pulmonary artery is the most common, with rare cases of myocardium perforation [37]. The failure to show improved outcome with the PAC, the delay in recognition of rapid changes when monitoring cardiac output, the costs of the advanced PAC and the complications associated with insertion, may all be responsible for the decline in popularity of PAC as a standard monitoring tool [28,34]. Diagnosis and treatment of portopulmonary hypertension (PPH) in patients undergoing LT remain the strongest indications for the insertion of a PAC [38].

Trans-Oesophageal Echocardiography

During the last decade, TEE has become increasingly popular for monitoring myocardial function, managing fluid therapy and identifying perioperative complications during LT. [39-45]. The principle advantage of TEE is that its real-time images provide immediate visual information about the structural nature of the heart and its dynamic function [44]. It is less adept at providing the numerical data that we are used to receiving from PAC, but in reality the information from the latter on cardiac filling gives the identical message to that provided by the real time images of TEE [44]. Among the factors that can influence pressure readings are intermittent positive pressure ventilation, pulmonary hypertension, valvular dysfunction and ventricular failure. TEE offers more accurate interpretation of myocardial wall tension than PAC pressure measurement [44]. (Tables 2 and 3)

Right ventricular failure is of particular importance during the reperfusion phase of liver transplantation. A significant advantage of TEE is identification of right ventricular failure by virtue of dynamic rather than pressure changes. The compliance of the right ventricle is such that it may dilate significantly before pressure begins to rise. Once dilated, the contractility of the right ventricle is markedly reduced. The PAC is unable to warn of this relative disability until there is severe failure. During the reperfusion period, or soon after, when the risk of right ventricular failure is very high, the imaging provided by TEE can be hugely important [40, 44].

Other advantages of TEE include the ability to re-assess cardiopulmonary status immediately prior to surgery when it can identify any changes that may have occurred since being listed for OLT, that may affect suitability [44]. TEE may also be of benefit in the occasional situation in which PAC cannot be placed. Finally, TEE allows the visualisation of large vessels such as the inferior vena cava and its probe can be used to assist in the placement of transcutaneous veno-venous bypass lines [45].

Negative aspects of TEE are that during LT, the presence of oesophageal varices and retraction of the stomach can make transgastric viewing technically difficult or impossible [39-41]. Another problem specific to TEE and LT is that movement of the operative field can affect the relative position of the heart, oesophagus and stomach. At certain times during the dissection of the native liver it can be difficult to obtain steady images [43].

The use of TEE as a monitoring tool during LT has slowly gained in popularity. A recent survey of high-volume LT centres (>50 LT per year) found that among 217 anaesthetists from 30/40 centres, 87% used TEE in some cases. Most were 'limited scope' users, although some performed a comprehensive TEE examination during LT [43]. Only 12% of users were board certified in the use of TEE [43].

Table 2. Comparison of the Pulmonary Artery Flotation Catheter Against Transoesophageal Echocardiography

	PAFC	TOE
Accuracy	Good. Traditionally considered gold standard. Possibly inaccurate immediately after caval clamping and reperfusion.	Good, but requires training and time to estimate left ventricular filling pressures and cardiac output numerically. "Global" visual assessment very rapid.
Precision	Good	Good, but relies on good view acquisition
Rapid response time / Continuous data	PA pressure reading continuous and rapidly updated. Cardiac output calculation slow (intermittent thermodilution) and not continuous. (Continuous CO PAFC equipment available)	Real time views continuously updated. Computer driven algorithms permit rapid calculation of pressure gradients and cardiac output. Dynamic appearance of cardiac structures instantaneous.
"Real Time" updating	Poor	Excellent
Reproducibility	Good	Good
Operator independent	Yes	Yes
Minimal risk to patient	Risks associated with venous cannulation, catheter flotation and wedging of PAFC.	Low risk. Relatively non-invasive.
Maximal information	Limited to numerical measurement and calculated parameters. Wedge pressure used to imply LVEDP can be misleading. Pressure potentially a poor surrogate for filling or wall tension.	No direct pressure measurements, but able to directly visualise structural as well as dynamic abnormalities. Filling represented visually and calculations possible to derive volume cardiac output and other parameters. Pulmonary artery pressure difficult to assess in absence of tricuspid regurgitation
Cost	Monitors integrated into standard monitoring equipment. Moderate unit cost of PAFC.	High set up cost, low unit cost. (cleaning of probe and protective sheath)

Abbreviations: LVEDP, Left Ventricular End Diastolic Pressure
Reproduced from [39] with permission.

The American Society of Echocardiography does not differentiate between the full and "limited-scope" skill levels, and recommends a training program involving 300 transthoracic echographic examinations, 25 oesophageal intubations and 50 TEE examinations within a six month period, followed by the use of TEE 50-75 times per year [43]. Implementing these recommendations would restrict the use of TEE for OLT considerably [43].

Table 3.

Complications of PAFC
1) Associated risks of venous cannulation
a) Haemorrhage
b) Arterial puncture
c) Arrhythmia
d) Myocardial puncture / rupture
e) Cardiac tamponade
f) Thoracic duct damage
g) Pneumothorax
h) Infection (medium to longer term complication)
2) Complications of pulmonary artery catheterisation
a) Arrhythmia
b) Myocardial puncture and cardiac tamponade
c) Knotting of PAFC
d) Pulmonary artery rupture
e) Right sided valvular damage
f) Risk of microshock
Complications of TOE
a) Dental trauma
b) Pharyngeal abrasion
c) Variceal bleeding*
d) Oesophageal rupture
e) Recurrent laryngeal nerve injury
f) Autonomic disturbance
g) Increased gastro-oesophageal reflux
h) Risk of microshock (less than PAFC)
*Oesophageal varices are generally considered to be a relative contraindication to TOE. Evaluation of the relative risks and benefits of TOE vs. PAFC is essential for all cases, with specific consideration required to the grade of varices present and bleeding history in the context of the of the anticipated advantages of TOE. A Medline search failed to identify any published adverse events relating to oesophageal varices and the insertion and manipulation of trans-oesophageal echocardiography probes.

Reproduced from [39] with permission.

Transcardiopulmonary Thermodilution (TCPID)

Transcardiopulmonary thermodilution (TCPID) is a technique that was introduced as a "minimally invasive" volumetric monitoring system [46,47]. The PiCCOplus (Pulsion Medical System; Munich Germany) system requires central venous and modified femoral or brachial arterial catheters. For determination of CO, a saline bolus is injected through the central venous catheter. The thermistor on the tip of the arterial PiCCO catheter measures the downstream temperature changes. The CO is calculated by means of the Stuart-Hamilton-equation from the area below the transpulmonary thermodilution curve.

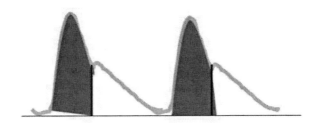

$$CO_{PCnew} = cal * HR * \int_{Systole} \left\{ \frac{P(t)}{SVR} + C(p) * \frac{dP}{dt} \right\} Dt$$

Legend: cal, specific calibration factor determined by transpulmonary thermodilution; CO, cardiac output; C(p), aortic compliance; dP/dt, shape of the pressure wave curve; HR, heart rate; P(t)/SVR, area under the pressure wave curve; SVR, systemic vascular resistance.

Figure 2. Principle of cardiac output assessment by pulse contour analysis using the PiCCOplus System.

From the Mean Transit time (MTt) and the Down Slope time (DSt) of the thermodilution curve, preload and lung water are determined (Figure 2) Simultaneously, the arterial pulse contour is analysed and the aortic compliance determined. With this technology, a pulse contour algorithm is calibrated, and this is used to calculate individual values for SV, CO and SVV, a clinically validated fluid responsiveness index in controlled mechanically ventilated patients [48-52]. The TCPID technique also allows estimation of preload indices such as intrathoracic blood volume (ITBV), extravascular lung water (EVLW) and global end diastolic volume (GEDV) [54-58]. (Table 4).

CCO measured with TCPID is in agreement with CO measurements obtained using PAC in different clinical settings [59-62]. During rapid haemodynamic change like those following cross-clamping of the inferior vena cava, and reperfusion, the algorithms faithfully follow change in cardiac output until it exceeds 30% when reliability begins to deteriorate. If a change of this magnitude is anticipated, calibration using the thermodilution technique is recommended.

A volumetric assessment of intravascular blood volume in cirrhotic patients during LT found that the hyperdynamic circulation of the cirrhotic patient coexists with hypovolemia [63-65]. Total blood volume index (TBVI) was markedly reduced compared to ITBVI probably because of the enlarged "third space" (intra and extravascular) associated with hepatic disease [64]. ITBV proved to be a better reflection of preload in hyperdynamic LT recipients (ITBVI vs. SVI, $r^2=0.55$), [65]. Statistically significant correlations were obtained from analysing preload data at predefined steps. A comparison between the single indicator thermodilution technique and the single TCPID technique during anaesthesia for LT [3] showed a good correlation between ITBVI and SVI, and CI, but in neither study was there any consistent correlation between PAOP and SVI, and CI. [64,65].

Table 4. Different characteristics of clinical available devices for hemodynamic monitoring (and diagnosis)

	ICO	CCO	Invasiveness	Major limitations	Accuracy	Additional information	Precision
PAC	+	+	+++	Well described complications Time limited insertion	Gold standard	PAOP, PAP, SvO$_2$	Good
PiCCO	+	+	++	Dedicated femoral catheter Arterial signal quality	Good	GEDVI,/ITBVI, EVLWI, SVV, PPV SPV	Good
LiDCOplus	+	+	+	Arterial signal quality Lithium injection	Good	SVV, PPV, SPV	Good
Vigileo	-	+	+	Arterial signal quality Arrhythmia	Low in Hyperdynamic patients	SVV, PPV, SPV ScvO$_2$	Low in Hyperdynamic patients
TEE	+*	-	+/-	Operator dependency, Intubated patients		Diagnostic assessment	Good, but relies on good view aquisition

Legend: ICO, intermittent cardiac output; CCO, continuous cardiac output; PAOP, pulmonary artery occlusion pressure; PAP pulmonary artery pressure; SvO$_2$ mixed venous oxygen saturation; systemic vascular resistance; PVR, pulmonary vascular resistance; GEDV, global end diastolic volume; ITBVI, intrathoracic blood volume; EVLW, extravascular lung water; SVV, stroke volume variation; SPV systolic pressure variation; PPV, pulse pressure variation; ScVO$_2$ central venous oxygen saturation. * only through off line calculation.

The strength of the correlation has confirmed the role of ITBVI as a preload index during episodes of major haemodynamic disturbance following clamping of the inferior vena cava, the release of vascular clamps, and graft reperfusion, bleeding and surgical manipulation [3].

It has been argued that circulating volume in general and cardiac output may affect the relationship between GEDV and ITBV. It may also be affected by compensatory venous/arteriolar vasoconstriction in the pulmonary, systemic and splanchnic circulations and the consequent redistribution of blood from the peripheral compartments more centrally. In patients receiving vasoconstrictors, it is possible to detect 'normal' ITBV due to blood volume centralisation despite a relative general hypovolemia [67].

Sakka demonstrated that EVLWI correlated well with survival and was an independent predictor of prognosis. Unfortunately EVLW, and its clinical application to date, lack definitive data [58]. Krenn and colleagues observed that a post-reperfusion increase in ITBVI was accompanied by an increase in pulmonary shunt without impairing oxygenation or altering the extravascular lung water index (EVLWI) [47].

Table 5. Intravascular volume and filling pressure relationships with cardiac index or stroke volume index in liver transplanted patients

Authors	Year	Ref	Patients	Device	Data analyzed	r²
De Wolf A	1993	20	20	PAC	RVEDVI/SVI	0.80
Della Rocca G	2001	70	32	PiCCO	ITBVI/CI PAOP/CI CVP/CI	0.37 0.07 0.02
			24	COLD	ITBVI/CI PAOP/CI CVP/CI	0.45 0.11 0.19
Della Rocca G	2001	69	9*	COLD	ITBVI/CI PAOP/CI CVP/CI	0.34 0.12 0.07
Della Rocca G	2002	71	60	PiCCO	ITBVI/SVI PAOP/SVI	0.55 0.015
Della Rocca G	2008	35	244	PAC	RVEDVI/SVI	0.30°
Della Rocca G	2009	51	20	TEE	LVEDAI/SVI RVEDVI/SVI	0.52° 0.60°

Legend: ITBVI, Intrathoracic Blood Volume Index; GEDVI, Global End Diastolic Volume Index; CI, Cardiac Index; SVI, Stroke Volume Index; CVP = Central Venous Pressure; PAOP = Pulmonary Arterial Occlusion Pressure; LVEDAI, Left Ventricular End Diastolic Area Index; RVEDAI, Right Ventricular End Diastolic Volume Index; TEE = Transesophageal Echogardiography; * nine patients undergoing LT for fulminant hepatic failure; ° r square of the multivariate model ($p<0.0001$).

LiDCO

Recently, new non-invasive cardiovascular monitoring technologies have been introduced and tested during LT. One device based on TPID technique for monitoring CO (LiDCOplus System, LiDCO Ltd, London, UK) needs only a standard peripheral arterial line plus a central or peripheral venous line [68-72]. An established dilution technique is used to define CO using lithium chloride (0.3 mmol; 2 ml) as indicator and a disposable lithium-selective electrode, positioned in the arterial pressure catheter tubing, serves as the sensor (COLi, LiDCO, London, UK). For each COLi measurement, a lithium bolus is given through a central intravenous catheter, whilst a battery-powered roller pump draws arterial blood through the lithium sensor. A lithium concentration washout curve is devised, from which the device derives the CO, and this in turn is used to calibrate a pressure waveform system (PulseCO) that estimates the nominal CO by a nonlinear transformation of the input analogue arterial pressure [73-75]. PulseCO measurements are based on harmonic waveform analysis (Fourier transformation) and integrate beat duration, ejection duration and mean arterial pressure. Compared with thermodilution, LiDCO is not temperature sensitive, but is influenced by electrolyte and haematocrit concentrations and the maximum recommended daily lithium dose of 3 mMols puts a limit on the number of calibration measurements that can be made. The accuracy and trending ability of the PulseCO algorithm following TCPID calibration, has been confirmed in different patient groups [73-75].

A comparison of the LiDCO monitor with bolus pulmonary artery catheter thermodilution showed good overall agreement between the two methods ($r^2 = 0.94$). In post-cardiac surgery patients the monitor was at least as accurate as bolus thermodilution, with significantly greater precision [68]. In ICU patients with a hyperdynamic circulation, continuous CO values determined using the LiDCO system showed good agreement with those obtained using intermittent pulmonary artery thermodilution [75]. So far, there has been only one study that has validated LiDCO in patients immediately following LT [75]. The study found good correlation between data observed with LiDCO and PAC and did not observe any significant variation in agreement at higher and lower CO levels [75].

Some centres have accumulated ten years' experience of continuous intra-operative haemodynamic monitoring during OLT with LiDCO. Patients with pulmonary hypertension were excluded and monitored with PAC [11]. Apart from being non-invasive, LiDCO monitoring provides haemodynamic data continuously through the procedure on a beat-to-beat basis and allows the data to be saved and analysed [69].

Lithium calibration cannot be performed in patients who have received atracurium as a neuromuscular blocker 30 min before calibration because it reacts with the lithium sensor, and the LiDCO system cannot be used in patients receiving lithium therapy. Arrhythmias may make pulse waveform analysis unreliable, as the heart rate can be miscalculated when very large changes are seen in the pressure waveform. Significant fluctuations in the compliance of the arterial vascular system may change the arterial pressure waveform and affect the accuracy of the pulse power analysis performed by PulseCO. Such changes are likely to occur in the operating room or in the ICU after surgery. Frequent recalibration provides a simple solution but is potentially time consuming. Available evidence suggests that calibration every 6-8 h is sufficient for accurate continuous PulseCO monitoring in the ICU setting [72].

Transoesophageal Echo-Dopler (ED)

Transoesophageal echo-Doppler (ED) is another non-invasive approach to continuous CO measurement. It is an ultrasound-based technique that measures blood velocity in the descending aorta using an oesophageal transducer [76], which is rotated to obtain a basic image of the aorta with the Doppler sensor. With this monitor it is possible to measure or derive cardiac index (CI), left ventricular (LV) ejection time interval indexed to the heart rate (a measure of LV filling), maximum acceleration (a measure of contractility and global ventricular function), peak velocity, and systemic vascular resistance (SVR). When compared with "gold standard" CO measurements obtained by thermodilution, the Doppler-derived CI values showed significant bias and only moderate clinical agreement in thoracic surgery, but clinically acceptable agreement was found during cardiac surgery [77,78].

There are three studies in LT patients that compared CO data obtained with ED with PAC [76,79,80]. Boucard et al compared CO during a 5 min hepatic vascular exclusion test performed at the end of the dissection phase and found no correlation [80]. In contrast,

Odenstedt, with data from 14 patients, found good correlation [76], but Perilli with data from 42 cirrhotic patients found that ED correlated poorly with PAC [79]. When the data was taken only from cirrhotic patients with a MELD score <15, the precision of the ED was in fact, comparable to that of PAC. Their suggestion was that ED should not replace PAC for monitoring severely cirrhotic patients undergoing LT, but in patients with MELD score <15, including many subjects with hepatocellular carcinoma, the device does have the potential to yield reliable data and could be used in place of PAC [79].

The main advantage of ED is that it is fairly simple and does not require any sonographic skills. Furthermore, all studies agree that its short response time and reliability in patients with relatively early chronic liver disease is important [76,79]. Against its use are the limitations described above and loss of the Doppler signal caused by diathermy, gastric tube and surgical traction [80].

Vigileo CO Monitoring

In contrast to the calibrated systems described above, the FloTrac sensor attached to the Vigileo device does not require external calibration, and it uses an algorithm to derive cardiac output from the arterial pressure wave (APCO). The system can use any arterial line already in situ, but the signal needs a specific transducer, the FloTrac. The algorithm gets all the information it needs to calculate the arterial impedance from the analysis of the arterial pressure waveform together with the patient's age, sex, height and weight. For APCO assessment the standard deviation of pulse pressure measured during time windows of 20 s is empirically correlated to the 'normal' stroke volume based on underlying patient data. Aortic compliance is also estimated using these data, whereas resistance is derived by analysing the actual pressure waveform characteristics.

The Vigileo system represents a genuine revolution in the field of pulse pressure analysis, being a real "plug and play" tool, but assessment of the performance of the algorithms (two versions of the software have already been released in less than three years) is still underway. To date the reception has been mixed, with some finding good agreement between the Vigileo system and intermittent thermodilution, whilst others have reported poor limits of agreement [81-89].

To our knowledge three studies investigate APCO accuracy and precision in OLT [90-92]. Biasis et.al failed to see good agreement between Vigileo/FloTrac CO and automatic thermodilution in patients undergoing LT, especially in Child-Pugh grade B and C patients with low systemic vascular resistance [91]. The device did show an acceptable bias and precision when compared with intermittent and continuous CO obtained with PAC in the postoperative period after LT [90]. Better agreement was seen when CO levels were lower than 8 L min^{-1} and showed a percentage error less than 25%. When CO was higher than 8 L min^{-1}, APCO underestimated CO in comparison with intermittent and continuous CO measurements [90.]. Biancofiore et al showed that during both the intra- and postoperative LT period, the measurement of CO by the Vigileo system underestimated CO and showed poor agreement with standard thermodilution CO measurements [92].

One interpretation of the above is that the arterial pressure waveform seen in LT patient is affected by the vasodilatation typically seen in cirrhosis, and this interferes with the waveform analysis. Similarly, vasoactive agents induce changes in vascular impedance and compliance with a subsequent impact on arterial pressure waveform. Intermittent cardiac output measurement may be less susceptible to these influences than APCO.

LiDCOrapid

The LiDCOrapid represents the newest arterial pulse wave analysis device. It uses a nomogram to make an estimate of the calibration factor used in the generalised equation used to scale and transform the nominal maximum aortic volume. The LiDCOrapid nomogram has been derived by the manufacturer from a multivariate analysis of the relationship between aortic volume and age, height, weight and body surface area. In the LiDCOrapid set-up the user only has to input these patient details into the monitor and the scaling factor is automatically estimated. The manufacturer claims that once the patient's details have been entered into the system, the monitor follows cardiac output trends. The bias and precision of the nomogram scaled version of the PulseCO$_{LiR}$ algorithm in 10 liver transplanted patients [93] was found to be acceptable measurements when compared to ICO and CCO but percentage error was 30% and 26% respectively.

Increasing attention has been given to the validation of less invasive monitoring tools in hyperdynamic patients, and yet these monitoring devices fail to be applicable for intraoperative monitoring during OLT. Nevertheless, testing their accuracy in this clinical situation is a further step towards their uptake in high-risk surgical patients and critical illness.

Conclusion

Traditional haemodynamic monitoring during liver transplantation is based on pulmonary artery catheter and trans-oesophageal echocardiography. The new developments in PAC technology offer the opportunity to monitor right heart pressures and preload indices with variables such as RVEDV and RVEF that give a better reflection of preload status than the "old" filling pressures. This advanced approach has only been studied in liver transplantation. TEE is receiving growing attention because it allows direct visualisation of heart structure, shape and function. The PiCCO system measures transpulmonary thermodilution cardiac output, but to this it adds a preload index through intrathoracic blood volume measurement, and monitors lung function status through extravascular lung water. Uncalibrated less invasive CO monitoring devices do not give reliably accurate information on cardiac output in the hyperdynamic conditions that are typically seen in most patients undergoing LT.

References

[1] Moller S, Henriksen JH. Cardiovascular complications in cirrhosis. *Gut* 2008;57:268-78
[2] Biancofiore G, Mandell MS, Della Rocca G. Perioperative considerations in patients with cirrhotic cardiomyopathy. *Curr. Opin. Anaesth.* 2010;23:128-92

[3] Della Rocca G, Costa MG, Coccia C, et al. Intravascular blood volume in cirrhotic patients. *Transplant. Proc.* 2001;33:1405-7
[4] Della Rocca G, Costa MG, Pompei L, Chiarandini P. The liver transplant recipient with cardiac disease. *Transplant. Proc.* 2008;40:1172-4
[5] Krenn CG, De Wolf AM. Current approach to intraoperative monitoring in liver transplantation. *Curr. Opin. Organ Transplant.* 2008;13:285-90
[6] Ripoll C, Catalina VM, Yotti R. Cardiac dysfunction during liver transplantation: incidence and preoperative predictors. *Transplantation* 2008;85:1766-72
[7] Schroeder RA, Collins BH, Tuttle-Newhall E. Intraoperative fluid management during ortothopic liver transplantation. *J. Cardiothorac. Vasc. Anest.* 2004;18:438-41
[8] De Wolf AM, Aggarwal S. Monitoring preload during liver transplantation. Liver Transpl 2008:14:268-9
[9] De Wolf AM. Pulmonary artery catheter: rest in peace? Not just quite yet. *Liver Transpl.* 2008;14:917-8
[10] Costa MG, Chiarandini P, Della Rocca G. Hemodynamics during liver transplantation. *Transplant. Proc.* 2007;39:1871-3
[11] Jankovic Z, Taylor, Duncan B, Kedilaya H, Sylvester D, Narayanan R, on behalf of the Leeds Liver Group. Haemodynamic changes during liver transplantation: predictive value for outcome and effect of marginal donors in Knudsen KH (editor): Liver transplantation: immunosuppression and complications. Novapublishers 2009
[12] Frezza EE, Mezghebe H. Indications and complications of arterial catheter use in surgical or medical intensive care units. Analysis of 4932 patients. *Am. Surg.* 1998;64(2):127–31.
[13] Dorman T, Breslow MJ, Lipsett PA, et al. Radial artery pressure monitoring underestimates central arterial pressure during vasopressor therapy in critically ill surgical patients. *Crit. Care Med.* 1998;26:1646–9.
[14] Arnal D, Garutti I, Perez-Pena J, Olmedilla L, Tzenkov IG. Radial to femoral arterial blood pressure differences during liver transplantation. *Anaesthesia* 2005;60:766–71
[15] Shin BS, Kim GS, Ko JS, Gwak MS, Yang M, Kim CS et al. Comparison of femoral arterial blood pressure with radial arterial blood pressure and noninvasive upper arm blood pressure in the reperfusion period during liver transplantation. *Transplant. Proc.* 2007;39(5):1326-8
[16] Scheuren K, Wente MN, Hainer C, Scheffler M, Lichtenstern C, Martin E, Schmidt J, Bopp C, Weigand MA. Left ventricular end-diastolic area is a measure of cardiac preload in patients with early septic shock. *Eur. J. Anaesthesiol.* 2009;26:759-65
[17] Raper R, Sibbald WJ. Misled by the wedge? The Swan-Ganz catheter and left ventricular preload. *Chest* 1986;89:427-34
[18] Kumar A, Anel R, Bunnell E, et al. Pulmonary artery occlusion pressure and central venous pressure fail to predict ventricular filling volume, cardiac performance, or the response to volume infusion in normal subjects. *Crit. Care Med.* 2004;32:691-9
[19] De Wolf A, Begliomini B, Gasior T, Kong Y, Pinsky MR. Right ventricular function during liver transplantation. *Anesth. Analg.* 1993;76:562-8
[20] Nishikawa T, Dohi S. Errors in the measurement of cardiac output by thermodilution. *Can. J. Anaesth.* 1993;40:142-53.

[21] Reuter DA, Huang C, Edrich T, Sherman SK, Eltzschig HK. Cardiac Output Monitoring Using Indicator-Dilution Techniques: Basics, Limits, and Perspectives. *Anesth. Analg.* 2010;110(3):799-811

[22] Yederman M. Continuous measurement of cardiac output with the use of stochastic system identification techniques. J Clin Monit 1990;6:322-32

[23] Greim CA, Roewer N, Thiel H, et al. Continuous cardiac output monitoring during adult liver transplantation: thermal filament technique versus bolus thermodilution. Anesth Analg 1997;85:483–8.

[24] Bottiger BW, Sinner B, Motsch J, Bach A, Bauer H, Martin E. Continuous versus intermittent cardiac output measurement during orthotopic *liver transplantation. Anaesthesia* 1997;52:207-14

[25] Bao FP, Wu J. Continuous versus bolus cardiac output monitoring during orthotopic liver transplantation. *Hepatobiliary Pancreatic Dis. Int.* 2008;7:138-44.

[26] Lazor MA, Pierce ET, Stanley GD, Cass JL, Halpern EF, Bode RH Jr. Evaluation of the accuracy and response time of STAT-mode continuous cardiac output. *J. Cardiothorac. Vasc. Anesth.* 1997;11(4):432-6

[27] Aranda M, Mihm FG, Garrett S, Mihm MN, Pearl RG. Continuous cardiac output catheters: delay in vitro response time after controlled flow changes. *Anesthesiology* 1998;89:1592-5

[28] Wiener RS, Welch HG. Trends in the use of the pulmonary artery catheter in the United States, 1993-2004. *JAMA* 2007;298:423-9

[29] Della Rocca G, Costa MG, Feltracco P. et al. Continuous right ventricular end diastolic volume and right ventricular ejection fraction during liver transplantation: a multicenter study. *Liver Transpl.* 2008;14:327-32

[30] Chang MC, Black CS, Meredith JW. Volumetric assessment of preload in trauma patients: addressing the problem of mathematical coupling. Shock 1996;6:326-9

[31] Nelson LD, Safcsak K, Cheatham ML, et al. Mathematical coupling does not explain the relationship between right ventricular end diastolic volume and cardiac output. *Crit. Care Med.* 2001;29:940-3

[32] Acosta F, Sansano T, Palenciano CG, et al. Does mixed venous oxygen saturation reflect the changes in cardiac output during liver transplantation? *Transplant. Proc.* 2002; 34:277.

[33] Dahmani S, Paugam-Burtz C, Gauss T, Alves M, Le Bihan E, Necib S, Belghiti J, Mantz J. Comparison of central and mixed venous saturation during liver transplantation in cirrhotic patients: a pilot study. *Eur. J. Anaesthesiol.* 2010; 27(8):714-9

[34] Connors AF, Speroff T, Dawson NV et al. The effectiveness of right heart catheterization in the initial care of critically ill patient. *JAMA* 1996;276:889-97.

[35] Harvey S, Harrison DA, Singer M, Ashcroft J, Jones CM, Elbourne D, Brampton W, Williams D, Young D, Rowan K, on behalf of the PAC-Man study collaboration. Assessment of the clinical effectiveness of pulmonary artery catheters in management of patients in intensive care (PAC-Man): a randomised controlled trial. *Lancet* 2005;366:472–7

[36] Gwak MS, Kim JA, Kim GS, Choi SJ, et al. Incidence of severe ventricular arrhythmias during pulmonary artery catheterization in liver allograft recipients. *Liver Transpl.* 2007;13:1451–4.

[37] Bossert T, Gummert JF, Bittner HB et al. Swan-Ganz catheter-induced severe complications in cardiac surgery: right ventricular perforation, knotting, and rupture of a pulmonary artery. *Journal of Cardiac Surgery* 2006; 21(3):292–5.

[38] Tam NL, He XS. Clinical management of portopulmonary hypertension. *Hepatobiliary Pancreat. Dis. Int.* 2007;6:464–9.

[39] Burtenshaw AJ, Isaac JL. The role of trans-oesophageal echocardiography for the perioperative monitoring during orthotopic liver transplantation. *Liver Transpl.* 2006;12:1577-83

[40] De Wolf A. Transesophageal echocardiography and orthotopic liver transplantation: general concepts. *Liver Transpl. Surg.* 1999;5:339-40

[41] Steltzer H, Blazek G, Gabriel A et al. Two-dimensional transesophageal echocardiography in early diagnosis and treatment of hemodynamic disturbances during liver transplantation. *Transplant. Proc.* 1991;23:1957-8

[42] Denault AY, Couture P, McKenty S, et al. Perioperative use of transoesophageal echocardiography by anesthesiologists: impact in non-cardiac surgery and in the intensive care unit. *Can. J. Anesth.* 2002;49:287-93

[43] Wax DB, Torrens A, Scher C, Leibowitz AB. Transesophageal echocardiography utilization in high-volume liver transplantation centers in the United States. *J. Cardiothorac. Vasc. Anesth.* 2008; 22(6):811-3

[44] Burtenshaw AJ, Isaac JL. The role of trans-oesophageal echocardiography for perioperative cardiovascular monitoring during orthotopic liver transplantation. *Liver Transplantation* 2006;12:1577-83.

[45] Thys DM, Abel MD, Brooker RF, Cahalan MK, Connis RT, Duke PG et al. Practice Guidelines for Perioperative Transesophageal Echocardiography. An Updated Report by the American Society of Anesthesiologists and the Society of Cardiovascular Anesthesiologists Task Force on ransesophageal Echocardiography. *Anesthesiology* 2010;112:1084-96

[46] Hofer CK, Furrer L, Matter-Esner S, Maloigne M, Klaghofer R, Genoni M et al. Volumetric preload measurement by thermodilution: a comparison with transesophageal echocardiography. *Br .J. Anaesth.* 2005;94:749-55

[47] De Simone R, Wolf I, Mottl-Link S, et al. Intraoperative assessment of right ventricular volume and function. *Eur. J. Cardiothor. Surg.* 2005;27:988-93

[48] Reuter DA, Felbinger TW, Kilger E, et al. Optimising fluid therapy in mechanically ventilated patients after cardiac surgery by on-line monitoring of left ventricular stroke volume variations - a comparison to aortic systolic pressure variations. *Br. J. Anaesth.* 2002;88:124–6

[49] Reuter DA, Felbinger TW, Schmidt C, et al. Stroke volume variations for assessment of cardiac responsiveness to volume loading in mechanically ventilated patients after cardiac surgery. *Intensive Care Med.* 2002;28:392-8

[50] Godie O, Hoke K, Goetz AE, Felbinger TW, Reuter DA, Reichart B, Friedl R, Hannekum A, Pfeiffer UJ. Reliability of a new algorithm for continuous cardiac output determination by pulse-contour analysis during hemodynamic instability. *Crit. Care Med.* 2002;30:52-8

[51] Felbinger TW, Reuter DA, Eltzschig HK, et al. Cardiac index measurements during rapid preload changes: a comparison of pulmonary artery thermodilution with arterial pulse contour analysis. *J. Clin. Anest.* 2005;17:241–248.

[52] www.pulsion.com
[53] Sakka SG, Bredle DL, Reinhart K, Meier-Hellmann A. Comparison between intrathoracic blood volume and cardiac filling pressures in the early phase of hemodynamic instability of patients with sepsis or septic shock. *J. Crit. Care* 1999;14:78-83.
[54] Gödje O, Peyerl M, Seebauer T, Lamm P, Mair H, Reichart B. Central venous pressure, pulmonary capillary wedge pressure and intrathoracic blood volumes as preload indicators in cardiac surgery patients. *Eur. J. Cardiothorac. Surg.* 1998;13:533-9.
[55] Hofer CK, Furrer L, Matter-Ensner S, Maloigne M, Klaghofer R, Genoni M et al. Volumetric preload measurement by thermodilution: a comparison with transesophageal echocardiography. *Br. J. Anaesth.* 2005; 94:749-55.
[56] Michard F, Alaja S, Zarka V, Bahloul M, Richard C, Teboul JL. Global end-diastolic volume as an indicator of cardiac preload in patients with septic shock. *Chest* 2003;124(5):1900-8
[57] Davey-Quinn A, Gedney JA, Whiteley SM, Bellamy MC. Extravascular lung water and acute respiratory distress syndrome. Oxygenation and outcome. *Anaesth Intensive Care* 1999;27:357-62.
[58] Sakka S, Klein M, Reinhart K, Meier-Hellmann. Prognostic value of extravascular lung water in critically ill patients. *Chest* 2002;122:2080-6.
[59] Della Rocca G, Costa MG, Pompei L, Coccia C, Pietropaoli P. Continuous and intermittent cardiac output measurement: pulmonary artery catheter versus aortic transpulmonary technique. *Br. J. Anaesth.* 2002;88(3):350-6
[60] Tzenkov GI, Arna Velasco D, Perez Pena JM, Olmedilla Arnal L, Garutti Martinez I, Sanz Fernanez J. Cardiac output by femoral arterial thermodilution-calibrated pulse contour analysis during liver transplantation: comparison with pulmonary artery thermodilution. *Transpl. Proc.* 2003 Aug;35(5):1920-2
[61] Sakka SG, Reinhart K, Meier-Hellmann A. Comparison of pulmonary artery and arterial thermodilution cardiac output in critically ill patients. *Intensive Care Med.* 1999;25:843-6.
[62] Rodig G, Prasser C, Keyl C, et al. Continuous cardiac output measurement: pulse contour analysis vs thermodilution technique in cardiac surgical patients. *Br. J. Anaesth.* 1999;82:525–30.
[63] Della Rocca G, Montecchi C, Costa MG, Coccia C, Di Marco P, Iappelli M, Rossi M, Pietropaoli P, Cortesini R. Circulating blood volume monitoring during liver transplantation for fulminant hepatic failure. *Transplant.Proc.* 2001;33:1478-81.
[64] Della Rocca G, Pompei L, Costa MG, Coccia C, Rossi M, Berloco PM, Pietropaoli P, Cortesini R. Hemodynamic-Volumetric Versus Pulmonary Artery Catheter Monitoring During Anesthesia for Liver Transplantation. *Transplant. Proc.* 2001;33:1394–6
[65] Della Rocca G, Costa MG, Coccia C, et al. Preload and hemodynamic assessment during liver transplantation. A comparison between pulmonary artery catheter and transpulmonary indicator dilution technique. *Eur. J. Anaesthesiol.* 2002;19:868-75
[66] Della Rocca G, Costa MG, Coccia C, et al. Continuous right ventricular end diastolic volume comparison with left ventricular end diastolic area. *Eur. J. Anaesthesiol.* 2009;26(4):272-8.
[67] Della Rocca G, Brondani A, Costa MG. Intraoperative hemodynamic monitoring during organ transplantation: what is new? Curr Opin Organ Transplant 2009,14:291–6

[68] Linton RA, Band DM, O'Brien TK, Jonas M, Leach R. Lithium dilution cardiac output measurement: a comparison with thermodilution. *Crit. Care Med.* 1997;25:1796-1800

[69] Kurita T, Morita K, Kato S, Kikura M, Horie M, Ikeda K. Comparison of the accuracy of the lithium dilution technique with the thermodilution technique for measurement of cardiac output. *Br. J. Anaesth.* 1997;79:770-5

[70] Mason D, O'Gray M, Woods JP, McDonell W. Assessment of lithium dilution cardiac output as technique for measurement of cardiac output in dogs. *Am. J. Vet. Res.* 2001;62(8):1255-61

[71] Linton RA, Jonas MM, Tibby SM, Murdoch IA, O'Brien TK, Linton NWF, Band DM. Cardiac output measured by lithium dilution and transpulmonary thermodilution in patients in a paediatric intensive care unit. *Intensive Care Med.* 2000;26:1507-11

[72] Pearse RM, Ikram K, Barry J. Equipment review: an appraisal of the LiDCO Plus method of measuring cardiac output. *Crit. Care.* 2004;8(3):190-5

[73] Pittman J, Bar-Yosef S, SumPing J, Sherwood M, Mark J. Continuous cardiac output monitoring with pulse contour analysis: A comparison with lithium indicator dilution cardiac output measurement. *Crit. Care Med.* 2005;33(9):2015-21

[74] Hamilton TT, Huber LM, Jessen ME. PulseCO™: A less-Invasive Method to Monitor Cardiac Output From Arterial Pressure After Cardiac Surgery. *Ann. Thorac. Surg.* 2002;74:S1408-12

[75] Costa MG, Della Rocca G, Chiarandini P et al. Continuous and intermittent cardiac output measurement in hyperdinamic conditions: pumonary artery catheter vs lithium dilution technique. *Intensive Care Med.* 2008;34:257-63

[76] Odenstedt H, Aneman A, Oi Y, Stevenson M, Stenqvist O, Lundin S. Descending aortic blood flow and cardiac output: A clinical and experimental study of continuous oesophageal echo-Doppler flowmetry. *Acta Anaesthesiol. Scand.* 2001;45:180-7

[77] Diaper J, Ellenberger C, Villiger Y, Robert J, Inan C, Tschopp JM, Licker M. Comparison of cardiac output as assessed by transesophageal echo-Doppler and transpulmonary thermodilution in patients undergoing thoracic surgery. *J. Clin. Anesth.* 2010;22(2):97-103

[78] Parra V, Fita G, Rovira I, Matute P, Gomar C, Pare C. Transoesophageal echocardiography accurately detects cardiac output variations: a prospective comparison with thermodilution in cardiac surgery. *Eur. J. Anaesthesiol.* 2008;25 (2):135-43

[79] Perilli V, Avolio AW, Sacco T, Modesti C, Gaspari R, Caserta R. et al. Use of an esophageal echo-Doppler device during liver transplantation: preliminary report. *Transplant. Proc.* 2008;41(1):198-200

[80] Boucaud C, Bouffard Y, Dumorttier J, Gaillac N, Sagnard P, Graber MC et al. Transoesophageal echo-Doppler vs. thermodilution cardiac output measurement during hepatic vascular exclusion in liver transplantation. *Eur. J. Anaesthesiol.* 2008;25:485-9

[81] Hofer CK, Ganter MT, Zollinger A. What technique should I use to measure cardiac output? *Curr. Opin. Crit. Care* 2007;13:308–317

[82] de Waal EEC, Kalkman CJ, Rex S, Buhre WF. Validation of a new arterial pulse contour-based cardiac output device. *Crit. Care Med.* 2007;35(8):1-6.

[83] Cannesson M, Artof Y, Rosamel P et al. Comparison of FloTrac™ cardiac output monitoring system in patients undergoing coronary artery bypass grafting with

pulmonary artery cardiac output measurements. *Eur. J. Anaesthesiol.* 2007;24(10):832-9.

[84] Sakka SG, Kozieras J, Thuemer O, van Hout N. Measurement of cardiac output: a comparison between transpulmonary thermodilution and uncalibrated pulse contour analysis. *Br. J. Anaesth.* 2007;99(3):337-42.

[85] Mayer J, Boldt J, Scholhorn T et al. Semi-invasive monitoring of cardiac output by a new device using arterial pressure waveform analysis: a comparison with intermittent pulmonary artery thermodilution in patients undergoing cardiac surgery. *Br. J. Anaesth.* 2007;98(2):176-82

[86] Opdam HI, Wan Li, Bellomo R. A pilot assessment of the FloTrac™ cardiac output monitoring system. *Intensive Care Med.* 2007;33(2):344-9

[87] Manecke GR, Auger WR. Cardiac output determination from the arterial pressure wave: clinical testing of a novel algorithm that does not require calibration. *J. Cardiothorac Vasc. Anesth.* 2007;21(1):3-7

[88] Hofer CK, Button D, Weibel L, Genoni M, Zollinger A. Uncalibrated radial and femoral arterial pressure waveform analysis for continuous cardiac output measurement: and evaluation in cardiac surgery patients. *J. Cardiothorac. Vasc. Anesth.* 2010;24(2):257-64

[89] Button D, Weibel L, Reuthebuch O et al Clinical evaluation of the FloTrac/Vigileo™ system and two established continuous cardiac output monitoring devices in patients undergoing cardiac surgery. *Br. J. Anaesth.* 2007;99(3):329-36.

[90] Della Rocca G, Costa MG, Chiarandini P et al. Arterial pulse cardiac output agreement with thermodilution in patients in hyperdynamic conditions. *J. Cardiothor. Vasc. Anesth.* 2008;22:681-7

[91] Biais M, Nouette-Gaulain K, Cottenceau V, Vallet A, Cochard JF, Revel P, Sztark F. Cardiac output measurement in patients undergoing liver transplantation: Pulmonary artery catheter versus uncalibrated arterial pressure waveform analysis. *Anesth. Analg.* 2008;106:1480–6

[92] Biancofiore G, Critchley LAH, Bindi L et al. Evaluation of an uncalibrated arterial pulse contour cardiac output monitoring system in cirrhotic patients undergoing liver surgery. *Br. J. Anesth.* 2009;102:47-54

[93] 93.Costa MG, Cecconi A, Shehu I, Chiarandini P, Pompei L, Della Rocca G. Uncalibrated arterial pulse analysis cardiac output obtained with LiDCORapid versus PAC thermodilution technique. *Intensive Care Med.* 2009; 35(S)

In: Cardiovascular Diseases and Liver Transplantation
Editor: Zoka Milan, pp. 259-273
ISBN: 978-1-61122-910-3
© 2011 Nova Science Publishers, Inc.

Chapter XVII

Cardiovascular Profile and Cardiac Complications Following Liver Transplantation

Aileen R Smith[1], George Therapondos[1], Tamer R Fouad[2] and Samuel S. Lee[3]*

[1]Multiorgan Transplant Program, University of Toronto and University Health Network, Toronto General Hospital, Canada
[2]Division of Gastroenterology/Hepatology, Menofiya University, Menofiya, Egypt
[3]University of Calgary Liver Unit, Calgary, Canada

Abstract

Cardiac events in the early post-operative period are common and may influence longer-term cardiac morbidity and even indicate potential mortality. Immunosuppressive therapy may have short-term cardiotoxic effects but is more likely to adversely affect cardiovascular risk factors such as hypertension, diabetes mellitus and dyslipidemia in the longer-term. This chapter will discuss hemodynamic profile post-liver transplant (LT), the early- and late-postoperative cardiovascular complications following LT, the cardiac problems associated with immunosuppression and prediction of post-operative cardiac complications.

Introduction

Cardiovascular (CV) complications are a leading cause of non-graft-related death in liver transplant recipients, accounting for 1 to 2.7% mortality in the first year post-transplant and

---

* Correspondence: George Therapondos, BSc, MB ChB, Director, Clinical Trials Unit, Assistant Professor of Medicine, Multiorgan Transplant Program, University of Toronto and University Health Network, Toronto General Hospital, Toronto, Ontario M5G 2N2, Tel: + 416 340 4248, Fax: + 416 340 4041, E-mail: george.therapondos@utoronto.ca.

21% of deaths in LT recipients surviving more than three years [1-6]. In the early-postoperative period hemodynamic changes, increased blood pressure and systemic vascular resistance impose major stress on the CV system; this may exacerbate pre-existing latent cardiac dysfunction (cirrhotic cardiomyopathy) or mild coronary artery disease (CAD) [7-10]. Cardiovascular disease in the late-post-LT population arises from a combination of pre-existing disease pre-LT and chronic exposure to immunosuppressive medication post-LT [11-15]. This chapter will discuss in detail the early and late CV complications following LT as well as the cardiac problems associated with immunosuppression and prediction of postoperative complications.

Cardiac Function Post-Liver Transplant

Cardiovascular abnormalities characteristic to end-stage liver disease gradually improve following LT. As previously reported, some LT patients already have other cardiovascular abnormalities, such as hypertension or coronary artery disease, and their post-operative recovery can be prolonged or less effective.

Several studies reported improvement in cardiovascular function post-LT occurring up to two years post-LT [16-19]. Piscaglia et al. [7] followed 28 LT patients prospectively (mean follow-up 17 months) and found that systemic, renal and most splanchnic circulatory alterations returned to normal post-LT. However, they reported markedly increased blood pressure and total peripheral resistance, which they explained with restoration of normal liver function combined with side effects of calcineurin inhibitor (CNI) immunosuppression.

Park et al. [19], who performed echocardiographic studies of cirrhotic patients before and after LT, also showed improvement in cardiac function expressed by reduction in the previously increased cardiac index by 35% at one to 13 months after transplantation.

Sampathkumar et al. [20] hypothesized that cirrhotic cardiomyopathy may be reversible post-LT, having observed a complete recovery in the seven patients in their series who developed postoperative myocardial depression. This potential for reversibility is also suggested by the correction of prolonged QT intervals after transplant [21].

Torregrossa et al. [22] compared echocardiography and stress ventriculography in LT recipients pre- and post-transplant; pre-LT patients had mildly increased ventricular wall thickness, diastolic dysfunction that worsened with ascites and physical stress, and abnormal systolic response to stress with limited exercise capacity. Patients were re-evaluated six to 12 months post-LT and demonstrated reversal of cardiac dysfunction.

However, there are studies reporting deterioration, although subclinical, of cardiac function following LT. Echocardiographic evidence of myocardial dysfunction has been reported in 1 to 20% of transplant recipients [7, 19]. Acosta et al. [23] demonstrated altered systolic or diastolic ventricular function in 20% of patients at 21 months post-LT; pre-transplant studies were within normal parameters. Although none of the patients presented with cardiac symptoms, and ejection fraction (EF) remained within normal limits, the number of patients with an EF< 60% increased. A significant decrease in diastolic function was reported, with mean values at the lower limits of normality and an increase in the number of patients with abnormal values. There were no significant differences between patients with or without alcoholic etiology pre- or post-transplant. Therapondos et al. [24] confirmed a deterioration of diastolic cardiac function three months after LT. This occurred in association with mildly increased ventricular hypertrophy but again there was no correlation with symptoms of cardiac failure.

Early Post-Operative Cardiac Complications

Retrospective reviews of CV outcomes following LT have shown intra-operative cardiovascular events, pre-existing heart disease, recipient age and advanced liver disease to be the most useful predictors of early post-LT CV complications [1, 9, 10, 25-29].

In the early post-operative period, substantial elevations in blood pressure and systemic vascular resistance impose major stress on the CV system; this probably results from0 restoration of normal liver function and portal pressure combined with the hypertensive side effects of immunosuppression [7, 11, 30, 31].

Dec et al. [1] performed a retrospective review of all liver recipients in their center from 1983 to 1992. They studied 146 patients and reported four cardiovascular deaths (one from previously unrecognized severe pulmonary hypertension, one from hypoxemia due to intrapulmonary shunting and two unexplained) during the first six months post-LT.

Pulmonary Edema

Pulmonary edema is the most frequent post-operative cardiac complication, affecting 9 to 56% of patients in the first post-operative month; it most commonly occurs within the first 24 to 72 hours post-transplant in association with large-volume blood loss and peri-operative transfusions [1, 32-34]. Pulmonary congestion is associated with impaired gas exchange, increased ventilation requirements and prolonged length of stay in the intensive care unit (ICU). This may have implications for oxygenation of the newly transplanted organ [35]. Plevak et al. [32] reported evidence of non-infective pulmonary infiltrates in 22% of LT recipients, either at initial or subsequent intensive care unit admissions, and Glanneman et al. identified pulmonary edema as the indication for reintubation during post-operative care in 2.7% of LT recipients [36]. A prospective study by Therapondos et al. [24] reported CV complications, most commonly pulmonary edema, in 25% of patients within three months of LT.

Other factors influencing the incidence of post-operative pulmonary edema include pulmonary function of the patient at the time of transplant. Patients with fulminant hepatic failure (FHF) have a high incidence (37%) of pulmonary edema [34,37]. Pulmonary edema in pediatric LT recipients is rarely reported; a review of 176 cases in Madrid described only seven cases, a probable reflection of differences in the preoperative hemodynamic status of this patient population in comparison with adult groups [38].

Snowden at al. [34] studied the incidence of radiological pulmonary edema post-LT and reported an overall incidence of 47% (16 out of 34 patients). Of these patients, three had evidence of edema immediately after surgery, and 10 had pulmonary edema at 24 hours that had not been present immediately after surgery. When comparing patients who developed edema later in the post-operative course with those who did not, there was no significant difference in fluid replacement, incidence of pleural effusions, physical characteristics or severity of liver disease between the two groups. There was a higher proportion of patients with more severe liver disease in the group that developed pulmonary edema, although this was not statistically significant.

Multivariate analyses have identified pulmonary edema as a major independent risk factor for the development of post-LT pneumonia. Closer radiographic monitoring is recommended for these recipients [39].

We must point out that all reports of this serious complication dated from up to a decade ago. We believe that with improvement of patient selection, pre-operative assessment and preparation, surgical technique and monitoring, as well as fast-tracking LT patients, pulmonary edema is a less common post-operative complication following LT.

Dilated Cardiomyopathy

Development of new dilated cardiomyopathy post-LT has been reported by two retrospective reviews; both reported association with pulmonary edema and spontaneous resolution, but a causative factor could not be identified [1, 20].

Dec et al. [1] identified new dilated cardiomyopathy in 3.4% of recipients following LT. This was more prevalent in older patients with pre-existing cardiac disease, and there was no impact on six months' survival.

A report from the Mayo Clinic [20] reviewed the records of 754 transplant recipients and identified seven patients who developed a reversible dilated cardiomyopathy in the first five days post-LT. The median age of the patients was 37, and none had a history of cardiac disease or significant intra-operative CV complications. Potential causes of myocardial dysfunction such as myocardial ischemia, thyroid dysfunction and electrolyte imbalances were excluded. Left ventricular ejection fraction (LVEF) decreased from a pre-operative median baseline of 60% to 20% post-LT, with four-chamber dilatation on echocardiogram. All patients received supportive ICU care and cardiac function subsequently improved, with LVEF increasing to a median of 50%. Patients were followed for a median duration of 15 months and showed no recurrence of cardiac failure.

Pulmonary Embolism

Sankey et al. [40] studied necropsy tissues from patients who died within 10 days of LT and identified massive pulmonary platelet thromboembolism as a common cause of sudden perioperative death in LT recipients. Patient numbers were small (six LT patients and 13 controls), and there are no recent studies investigating this phenomenon. Its wider implications are unknown.

Myocardial Infarction

Myocardial infarction is a relatively rare phenomenon in the early post-LT period, probably reflecting the extensive pre-operative cardiac evaluation to screen patients for CAD.

Post-operative myocardial ischemic events have been reported in 3 to 7% of LT recipients [1, 41, 42].

However, Rubin et al. [38] found a higher incidence (13%) of symptomatic ischemic electrocardiography changes (T-wave or ST-segment changes) in a group of 45 consecutive patients undergoing LT.

Long-Term Cardiovascular Risk

The long-term cardiac risks arise from a combination of CAD and chronic exposure to immunosuppressant medication [11-15]. Prevalence of CV risk factors in the post-LT population has risen in recent decades as LT survival rates have improved; whether this has been accompanied by a higher incidence of atherosclerotic complications in comparison to the general population remains controversial. Two long-term outcome studies showed no significant difference in the incidence of atherosclerotic cardiovascular disease post-LT compared to the age- and gender-matched general population [13, 44], although hypertension and diabetes were more frequent in LT population [44]. In contrast to these data, Johnston et al. [15] calculated that the relative risk of ischemic cardiac events was 3.07, with the relative risk of cardiac death at 2.56 when compared with a non-transplant age and gender-matched population. In that study patients with evidence of heart disease and smokers were excluded. The researchers found that moderate hypertension and hyperlipidemia were more detrimental in LT recipients compared to non-transplant patients, and recommended that risk factor modification should be a priority in this population.

Recent publications report CV event rates of 9% at five years, rising to 24% at 10 years post-transplant, with up to 21% of deaths in long-term survivors being attributed to CV disease [5, 45, 46]. A prospective series analyzing graft loss in 1,174 patients surviving at least one year post-LT reported a cardiovascular mortality of 2.6% [4]. Pruthi et al. [5] reported similar results, identifying a CV cause of death in 2.6% (8 out of 299) of patients who survived more than three years post-transplant. This represented 21% of all deaths in this group, which is similar to Neuberger [6], who identified cardiovascular death as the most common cause of death (22%) in 617 adult liver patients five or more years after LT.

Liver graft recipients are at an increased risk for hypercholesterolemia, hypertension and diabetes, and the development of post-transplant metabolic syndrome has been reported to occur in 43 to 58% of LT recipients [47]. The exact prevalence of new-onset diabetes mellitus (NODM) post-LT is unclear due to differences in diagnostic criteria among published studies; a higher prevalence in patients receiving tacrolimus-based immunosuppression, 15.3 to 18.2%, has been recognized in comparison with those on cyclosporine, 5.7 to 7.7% [48]. The prevalence of hypertension following liver transplantation has been reported to range from 62 to 69% in patients followed for at least one year after LT, with a rise in the incidence of hypertension from 19% pre-transplantation to 64.2% post-transplantation [47]. Obesity develops in 21 to 43% of patients post-LT, and the prevalence of dyslipidemia ranges from 66 to 85% [47].

A prospective 10-year follow-up study performed by Guckelberger et al. [12] demonstrated a clear correlation between elevated CV risk factors and the incidence of cardiac events post-transplant. Early post-operative complications such as hypotension, myocardial infarction, pulmonary embolism, and arrhythmias may also contribute to an increased risk of late onset cardiovascular disease. Dec et al. [1] reported a reduction in the five-year survival of patients who suffered cardiac events during their early post-transplantation course.

Cardiotoxicity Associated with Immunosuppression

Tacrolimus-Related Cardiotoxicity

Cardiotoxic side effects related to tacrolimus were originally described in animal studies involving rabbits and baboons [49]. The first human cases were reported in pediatric liver transplants [49-53].

Tacrolimus cardiotoxicity has also been reported in adult patients. Dollinger et al. [54] performed post-operative 2D-echocardiograms on 12 LT recipients, four of whom were found to have abnormal echocardiograms (two developed LVH and one had LV dysfunction). Of these four, only one patient developed an unexplained cardiomyopathy after a protracted intensive care unit admission with prolonged sepsis. This patient was the only recipient in the study group to have received tacrolimus intravenously, and the cardiomyopathy resolved following the change of immunosuppression to cyclosporine.

Nakata et al. [55] reported LVH in 40% (13 out of 32) of living donor LT recipients within two weeks of transplantation; LV wall thickening occurred in association with tacrolimus levels >15 ng/mL. Left ventricular thickness returned to normal by four weeks post-LT, and all affected patients were asymptomatic. Therapondos et al. [24] performed a prospective study comparing cardiac function in patients receiving tacrolimus or cyclosporine immunosuppression post-LT; tacrolimus therapy was associated with increased posterior wall thickness, reduced heart rate variability and higher serum brain atrial natriuretic peptide (BNP) but this did not translate to an increase in cardiac clinical events. Tacrolimus levels in this study were maintained below15 ng/mL.

Several studies refute the evidence for tacrolimus cardiotoxicity. Autopsy study by Khanna et al. [56] examined cardiac findings post-mortem in adults and children following LT and tacrolimus therapy and compared their findings with autopsies of patients who died of ESLD without transplantation. The mean weight of the heart in both groups was similar, but was higher than in the normal population. These results were comparable to an echocardiographic study by Park et al. [56], who concluded that LVH was associated with the hemodynamic changes seen in cirrhosis rather than tacrolimus therapy. Another autopsy study [57] compared hearts from LT recipients receiving tacrolimus to those of recipients receiving cyclosporine and a non-transplanted control group. Cardiomegaly with preferential septal hypertrophy was found to be common at autopsy in both adult and pediatric LT patients, but there was no demonstrable difference in cardiac findings between the tacrolimus or cyclosporine groups.

Cyclosporine

Although most reports describe tacrolimus-associated HCM, there are reports of LVH caused by cyclosporine in heart and bone marrow transplant recipients [58, 59].

Long-Term Cardiovascular Risk Associated with Immunosuppression

In current clinical practice, tacrolimus is prescribed more commonly than cyclosporine. Despite the association with HCM and cardiac failure in the early post-operative period, these occurrences are relatively rare and, in the longer term, tacrolimus appears to have a more favorable CV risk profile. An evaluation of CV risk after transplantation at one year post-LT found that tacrolimus was associated with a less adverse risk profile in comparison to cyclosporine [60]. Another group investigated the incidence of hypertension, hyperlipidemia, DM and CV disease in two cohorts of LT recipients who received either tacrolimus or cyclosporine. At three years post-LT, 18% of patients had evidence of CV disease in the cyclosporine group, compared with 0% in the tacrolimus group [61].

Assessment of individual risk factors reveled a higher prevalence of hypertension, hyperlipidemia and weight gain in patients receiving cyclosporine compared with tacrolimus [12, 62-66]. In general, it is accepted that development of post-transplant DM appears to occur more frequently with tacrolimus [65,66], although some studies have found similar results between cyclosporin and tacrolimus-based immunosuppression [60,63].

Addition of mycophenolate mofetil (MMF) as a CNI-sparing agent may improve hypertension, DM and dyslipidemia, and the use of MMF with low-dose CNI or low-dose corticosteroids is associated with low risk of rejection [68-70].

Conversion from CNI to sirolimus-based immunosuppression reduces hypertension and DM but may result in higher rates of dyslipidemia [71]. The University of Miami experience showed a 55.2% rate of dyslipidemia in patients receiving sirolimus with most patients required lipid-lowering therapy [72].

Infections

Chronic exposure to immunosuppression results in increased susceptibility to unusual opportunistic infections. Cytomegalovirus (CMV) infection occurs in 19 to 29% of LT recipients; most commonly it manifests as asymptomatic antigenemia or an infectious mononucleosis-type syndrome [73]. CMV myocarditis has been described in two LT recipients: One presented with an influenza-type syndrome and was found to have myocarditis on echocardiography and magnetic imaging [74], while the second developed biventricular failure but enjoyed a full recovery following ganciclovir treatment [75]. Purulent pericarditis due to Legionella pneumophila [76] and infective endocarditis have also been described [77].

Transmission of Chagas disease (Trypanosoma cruzi infection), which led to cardiomyopathy has been reported in two LT patients [78,79]. Souza et al. [80] reported a single case of acute chagasic myocardiopathy 10 months after LT. The patient presented with symptoms and signs of chronic heart failure, and echocardiogram revealed ejection fraction of 35% and moderate pulmonary hypertension. The patient responded to treatment with benzonidazole.

Prediction of Postoperative Cardiac Complications

In our recent study of 197 patients who had LT [10], 82 patients (42%) suffered one or more cardiac complications during 6 months after LT, and pulmonary edema was the commonest complication. Most of the routine tests that are commonly used for liver transplantation were studied, including the widely-used MELD score [81-83]. In addition, we examined two new modifications of the MELD score, the MELD-Na[84,85] and integrated-MELD (i-MELD) [86], which were devised to increase the efficacy of the original MELD. By univariate analysis, the following parameters were significantly related to occurrence of cardiovascular events: intraoperative cardiovascular event; previous history of cardiac disease or hypertension; increased MELD, MELD-Na and i-MELD; and increased amount of intraoperative transfused blood and plasma. By multivariate analysis, after adjusting for age and sex, independent predictors of cardiovascular complications were intraoperative cardiovascular event (adjusted odds ratio [aOR]; 95% CI: 4.71, 1.71-13.01); preoperative history of cardiac disease (2.45, 0.96-6.27) or hypertension (6.08, 2.21-16.76); and i-MELD score (1.06, 1.01-1.12). No other variable among the following were predictive: age, sex, indication for LT, weight, height, body mass index, history of smoking, alcohol consumption, PROCAM risk score [87], for prediction of CAD, pre-LT investigations, chest X-ray, ECG, any cardiac chamber enlargement, E deceleration time, E/A ratio, coronary angiography, pulmonary arterial pressure, MIBI scan, intraoperative crystalloid fluid transfusion, surgical technique (standard, venovenous shunt or preservation of the inferior vena cava), intraoperative graft variables (cadaveric vs living or cold ischemia and rewarming times) or type of immunosuppressive treatment (neither tacrolimus vs cyclosporine).

As for the ability to predict advanced liver disease (as estimated by i-MELD), we believe that it is most likely due to the known correlation between the degree of liver failure and the extent of cardiovascular anomalies, particularly cirrhotic cardiomyopathy, peripheral vasodilatation, and hyperdynamic circulation [88,89]. Studies suggested a direct correlation between degree of liver failure and severity of cirrhotic cardiomyopathy [90,91].

Because the serum sodium level has been reported to be significantly associated with mortality in those awaiting liver transplantation [84], it was added to the original MELD score to compensate for the latter's inability to account for those patients with refractory ascites with low MELD scores. This addition made the MELD-Na score superior to the original MELD score in survival prediction [85,92,93]. Age is another parameter that was introduced recently by Luca and colleagues [86] .They studied the inclusion of age and serum sodium levels to the original MELD score and demonstrated that this integrated MELD was superior to the original MELD in predicting mortality in patients undergoing TIPS. In our study, liver disease severity scoring systems, i.e., MELD, MELD-Na and i-MELD, were all significantly associated on univariate analysis with cardiovascular complications after LT, but the i-MELD was the only scoring system to independently predict cardiovascular complications. The most obvious explanation is that older cirrhotic patients with poor liver reserve have a greater risk of cardiovascular complications.

A recent study by Coss et al. examined predictive factors for late cardiovascular events including symptomatic angina, myocardial infarction, and overt congestive heart failure [94]. By using a retrospective-prospective design, 230 transplant recipients were followed for an average of 8 years. In this study, the following factors predicted cardiovascular events on multivariate analysis: age, diabetes, smoking, history of previous cardiovascular disease, and most intriguingly, a serum troponin I level >0.07ng/mL. This study is the first to report that a single serum test may be a useful predictive marker; these results need confirmation in larger prospective trials.

Conclusion

Liver transplantation imposes major stresses on the cardiovascular system of patients with cirrhosis. The underlying hemodynamic and cardiac status of these patents will determine their response to peri-operative stress; unfortunately, screening tests to identify patients with a higher risk potential for CV complications following LT remain unsatisfactory. These complications usually occur in older persons with a history of pre-transplant cardiovascular conditions and advanced liver failure.

Minor intra-operative morbidity and early cardiac complications are relatively common and may have an impact on longer-term cardiac problems. Major cardiac events, such as myocardial infarction or pulmonary embolism, may occur peri-operatively and in the early post-operative period but are much less common within the first few months. Immunosuppressive therapy, both CNI inhibitors and corticosteroids, may cause short-term cardiac complications but most importantly affect CV risk factors and have implications for CV disease in the long-term. As transplant recipient survival improves, further studies to determine optimal management of the long-term medical complications of LT are urgently required. In the meantime, our care of LT recipients should pay particular attention to cardiovascular screening, risk factor modification and appropriate tailoring of immunosuppression.

References

[1] Dec GW, Kondo N, Farrell ML, Dienstag J, Cosimi AB, Semigran MJ. Cardiovascular complications following liver transplantation. *Clin. Transplant* .1995;9(6):463-71.

[2] Rabkin JM, de La Melena V, Orloff SL, Corless CL, Rosen HR, Olyaei AJ. Late mortality after orthotopic liver transplantation. *Am. J. Surg.* 2001;181(5):475-9.

[3] Clavien PA, Camargo CA Jr, Croxford R, Langer B, Levy GA, Greig PD. Definition and classification of negative outcomes in solid organ transplantation. Application in liver transplantation. *Ann. Surg* .1994;220 (2):109-20.

[4] Abbasoglu O, Levy MF, Brkic BB, Testa G, Jeyarajah DR, Goldstein RM et al. Ten years of liver transplantation: an evolving understanding of late graft loss. *Transplantation* 1997;4(12):1801-7.

[5] Pruthi J, Medkiff KA, Esrason KT, Donovan JA, Yoshida EM, Erb SR et al. Analysis of causes of death in liver transplant recipients who survived more than 3 years. *Liver Transpl.* 2001;7 (9):811-5.
[6] Neuberger J. Liver transplantation. *J. Hepatol.* 2000;32(1Suppl):198-207.
[7] Piscaglia F, Zironi G, Gaiani S, Mazziotti A, Cavallari A, Gramantieri L et al. Systemic and splanchnic hemodynamic changes after liver transplantation for cirrhosis: a long-term prospective study. *Hepatology* 1999;30(1):58-64.
[8] Navasa M, Feu F, García-Pagán JC, Jiménez W, Llach J, Rimola A et al. Hemodynamic and humoral changes after liver transplantation in patients with cirrhosis. *Hepatology* 1993;17(3):355-60.
[9] Myers RP, Lee SS. Cirrhotic cardiomyopathy and liver transplantation. *Liver Transpl.* 2000;(4 Suppl 1):S44-52.
[10] Fouad TR, Abdel-Razek WM, Burak KW, Bain VG, Lee SS. Prediction of cardiac complications after liver transplantation. *Transplantation* 2009; 7(5):763-70.
[11] Therapondos G, Flapan AD, Plevris JN, Hayes PC. Cardiac morbidity and mortality related to orthotopic liver transplantation. *Liver Transpl.* 2004;10(12):1441-53.
[12] Guckelberger O, Bechstein WO, Neuhaus R, Luesebrink R, Lemmens HP, Kratschmer B et al. Cardiovascular risk factors in long-term follow-up after orthotopic liver transplantation. *Clin. Transplant.* 1997;11(1):60-5.
[13] Sheiner PA, Magliocca JF, Bodian CA, Kim-Schluger L, Altaca G et al. Long-term medical complications in patients surviving > or = 5 years after liver transplant. *Transplantation* 2000; 69(5):781-9.
[14] Reich D, Rothstein K, Manzarbeitia C, Muñoz S. Common medical diseases after liver transplantation. *Semin. Gastrointest. Dis.* 1998;9(3):110-25.
[15] Johnston SD, Morris JK, Cramb R, Gunson BK, Neuberger J. Cardiovascular morbidity and mortality after orthotopic liver transplantation. *Transplantation* 2002;73(6):901-6.
[16] Hadengue A, Lebrec D, Moreau R, Sogni P, Durand F, Gaudin C et al. Persistence of systemic and splanchnic hyperkinetic circulation in liver transplant patients. *Hepatology* 1993;17 (2):175-8.
[17] Henderson JM, Mackay GJ, Hooks M, Chezmar JL, Galloway JR, Dodson TF, Kutner MH. High cardiac output of advanced liver disease persists after orthotopic liver transplantation. *Hepatology* 1992;15(2):258-62.
[18] Gadano A, Hadengue A, Widmann JJ, Vachiery F, Moreau R, Yang S et al. Hemodynamics after orthotopic liver transplantation: study of associated factors and long-term effects. *Hepatology* 1995;22(2):458-65.
[19] Park SC, Beerman LB, Gartner JC, Zitelli BJ, Malatack JJ, Fricker FJ et al. Echocardiographic findings before and after liver transplantation. *Am. J. Cardiol.* 1985;55(11):1373-8.
[20] Sampathkumar P, Lerman A, Kim BY, Narr BJ, Poterucha JJ, Torsher LC, Plevak DJ. Post-liver transplantation myocardial dysfunction. *Liver Transpl. Surg.* 1998;4(5):399-403.
[21] Garcia GM, Hernandez-Madrid A, Lopez-Sanroman A, Candela A, Nuno J, Barcena R. Reversal of QT interval electrocardiographic alterations in cirrhotic patients undergoing liver transplantation. *Transplant Proc.* 1999;31:2366–7.

[22] Torregrosa M, Aguadé S, Dos L, Segura R, Gónzalez A, Evangelista A et al. Cardiac alterations in cirrhosis: reversibility after liver transplantation. *J. Hepatol.* 2005;42(1):68-74

[23] Acosta F, De La Morena G, Villegas M, Sansano T, Reche M, Beltran R et al. Evaluation of cardiac function before and after liver transplantation. *Transplant Proc.* 1999;31(6):2369-70.

[24] Therapondos G, Flapan AD, Dollinger MM, Garden OJ, Plevris JN, Hayes PC. Cardiac function after orthotopic liver transplantation and the effects of immunosuppression: a prospective randomized trial comparing cyclosporin (Neoral) and tacrolimus. *Liver Transpl*. 2002;8(8):690-700.

[25] Eagle KA, Berger PB, Calkins H, Chaitman BR, Ewy GA, Fleischmann KE et al. ACC/AHA Guideline Update for Perioperative Cardiovascular Evaluation for Noncardiac Surgery--Executive Summary. A report of the American College of Cardiology/American Heart Association Task Force on Practice Guidelines (Committee to Update the 1996 Guidelines on Perioperative Cardiovascular Evaluation for Noncardiac Surgery). *Anesth. Analg.* 2002;94(5):1052-64.

[26] Aggarwal S, Kang Y, Freeman JA, Fortunato FL, Pinsky MR. Postreperfusion syndrome: cardiovascular collapse following hepatic reperfusion during liver transplantation. *Transplant. Proc*. 1987;19(4 Suppl 3):54-5.

[27] Krowka MJ, Plevak DJ, Findlay JY, Rosen CB, Wiesner RH, Krom RA. Pulmonary hemodynamics and perioperative cardiopulmonary-related mortality in patients with portopulmonary hypertension undergoing liver transplantation. *Liver Transpl.* 2000;6(4):443-50.

[28] Ginés P, Quintero E, Arroyo V, Terés J, Bruguera M, Rimola A et al. Compensated cirrhosis: natural history and prognostic factors. *Hepatology* 1987;7(1):122-128.

[29] Saab S, Wang V, Ibrahim AB, Durazo F, Han S, Farmer DG et al. MELD score predicts 1-year patient survival post-orthotopic liver transplantation. *Liver Transpl.* 2003;9(5):473-6.

[30] Soresi M, Bascone F, Magliarisi C, Campagna P, Di Giovanni G et al. Hemodynamic changes in splanchnic circulation after orthotopic liver transplantation in patients with liver cirrhosis. *Abdom. Imaging* 2002;27(5):541-5.

[31] Textor SC, Wiesner R, Wilson DJ, Porayko M, Romero JC, Burnett JC Jr et al. Systemic and renal hemodynamic differences between FK506 and cyclosporine in liver transplant recipients. *Transplantation* 1993;55(6):1332-9.

[32] Plevak DJ, Southorn PA, Narr BJ, Peters SG. Intensive-care unit experience in the Mayo liver transplantation program: the first 100 cases. *Mayo Clin. Proc.* 1989;64(4):433-45.

[33] Donovan CL, Marcovitz PA, Punch JD, Bach DS, Brown KA, Lucey MR, Armstrong WF. Two-dimensional and dobutamine stress echocardiography in the preoperative assessment of patients with end-stage liver disease prior to orthotopic liver transplantation. *Transplantation* 1996;61(8):1180-1188.

[34] Snowden CP, Hughes T, Rose J, Roberts DR. Pulmonary edema in patients after liver transplantation. *Liver Transpl.* 2000;6 (4):466-70.

[35] Levy MF, Greene L, Ramsay MA, Jennings LW, Ramsay KJ, Meng J et al. Readmission to the intensive care unit after liver transplantation. *Crit. Care Med.* 2001;29(1):18-24.

[36] Glanemann M, Kaisers U, Langrehr JM, Schenk R, Stange BJ, Müller AR et al. Incidence and indications for reintubation during postoperative care following orthotopic liver transplantation. *J. Clin. Anesth* .2001;13(5): 377-82.

[37] Kim EK, Shim TS, Lim CM, Lee SD, Kim WS, Kim DS, Kim WD. Child-Pugh class C liver cirrhosis is an independent prognostic factor in patients with ARDS. *Crit. Care and Shock* 2003;6: 198 – 207.

[38] Garcia S, Ruza F, Gonzalez M, Roque J, Frias M, Calvo C et al. Evolution and complications in the immediate postoperative period after pediatric liver transplantation: our experience with 176 transplantations. *Transplant. Proc.* 1999;31 (3):1691-5.

[39] Golfieri R, Giampalma E, Morselli Labate AM, d'Arienzo P, Jovine E, Grazi GL et al. Pulmonary complications of liver transplantation: radiological appearance and statistical evaluation of risk factors in 300 cases. *Eur. Radiol.* 2000;10(7):1169-83.

[40] Sankey EA, Crow J, Mallett SV, Alcock RJ, More L, Burroughs AK, Rolles K. Pulmonary platelet aggregates: possible cause of sudden peroperative death in adults undergoing liver transplantation. *J. Clin. Pathol* .1993;46(3):222-7.

[41] Safadi A, Homsi M, Maskoun W, Lane KA, Singh I, Sawada SG, Mahenthiran J. Perioperative risk predictors of cardiac outcomes in patients undergoing liver transplantation surgery. *Circulation* 2009;120(13):1189-94.

[42] Umphrey LG, Hurst RT, Eleid MF, Lee KS, Reuss CS, Hentz JG et al. Preoperative dobutamine stress echocardiographic findings and subsequent short-term adverse cardiac events after orthotopic liver transplantation. *Liver Transpl* 2008;14(6):886-92.

[43] Rubin DA, Schulman DS, Edwards TD, Starzl TE, Curtiss EI. Myocardial ischemia after orthotopic liver transplantation. *Am. J. Cardiol.* 1994;74(1):5-56.

[44] Fernández-Miranda C, Sanz M, dela Calle A, Loinaz C, Gómez R, Jiménez C et al. Cardiovascular risk factors in 116 patients 5 years or more after liver transplantation. *Transpl. Int.* 2002;15(11):556-62.

[45] Mazuelos F, Abril J, Zaragoza C, Rubio E, Moreno JM, Turrión VS, Cuervas-Mons V. Cardiovascular morbidity and obesity in adult liver transplant recipients. *Transplant. Proc* .2003;35(5):1909-10.

[46] Ciccarelli O, Kaczmarek B, Roggen F, DeReyck C, Goffette P, Danse E et al. Long-term medical complications and quality of life in adult recipients surviving 10 years or more after liver transplantation. *Acta Gastroenterol. Belg.* 2005;68(3):323-30.

[47] Pagadala M, Dasarathy S, Eghtesad B, McCullough AJ. Posttransplant metabolic syndrome: an epidemic waiting to happen. *Liver Transpl* 2009;15(12):1662-70.

[48] Heisel O, Heisel R, Balshaw R, Keown P. New onset diabetes mellitus in patients receiving calcineurin inhibitors: a systematic review and meta-analysis. *Am. J. Transplant.* 2004;4(4):583-595.

[49] Atkison P, Joubert G, Barron A, Grant D, Paradis K, Seidman E et al. Hypertrophic cardiomyopathy associated with tacrolimus in paediatric transplant patients. *Lancet* 1995;345(8954):894-6.

[50] Whitington PF, Alonso EM, Piper JB. Pediatric liver transplantation. *Semin. Liver Dis.* 1994;14(3):303-17.

[51] Scott JS, Boyle GJ, Daubeney PE, Miller SA, Law Y, Pigula F et al. Tacrolimus: a cause of hypertrophic cardiomyopathy in pediatric heart transplant recipients? *Transplant. Proc.* 1999; 31(1-2):82-3.

[52] Baruch Y, Weitzman E, Markiewicz W, Eisenman A, Eid A, Enat R. Anasarca and hypertrophic cardiomyopathy in a liver transplant patient on FK506: relieved after a switch to Neoral. *Transplant. Proc.* 1996;28(4):2250-1.

[53] Pappas PA, Weppler D, Pinna AD, Rusconi P, Thompson JF, Jaffe JS, Tzakis AG. Sirolimus in pediatric gastrointestinal transplantation: the use of sirolimus for pediatric transplant patients with tacrolimus-related cardiomyopathy. *Pediatr. Transplant.* 2000;4(1): 45-9.

[54] Dollinger MM, Plevris JN, Chauhan A, MacGilchrist AJ, Finlayson ND, Hayes PC. Tacrolimus and cardiotoxicity in adult liver transplant recipients. *Lancet* 1995;346(8973):507.

[55] Nakata Y, Yoshibayashi M, Yonemura T, Uemoto S, Inomata Y, Tanaka K et al. Tacrolimus and myocardial hypertrophy. Transplantation. 2000;69(9):1960-1962Cox TH, Baillie GM, Baliga P. Bradycardia associated with intravenous administration of tacrolimus in a liver transplant recipient. *Pharmacotherapy* 1997;17(6):1328-30.

[56] Khanna A, Jain A, Ziady G, Demetris AJ, Fung JJ, Kramer D, Starzl TE. Cardiac changes at autopsy in adult liver transplant recipients under tacrolimus. *Transplant. Proc.* 1997;29 (1-2):532-3.

[57] Roberts CA, Stern DL, Radio SJ. Asymmetric cardiac hypertrophy at autopsy in patients who received FK506 (tacrolimus) or cyclosporine A after liver transplant. *Transplantation* 2002;74(6):817-21.

[58] Schwitter J, De Marco T, Globits S, Sakuma H, Klinski C, Chatterjee K et al. Influence of felodipine on left ventricular hypertrophy and systolic function in orthotopic heart transplant recipients: possible interaction with cyclosporine medication. *J. Heart. Lung. Transplant* .1999;18(10):1003-13.

[59] Espino G, Denney J, Furlong T, Fitzsimmons W, Nash RA. Assessment of myocardial hypertrophy by echocardiography in adult patients receiving tacrolimus or cyclosporine therapy for prevention of acute GVHD. *Bone Marrow Transplant.* 2001;28(12):1097-103.

[60] Canzanello VJ, Schwartz L, Taler SJ, Textor SC, Wiesner RH, Porayko MK, et al. Evolution of cardiovascular risk after liver transplantation: a comparison of cyclosporine A and tacrolimus (FK506). *Liver Transpl. Surg.* 1997;3:1–9.

[61] Rabkin JM, Corless CL, Rosen HR, Olyaei AJ. Immunosuppression impact on long-term cardiovascular complications after liver transplantation. *Am. J. Surg.*2002;183:595 –9.

[62] Jindal RM, Popescu I, Emre S, Boccagni P, Miller CM. Serum lipid changes in liver transplant recipients in a prospective trial of cyclosporine versus FK506. *Transplantation* 1994; 57: 1395.

[63] Loss M, Winkler A, Schneider C, Brinkmann C, Manns M, Ringe B and Pichlmayr R. Influence of long-term cyclosporine or FK506 therapy on glucose and lipid metabolism in stable liver graft recipients. *Transplant Proc* .1995; 27: 1136.

[64] Mells G, Neuberger J. Long-term care of the liver allograft recipient. *Semin. Liver Dis.* 2009;29:102–20.

[65] Hjelmesaeth J, Hartmann A, Kofstad J, Stenstrøm J, Leivestad T, Egeland T, Fauchald P. Glucose intolerance after renal transplantation depends on prednisolone dose and recipient age. *Transplantation* 1997;64: 979–83.

[66] Devlin J, Wong P, Williams R, Neuhaus P, McMaster P, Calne R. et al. Renal complications and development of hypertension in the European study of FK506 and cyclosporine in primary liver transplant recipients. *Transpl Int* 1994;7:S22–S26.

[67] Neal DAJ, Tom BDM, Luan J, Wareham NJ, Gimson AES, Delriviere LD, Byrne CD, Alexander GJM. Is there disparity between risk and incidence of cardiovascular disease after liver transplant? *Transplantation* 2002;77: 93-9.

[68] Herrero JI, Quiroga J, Sangro B, Girala M, Gómez-Manero N, Pardo F et al. Conversion of liver transplant recipients on cyclosporine with renal impairment to mycophenolate mofetil. *Liver Transpl. Surg.* 1999;5:414–20.

[69] Moreno JM, Rubio E, Gomez A, Lopez-Monclus J, Herreros A, Revilla J, et al. Effectiveness and safety of mycophenolate mofetil as monotherapy in liver transplantation. *Transplant. Proc* .2003;35:1874–6.

[70] Schlitt HJ, Barkmann A, Boker KH, Schmidt HH, Emmanouilidis N, Rosenau J et al. Replacement of calcineurin inhibitors with mycophenolate mofetil in liver-transplant patients with renal dysfunction: a randomized controlled study. *Lancet* 2001;357:587–91.

[71] Kreis H, Oberbauer R, Campistol JM, Mathew T, Daloze P, Schena FP, et al, for the Rapamune Maintenance Regimen Trial. Long-term benefits with sirolimus-based therapy after early cyclosporine withdrawal. *J. Am. Soc. Nephrol* .2004;15:809–17.

[72] Neff GW, Montalbano M, Tzakis AG. Ten years of sirolimus therapy in orthotopic liver transplant recipients. *Transplant. Proc.* 2003;35(Suppl):209S–216S.

[73] Humar A, Snydman D; AST Infectious Diseases Community of Practice. Cytomegalovirus in solid organ transplant recipients. *Am. J. Transplant* .2009;9(Suppl 4):S78-86.

[74] Roubille C, Brunel AS, Gahide G, Vernhet Kovacsik H, Le Quellec A. Cytomegalovirus (CMV) and acute myocarditis in an immunocompetent patient. *Intern Med.* 2010;49(2):131-3.

[75] Stack WA, Mulcahy HE, Fenelon L, Hegarty JE. Cytomegalovirus myocarditis following liver transplantation. *Postgrad. Med. J* .1994;70:658–60.

[76] Greenberg ML, Niebulski HI, Uretsky BF, Salerni R, KleinHA, Forstate WJ, et al. Occult purulent pericarditis detected by indium-111 leukocyte imaging. *Chest* 1984;85:701–3.

[77] Hearn CJ, Smedira NG. Pulmonic valve endocarditis after orthotopic liver transplantation. *Liver Transpl .Surg.* 1999;5: 456–7.

[78] Angelis M, Cooper JT, Freeman RB. Impact of donor infections on outcome of orthotopic liver transplantation. *Liver Transpl* 2003;9: 451–62.

[79] Chagas disease after organ transplantation—United States, 2001. MMWR Morb Mortal Wkly Rep 2002;51:210–2.

[80] Souza FF, Castro-E-Silva O, Marin Neto JA, Sankarankutty AK, Teixeira AC, Martinelli AL et al. Acute chagasic myocardiopathy after orthotopic liver transplantation with donor and recipient serologically negative for Trypanosoma cruzi: a case report. *Transplant Proc* 2008;40(3):875-8.

[81] Kamath PS, Wiesner RH, Malinchoc M, Kremers W, Therneau TM, Kosberg CL, D'Amico G et al. A model to predict survival in patients with end-stage liver disease. *Hepatology* 2001;33:464-70.

[82] Freeman RB, Rohrer RJ, Katz E, Lewis WD, Jenkins R, Cosimi AB, Delmonico F et al. Preliminary results of a liver allocation plan using a continuous medical severity score that de-emphasizes waiting time. *Liver Transpl.* 2001;7:173-8.

[83] Saab S, Wang V, Ibrahim AB, Durazo F, Han S, Farmer DG et al. MELD score predicts 1-year patient survival post-orthotopic liver transplantation. *Liver Transpl.* 2003;9:473-6

[84] Biggins SW, Rodriguez HJ, Bacchetti P, Bass NM, Roberts JP, Terrault NA. Serum sodium predicts mortality in patients listed for liver transplantation. *Hepatology* 2005;41:32-9.

[85] Ruf AE, Kremers WK, Chavez LL, Descalzi VI, Podesta LG, Villamil FG. Addition of serum sodium into the MELD score predicts waiting list mortality better than MELD alone. *Liver Transpl.* 2005;11:336-43.

[86] Luca A, Angermayr B, Bertolini G, Koenig F, Vizzini G, Ploner M et al. An integrated MELD model including serum sodium and age improves the prediction of early mortality in patients with cirrhosis. *Liver Transpl.* 2007;13:1174-80.

[87] Assmann G, Cullen P, Schulte H. Simple scoring scheme for calculating the risk of acute coronary events based on the 10-year follow-up of the prospective cardiovascular Munster (PROCAM) study. *Circulation* 2002;105:310-15.

[88] Baik SK, Fouad TR, Lee SS. Cirrhotic cardiomyopathy. *Orphanet. J. Rare Dis.* 2007;2:15.

[89] Algahtani SA, Fouad TR, Lee SS. Cirrhotic cardiomyopathy. *Semin. Liver Dis.* 2008;28:59-69

[90] Torregrosa M, Aguade S, Dos L, Segura R, Gonzales A, Evangelista A et al. Cardiac alterations in cirrhosis: reversibility after liver transplantation. *J. Hepatol* .2005; 42:68-74

[91] Pozzi M, Carugo S, Boari G, Pecci V, de Ceglia S, Maggiolini S, et al. Evidence of functional and structural cardiac abnormalities in cirrhotic patients with and without ascites. *Hepatology* 1997;26:1131-7.

[92] Young AL, Rajagenashan R, Asthana S, Peters CJ, Toogood GJ, Davies MH, Lodge JP, Pollard SG, Prasad KR. The value of MELD and sodium in assessing potential liver transplant recipients in the United Kingdom. *Transpl. Int.* 2007;20:331-7.

[93] Wong VW, Chim AM, Wong GL, Sung JJ, Chan HL. Performance of the new MELD-Na score in predicting 3-month and 1-year mortality in Chinese patients with chronic hepatitis B. *Liver Transpl* .2007;13:1228-35

[94] Coss E, Watt KDS, Pedersen J, Dierkhising R, Heimbach JK, Charlton MR. Predictors of cardiovascular events after liver transplantation: a role for pretransplant serum troponin levels. *Liver Transpl* .2010;16(8): 990-8

Acknowledgments

Thanks to all authors for hard work and good quality chapters delivered mainly on time.

Thanks to Dr Gordon Lyons who did perfect language editing and rescued one particular book chapter.

I owe a great deal to Matthew Hockney who did all tables and most figures and Kerry Munro who did language editing of several chapters.

Thanks Barbara Rupnik for helping with technical work.

Thanks so all members of Leeds Liver Group for inspiring and supporting me to finish this work.

Index

A

access, 39, 47, 162, 180, 206
accounting, 259
acid, 8, 60
acidosis, 79, 90
action potential, 51
acute hypertensive episodes, xvi, 217
acute lymphoblastic leukemia, 166
acute renal failure, 146
acute respiratory distress syndrome, 256
adaptation, 177
adenosine, 24, 36
adenosine triphosphate, 24
adjustment, 62
adolescents, 52
adrenaline, 13, 24
adrenoceptors, 9, 24
adults, 52, 80, 100, 120, 126, 127, 133, 136, 152, 153, 160, 164, 185, 192, 213, 231, 264, 270
advancements, 164
adverse effects, xiii, 88, 99
aerobic capacity, 45, 209, 214
aetiology, xii, 67
age, 14, 32, 33, 43, 50, 55, 56, 103, 115, 120, 132, 150, 158, 160, 180, 181, 189, 196, 199, 204, 210, 251, 252, 261, 262, 263, 266, 267, 271, 273
aggression, 159
aggressiveness, 51
agonist, 108
air embolism, 61
alanine, 126
alanine aminotransferase, 126
albumin, 4, 17, 22, 25, 29, 181
alcohol abuse, 189
alcohol consumption, 33, 266
alcohol use, 106
alcoholic cardiomyopathy, 56
alcoholic cirrhosis, 17, 25, 27, 33, 176, 177
alcoholic liver disease, 132
alcoholism, 43, 106, 130
aldosterone, xvi, xxi, 2, 7, 13, 14, 22, 178, 217, 219, 231
algorithm, xii, 35, 67, 77, 90, 163, 164, 200, 241, 247, 250, 251, 252, 255, 258
ALT, 126, 129, 132
alveoli, 207
alveolus, 212
American Heart Association, xix, 43, 45, 47, 62, 150, 194, 199, 269
amino, 8
amyloid deposits, 149
amyloidosis, 136, 144, 148, 153, 155
anastomosis, 142, 145, 149
anatomy, 41, 86, 140
anesthesiologists, xvi, 217, 218, 228, 255
aneurysm, 208, 209, 214
angina, 43, 72, 100, 101, 267
angiogenesis, 7, 163
angiography, 32, 37, 38, 39, 41, 46, 118, 161, 183, 197, 198, 203, 266
angioplasty, 41, 102, 234
angiotensin converting enzyme, 70
angiotensin II, 9, 10, 14, 17, 23, 24, 25, 70, 162, 178, 219
angiotensin II receptor antagonist, 25, 70, 219
angiotensin receptor blockers, 164
ankylosing spondylitis, 73
antibiotic, 78, 79
antibody, xx, 145, 159, 164
anticancer treatment, xiv, 157, 158, 160, 163
anticoagulant, 57, 65, 148, 227
anticoagulation, 58, 64, 71, 76, 78, 79, 80, 143
antihypertensive agents, 229
antioxidant, 14, 162

antitumor, 158, 159, 162, 164, 165, 166
aorta, 100, 163, 250
aortic regurgitation, 73, 74
aortic stenosis, 72, 73, 80, 100, 140, 143
aortic valve, 71, 72, 74, 75, 80, 102, 143, 152
apoptosis, 160, 163, 167
ARDS, 270
Argentina, 136
arrhythmia, 50, 51, 52, 55, 60, 61, 62, 194
arterial blood gas, 185, 202, 207
arterial hypertension, xx, 16, 19, 33, 94, 95, 96, 221, 231, 232, 233, 234, 235
arteries, 16, 24, 107
arterioles, xii, 16, 83, 84, 85, 87, 91
arteriovenous shunt, 17
artery, xi, xii, xiii, xv, xix, xx, 12, 13, 20, 26, 31, 39, 41, 43, 46, 47, 50, 56, 60, 65, 78, 79, 83, 84, 92, 95, 102, 106, 108, 113, 117, 122, 133, 135, 143, 150, 151, 163, 193, 195, 196, 197, 211, 222, 235, 240, 241, 243, 248, 250, 252, 253, 254, 255, 256, 257, 258
ascites, xv, 2, 6, 8, 11, 14, 17, 21, 24, 25, 26, 27, 28, 30, 68, 70, 78, 130, 131, 136, 141, 169, 170, 172, 174, 175, 176, 177, 178, 260, 266, 273
aspartate, 126
assessment, xiii, xv, xvi, 28, 34, 35, 36, 39, 40, 44, 45, 46, 50, 51, 52, 56, 58, 68, 69, 84, 86, 89, 93, 94, 106, 137, 152, 166, 173, 193, 194, 195, 196, 198, 201, 202, 209, 210, 214, 215, 228, 231, 234, 235, 247, 251, 254, 255, 256, 258, 262, 269
asymptomatic, xvi, 74, 76, 100, 101, 105, 201, 202, 211, 219, 264, 265
atherosclerosis, xiv, 43, 72, 139
atherosclerotic vascular disease, 48
atmospheric pressure, 180
atria, 183
atrial fibrillation, xii, 49, 50, 56, 57, 59, 60, 64, 65, 69, 72, 74, 75, 76, 117, 219
atrial septal defect, 91
atrium, 183
auscultation, 195
autoimmune hepatitis, 85, 107
autonomic nervous system, 2, 15
autopsy, 56, 72, 127, 134, 264, 271
avoidance, 65, 73, 74, 90, 107, 119, 141, 160, 197
awareness, 74, 219
Azathioprine, 146

baroreceptor, xi, 1, 16
base, 60, 102, 159, 207
base pair, 159
beneficial effect, 19, 42, 70, 236
benefits, 57, 61, 116, 176, 227, 272
benign, 55
beta blocker, xvi, 54, 57, 162, 217, 218, 219
beverages, 44
bias, 32, 115, 243, 250, 251, 252
bicarbonate, 207
bicuspid, 72, 73
bile, 11, 184, 190
bile acids, 11
bile duct, 184, 190
biliary cirrhosis, 23, 25, 184, 190
bilirubin, 71, 126, 129, 132, 141, 186
bioavailability, 119
biological markers, 161
biomarkers, 85
biopsy, 128, 132, 133, 137, 148, 160, 165, 166
bleeding, xvi, 9, 22, 57, 58, 61, 70, 71, 129, 130, 135, 141, 143, 145, 163, 167, 218, 227, 228, 229, 235, 240, 248
blood, xiv, xv, xx, xxi, 2, 3, 4, 6, 7, 8, 9, 10, 12, 13, 14, 16, 18, 19, 22, 24, 26, 28, 29, 30, 34, 38, 59, 60, 70, 74, 78, 79, 84, 85, 94, 108, 109, 130, 142, 145, 158, 161, 169, 170, 172, 173, 174, 178, 179, 180, 204, 212, 219, 228, 230, 236, 240, 241, 242, 243, 247, 248, 249, 250, 252, 253, 256, 257, 260, 261, 266
body fluid, 22
body mass index (BMI), xix, 114, 115, 116, 117, 120, 121, 122, 210, 266
body size, 14
body weight, 116, 119, 121, 223
bone, 85, 237, 265
bradyarrhythmia, 50, 108
bradycardia, 54, 56, 60, 74, 158
bradykinin, 60
brain, xi, 1, 2, 3, 10, 12, 15, 26, 30, 52, 63, 94, 181, 264
breakdown, 159
breast cancer, 158, 159, 165, 166, 167
breathing, 181
bronchial asthma, 186
bundle branch block, 86, 158
bypass graft, xix

B

bacteria, 184
balloon angioplasty, 41
barbiturates, 53

C

Ca^{2+}, 184
cachexia, 121, 132

CAD, xi, xix, 31, 32, 33, 34, 35, 36, 37, 38, 39, 40, 41, 42, 114, 116, 117, 118, 140, 141, 194, 195, 196, 197, 198, 203, 260, 262, 263, 266
cadaver, 115, 236
Cairo, vii, 157, 165
calcification, 39, 46, 72, 117, 122
calcitonin, 6, 13, 15, 22, 23, 24
calcium, xvi, 26, 46, 51, 57, 63, 70, 75, 87, 101, 107, 111, 118, 160, 165, 217, 231, 236
calcium channel blocker, xvi, 51, 57, 70, 75, 87, 217, 236
calibration, 247, 250, 251, 252, 258
cancer, xiii, 113, 115, 116, 117, 119, 123, 159, 161, 162, 163, 164, 165, 166, 214
candidates, xi, xii, xiv, xv, xvi, 6, 29, 31, 32, 33, 35, 36, 37, 38, 39, 41, 42, 43, 45, 46, 50, 51, 60, 77, 83, 86, 94, 95, 96, 103, 116, 117, 118, 119, 123, 126, 137, 139, 140, 144, 150, 179, 180, 186, 189, 190, 191, 192, 193, 194, 195, 196, 197, 199, 201, 202, 203, 210, 211, 212, 213, 214
cannabinoids, 6, 11, 23
capillary, 6, 11, 12, 18, 23, 132, 163, 190, 208, 212, 256
carbon, xxi, 11, 13, 15, 30, 86, 181, 206
carbon dioxide, xxi, 86, 206
carbon monoxide, 11, 13, 15, 30, 181
carcinogenesis, 167
carcinoid syndrome, 76
carcinoma, 163, 164, 167
cardiac arrest, 50, 60, 228
cardiac arrhythmia, 62
cardiac catheterization, 38, 46, 105, 106, 118
cardiac involvement, 148
cardiac muscle, 159, 161, 162
cardiac operations, 111, 134, 140, 150
cardiac output, xvii, xix, 2, 3, 4, 7, 8, 9, 10, 11, 12, 16, 19, 25, 28, 59, 69, 70, 78, 85, 86, 88, 89, 90, 91, 92, 107, 108, 126, 141, 161, 170, 173, 174, 177, 181, 196, 212, 227, 239, 241, 242, 243, 244, 247, 248, 251, 252, 253, 254, 255, 256, 257, 258, 268
cardiac reserve, xi, 1
cardiac risk, 33, 35, 42, 44, 45, 46, 48, 121, 194, 195, 200, 213, 235, 263
cardiac risk factors, 33, 195
cardiac surgery, xiii, xiv, 35, 36, 38, 40, 41, 45, 46, 47, 48, 56, 59, 80, 88, 99, 104, 107, 108, 109, 111, 129, 133, 134, 139, 140, 143, 149, 150, 151, 152, 194, 234, 235, 250, 255, 256, 257, 258
cardiac tamponade, 141
cardiogenic shock, 126
cardiologist, 198, 229

cardiomyopathy, xi, xii, xiii, xv, xvi, xx, 1, 3, 10, 11, 12, 20, 21, 22, 24, 25, 26, 34, 38, 49, 50, 52, 60, 61, 75, 83, 84, 86, 88, 91, 94, 99, 100, 105, 110, 111, 132, 148, 155, 158, 159, 160, 161, 162, 165, 166, 176, 193, 194, 202, 208, 212, 217, 218, 219, 230, 237, 252, 260, 264, 265, 266, 268, 270, 271, 273
cardiopulmonary bypass, 70, 129, 135, 136, 145, 151, 154
Cardiopulmonary exercise testing, xvi, xix, 201, 202, 203, 213, 214, 215
cardiorespiratory disease, 202, 203
cardiovascular disease, xiii, 48, 113, 115, 117, 118, 123, 170, 194, 218, 230, 237, 240, 263, 264, 267, 272
cardiovascular function, 210, 260
cardiovascular morbidity, 32, 34, 35, 195
cardiovascular risk, xii, xvii, 31, 34, 35, 39, 47, 117, 122, 195, 197, 198, 214, 235, 259, 271
cardiovascular system, 10, 32, 33, 230, 267
carotid duplex, 118
case study, 224
catecholamines, 9, 10
catheter, xx, 51, 60, 78, 87, 88, 102, 108, 163, 222, 241, 242, 243, 246, 249, 250, 252, 253, 254, 256, 257, 258
CCA, 105
cell death, 159, 162
central nervous system, 15
centralisation, 248
cerebral blood flow, 19, 30
cerebral hemorrhage, 187
cerebrovascular disease, 35, 195, 196, 237
Chagas disease, 265, 272
challenges, xii, xvii, 49, 57, 73, 79, 107, 132, 239
channel blocker, xvi, xix, 58, 70, 218, 221, 229, 231
chemical, 222
chemical stability, 222
chemicals, 141
chemotherapeutic agent, xiv, 157, 158, 159, 160, 161, 162, 163, 164
chemotherapy, xiv, 157, 158, 159, 160, 161, 162, 163, 164, 166
Chicago, 241
children, 52, 63, 115, 153, 166, 264
cholestasis, 126, 132, 136
cholesterol, 119, 132
Chronic liver injury, xiii, 125
chronic obstructive pulmonary disease, 186, 227
chronic renal failure, 146
ciclosporin, xvi, 218, 229, 230
circulation, xi, xii, xiv, 1, 2, 3, 5, 6, 9, 10, 12, 16, 19, 20, 21, 22, 23, 24, 27, 30, 79, 83, 84, 107, 135,

146, 154, 169, 170, 172, 173, 181, 206, 212, 240, 241, 243, 247, 250, 266, 268, 269
cirrhosis, xi, xii, xiii, xv, xvi, 1, 2, 3, 4, 5, 6, 7, 8, 9, 10, 11, 12, 13, 14, 15, 16, 17, 18, 19, 20, 21, 22, 23, 24, 25, 26, 27, 28, 29, 30, 32, 43, 46, 52, 55, 61, 62, 63, 64, 76, 83, 86, 93, 94, 96, 111, 116, 123, 125, 126, 127, 129, 130, 131, 132, 133, 134, 136, 137, 140, 141, 143, 144, 150, 151, 163, 170, 172, 173, 176, 177, 178, 179, 183, 184, 190, 192, 193, 199, 214, 217, 218, 219, 230, 231, 251, 252, 264, 267, 268, 269, 273
cirrhotic cardiomyopathy, xi, xii, xv, xvi, 1, 3, 10, 11, 12, 22, 24, 26, 34, 38, 49, 50, 52, 61, 83, 84, 86, 88, 91, 176, 193, 194, 202, 208, 212, 217, 218, 219, 230, 252, 260, 266
classes, 70, 221, 222
classification, 34, 56, 141, 163, 221, 223, 267
clinical application, 241, 248
clinical assessment, 69
clinical diagnosis, 132
clinical examination, 164, 203
clinical judgment, 118
clinical presentation, xiv, 86, 125, 134
clinical symptoms, xii, 83
clinical trials, 167, 185
CO2, 204, 206, 207
coagulopathy, 78, 126, 129, 141, 142, 145, 148
collaboration, 45, 199, 254
collagen, 127
collateral, 9, 23, 219
colorectal cancer, 123
combination therapy, xvi, 217, 224, 227
combined heart and liver transplantation (CHLT), xiv, 139
common bile duct, 184
communication, 183
community, 119
comorbidity, 213
compliance, 2, 4, 8, 13, 14, 16, 21, 22, 23, 24, 26, 27, 73, 244, 247, 250, 251, 252
complications, xi, xii, xiii, xiv, xv, xvi, xvii, 1, 9, 14, 20, 21, 34, 35, 36, 38, 42, 43, 44, 49, 50, 56, 57, 58, 60, 61, 69, 70, 71, 84, 96, 104, 105, 109, 113, 115, 116, 117, 118, 119, 120, 121, 122, 123, 129, 130, 133, 140, 153, 165, 169, 170, 173, 175, 176, 178, 193, 196, 198, 199, 200, 202, 203, 204, 208, 209, 214, 217, 218, 219, 229, 230, 243, 244, 252, 253, 255, 259, 261, 262, 263, 264, 266, 267, 268, 270, 271, 272
compounds, 221
computed tomography, xxi, 30, 36, 46, 103, 118, 132, 183
conduction, 51, 159

congenital heart disease, 131, 144
congestive heart failure, 55, 75, 117, 137, 141, 158, 164, 170, 176, 177, 212, 219, 267
Congress, iv
consensus, xii, xvii, 49, 61, 109, 194, 197, 202, 240
construction, 142
consulting, 198
consumption, xx, xxi, 33, 44, 204, 205, 206, 221
contamination, 142
contour, 243, 247, 255, 256, 257, 258
control group, 38, 264
controlled trials, 120, 222, 223, 224
controversial, 32, 40, 52, 57, 228, 263
controversies, 198
COPD, xix, 55, 227
cor pulmonale, 93
coronary angioplasty, xxi, 40, 47
coronary arteries, 32, 72
coronary artery bypass graft, 40, 47, 140, 150, 151, 257
coronary artery disease, xiii, xv, 32, 34, 37, 38, 43, 44, 46, 50, 54, 55, 63, 113, 114, 116, 117, 140, 150, 152, 193, 194, 195, 199, 202, 213, 215, 260
Coronary artery disease (CAD), xi, 31
coronary bypass surgery, 47
coronary heart disease, 43, 44, 46
correlation, 114, 127, 132, 183, 190, 241, 247, 248, 250, 261, 263, 266
correlations, 134, 247
corticosteroids, 230, 265, 267
cost, 204, 229
cough, 74, 219
coumarins, 57
CPB, xix, 70, 73, 75, 135, 141, 142, 145
creatinine, 186
cure, xiv, xix, 157, 158
cycling, 204
cyclophosphamide, 158
cyclosporine, 146, 236, 237, 263, 264, 265, 266, 269, 271, 272
cystic duct, 145
cystic fibrosis, 154
cytochrome, 227
cytokines, xiii, 19, 125, 127, 129, 134

D

database, 61, 88, 96, 97, 115, 116, 120, 121, 144, 192
deaths, 35, 42, 104, 120, 122, 130, 142, 174, 210, 260, 261, 263
defects, 9, 14, 159, 212
defibrillation, 55

defibrillator, 58
degradation, 6, 7, 224
dehiscence, 115
denial, 39
Denmark, viii, 1
deposition, 127, 144, 148, 149
depression, 45, 141, 260
depth, 58
detectable, 107
detection, xv, 46, 53, 58, 165, 170, 183, 191, 204, 213
developed countries, 71
deviation, 145
diabetes, xiii, xvii, 33, 35, 37, 55, 56, 113, 114, 116, 117, 119, 120, 121, 122, 123, 195, 196, 259, 263, 267, 270
diagnostic criteria, 84, 180, 263
diarrhea, 222
diastole, 75, 76, 100
diastolic functions, xi, 1, 19
diastolic pressure, 11
diffusion, 29, 180, 212
digoxin, xvi, 70, 75, 76, 217, 234
dilated cardiomyopathy, 52, 143, 144, 160, 164, 165, 262
dilation, 75, 86, 127
direct bilirubin, 130
direct measure, 69, 108
disability, 50, 244
discomfort, 222
discrimination, 18
disease progression, 72
diseases, xii, xiv, 67, 73, 116, 117, 133, 139, 140, 143, 268
disorder, xiii, 99, 126, 148, 185
dispersion, xxi, 12, 28, 52, 62, 63, 64
distribution, 2, 3, 12, 16, 22, 127, 163, 191, 214
diuretic, 87
diuretics, xvi, 70, 74, 75, 76, 217, 219, 229
DNA, 159
DNA damage, 160
dogs, 257
donors, 149, 154, 253
Doppler echocardiogram, xiii, 12, 83
dosage, 62
dosing, 71
down-regulation, 9, 24
drainage, 129, 141, 142
drug interaction, 158, 230
drug therapy, xvi, 87, 217
drugs, xiv, 9, 14, 53, 57, 60, 61, 88, 108, 157, 158, 159, 165, 218, 220, 225, 227, 228, 229, 237
dumping, 170

durability, 129
dyslipidemia, xvii, 230, 259, 263, 265
dyspnea, 106, 154, 185, 222

E

echocardiogram, xiii, xv, 12, 56, 83, 107, 183, 193, 196, 262, 266
echocardiography, xiii, xv, xix, xxi, 36, 37, 43, 44, 45, 46, 51, 69, 72, 78, 79, 80, 84, 86, 89, 94, 100, 101, 102, 105, 106, 107, 108, 110, 111, 142, 150, 152, 160, 161, 164, 179, 181, 183, 186, 187, 190, 197, 199, 202, 203, 210, 213, 252, 255, 256, 257, 260, 265, 269, 271
edema, 141, 224, 261, 269
editors, 21, 22
Egypt, vii, 114, 157, 259
electrocardiogram, xv, 86, 158, 193, 196, 202
electrolyte, 50, 52, 58, 60, 79, 250, 262
electrolyte imbalance, 262
e-mail, 169
emboli, 183
embolism, 50, 148, 154
embolization, 183
emergency, 209
emission, xxi, 30, 36, 103
encephalopathy, 19, 30, 69
encouragement, 204
endocarditis, 71, 74, 78, 80, 143, 265, 272
endocrine, 23
endothelial cells, 6, 23, 184, 221, 223, 229, 236
endothelial dysfunction, xii, 23, 83, 85, 89, 91
endothelium, 6, 85, 88, 90, 177
endotoxins, 11
endotracheal intubation, 54
end-stage liver disease (ESLD), xiii, xiv, 49, 99, 104, 139, 194
energy, 204
enlargement, 74, 266
environment, 91
enzyme, xvi, xix, 70, 162, 164, 217, 219, 224
enzyme inhibitors, xvi, 70, 162, 164, 217, 219
enzymes, 88, 137
epidemic, 270
epidemiology, 167
epinephrine, 108
equilibrium, 212
equipment, 61, 204
ERA, xix
esophageal varices, 227
esophagus, 214
ester, 185, 191
estrogen, 85

ETA, 234
ethanol, 163
ethical issues, 40
etiology, xii, 25, 33, 50, 56, 63, 83, 85, 91, 127, 132, 159, 260
Europe, 55, 164, 213
evidence, xiii, xv, xvi, 6, 9, 12, 20, 22, 27, 38, 39, 40, 42, 44, 50, 51, 56, 57, 60, 61, 68, 69, 71, 74, 80, 84, 148, 163, 173, 174, 176, 179, 186, 187, 194, 197, 198, 201, 207, 209, 211, 219, 221, 222, 223, 224, 240, 250, 260, 261, 263, 264, 265
examinations, 245
excision, 149
exclusion, 250, 257
excretion, 16, 17, 27, 229
exercise, xvi, xix, xx, 11, 14, 25, 27, 35, 36, 45, 46, 51, 57, 68, 94, 185, 195, 198, 200, 201, 202, 203, 204, 205, 206, 207, 208, 209, 210, 212, 213, 214, 215, 222, 223, 224, 227, 228, 234, 260
exertion, 86, 105, 106
experimental condition, 91
exposure, 130, 142, 163, 260, 263, 265
extraction, 11

F

factor analysis, 134
fairness, 117
false positive, 34, 36, 38, 197, 202
familial hypercholesterolemia, 144, 153, 154
family history, 37, 195, 196
FDA, 159
fever, 74
fiber, 158
fibrillation, 55, 56, 60, 64, 76, 117
fibrinolysis, 58, 143
fibrinolytic, 228
fibrosis, xiii, 9, 12, 85, 87, 125, 126, 127, 128, 131, 132, 133, 134, 137, 160, 186
filament, 241, 254
filtration, 2, 6, 16, 46
fitness, 204, 214
flight, 195
fluctuations, 250
fluid, 4, 5, 7, 14, 16, 70, 78, 79, 109, 114, 129, 141, 219, 227, 240, 241, 244, 247, 253, 255, 262, 266
fluid balance, 129
foramen, 213
foramen ovale, 213
force, 48
formation, 6, 160, 162
formula, 52
France, 192

free radicals, 159, 162
freedom, 147
fresh frozen plasma, 142

G

gastrointestinal tract, xi, 1
gel, 125
general anesthesia, 55
general knowledge, 51
Germany, 246
glucose, 271
grades, 183
grading, 72
growth, 85, 88, 119, 159, 162, 163, 165, 167, 174, 185, 231
growth factor, 88, 119, 159, 163, 165, 167, 185
guidance, 107, 118
guidelines, xii, xvi, 31, 35, 36, 38, 39, 40, 42, 43, 45, 48, 57, 58, 60, 62, 86, 94, 133, 176, 193, 194, 196, 197, 198, 200, 228

H

haemodynamic changes, xi, 1, 3, 6, 7, 28, 63, 195
half-life, 58, 87
harmful effects, 159, 164
hazards, xvii, 163, 239
HE, 62, 272
headache, 87, 222
health, xiii, 114, 119, 140
heart and lung transplant, 236
heart disease, xii, 35, 43, 50, 51, 56, 61, 67, 68, 72, 79, 80, 127, 144, 195, 196, 219, 261, 263
heart failure, xiii, xvi, xix, 11, 20, 35, 56, 68, 72, 74, 75, 76, 84, 93, 100, 117, 125, 126, 127, 128, 129, 130, 131, 132, 133, 134, 135, 136, 137, 158, 165, 166, 178, 195, 196, 206, 214, 215, 218, 219, 220, 221, 230, 231, 266
heart rate, 2, 4, 7, 11, 12, 14, 16, 19, 26, 27, 28, 38, 51, 56, 57, 58, 59, 60, 63, 76, 108, 109, 173, 203, 205, 212, 241, 247, 250, 264
heart transplantation, xiv, xix, xx, 115, 125, 127, 130, 131, 133, 135, 136, 137, 144, 146, 147, 148, 149, 152, 153, 154
heart valves, 71, 80
height, 210, 251, 252, 266
heme, 184, 185
heme oxygenase, 184, 185
hemochromatosis, 136, 144, 153
hemodialysis, 89
hemoglobin, 223

hemorrhage, 141, 219
hemostasis, 64, 142, 145
hepatic encephalopathy, 2, 3, 19, 27, 69
hepatic failure, 19, 30, 64, 70, 130, 144, 249, 256, 261
hepatic fibrosis, xiii, 125, 126, 127, 132, 133, 134, 137
hepatic stellate cells, 9
hepatic transplant, 81, 215
hepatitis, 33, 44, 106, 126, 132, 133, 134, 144, 273
hepatocarcinogenesis, 163
hepatocellular carcinoma, 158, 159, 163, 164, 167, 251
hepatocytes, 161
hepatomegaly, 74, 131, 142
hepatopulmonary syndrome, xi, xv, 1, 2, 3, 18, 20, 29, 68, 85, 93, 180, 181, 189, 190, 191, 192, 193, 196, 202, 218
hepatorenal syndrome, xi, 1, 2, 3, 21, 22, 23, 28, 174, 175, 218
heterogeneity, 52
high risk patients, 38
history, xii, xiv, xv, xx, 35, 51, 67, 69, 70, 72, 74, 75, 76, 77, 134, 157, 159, 160, 161, 189, 193, 195, 202, 262, 266, 267, 269
HLA, 145, 146, 154
HO-1, 93
homeostasis, 23, 165, 176, 177
homogeneity, 186
hormones, 9, 119, 174
hospitalization, 120, 126
human, 17, 23, 146, 154, 159, 165, 264
Hunter, 26
hydrogen, 159
hydrogen peroxide, 159
hypercholesterolemia, 122, 136, 153, 154, 263
hyperdynamic circulation, xi, 1, 2, 3, 6, 10, 19, 20, 21, 22, 23, 27, 69, 79, 84, 107, 170, 173, 247, 250, 266
hyperemia, 24
hyperglycemia, 230
hyperinsulinemia, 119
hyperkalemia, 55
hyperlipidemia, xiii, xvi, 113, 114, 115, 117, 119, 218, 229, 230, 237, 263, 265
hypertension, xi, xii, xiii, xv, xvi, xvii, xx, 1, 2, 16, 19, 22, 29, 30, 37, 55, 56, 72, 74, 83, 84, 90, 91, 93, 94, 95, 96, 97, 100, 113, 115, 117, 118, 119, 122, 141, 143, 158, 176, 177, 178, 191, 192, 193, 195, 196, 200, 212, 217, 218, 219, 221, 222, 229, 230, 231, 232, 233, 234, 235, 236, 237, 244, 255, 259, 260, 263, 265, 266, 269, 272
hyperthyroidism, 55, 56

hypertrophic cardiomyopathy, 51, 109, 110, 111, 131, 230, 237, 270, 271
Hypertrophic obstructive cardiomyopathy (HOCM), xiii, 99, 100
hypertrophy, 12, 19, 69, 72, 73, 74, 84, 85, 100, 103, 110, 134, 174, 178, 219, 261, 264, 271
hyperventilation, 30
hypokalemia, 52
hypomagnesemia, 50, 52, 64
hypotension, xvi, 10, 16, 17, 23, 41, 44, 56, 73, 78, 88, 104, 108, 109, 111, 127, 158, 194, 217, 219, 224, 243, 264
hypotensive, 104
hypothermia, 50, 60, 64, 90, 141, 240
hypothesis, 2, 6, 20, 22, 87, 208
hypovolemia, 60, 108, 247, 248
hypoxemia, xv, 86, 179, 183, 184, 185, 186, 189, 191, 261
hypoxia, xiii, 41, 90, 125, 127, 167

I

ideal, 57
identification, xii, xv, 31, 33, 34, 39, 63, 70, 193, 206, 240, 244, 254
identity, 145
idiopathic, 73, 144, 186, 221, 233
image, 100, 161, 250
images, 244
imaging modalities, 137
immobilization, 148
Immunosuppressants, xvi, 218
immunosuppression, xvii, 65, 146, 154, 253, 259, 260, 261, 263, 264, 265, 267, 269
immunosuppressive agent, xvi, 48, 131, 146, 217, 218, 220, 229, 230
immunotherapy, 154
implants, 130
improvements, 140, 158, 223
in vitro, 254
incidence, xii, xiv, xvi, 33, 38, 43, 49, 50, 56, 59, 60, 61, 71, 76, 104, 115, 121, 123, 130, 139, 140, 146, 148, 165, 218, 228, 236, 253, 261, 263, 265, 272
increased workload, 84
indium, 272
individuals, 32, 33, 39, 100, 101, 104, 109, 209
induction, 54, 55, 63, 64, 146
infarction, xx, 35, 104, 196, 262
infection, xvi, 17, 87, 106, 129, 130, 187, 217, 219, 222, 265
infectious mononucleosis, 265

inferior vena cava, 73, 78, 79, 153, 194, 240, 244, 247, 248, 266
inflammation, 76, 132
inhaler, 88
inhibition, 9, 23, 24, 184, 185
inhibitor, 17, 58, 64, 71, 80, 87, 88, 146, 162, 163, 184, 185, 219, 223, 224, 260
initiation, 20, 88, 90, 142
injections, 183
injury, iv, xiii, 34, 44, 90, 125, 126, 131, 132, 135, 164, 166
insertion, xiv, 11, 19, 20, 60, 78, 169, 170, 171, 172, 173, 174, 176, 228, 229, 244
insulin, 115, 118, 119, 122
insulin resistance, 115, 118
integration, 204
integrity, 17
intensive care unit, 70, 78, 96, 140, 142, 253, 255, 257, 261, 264, 269
interdependence, 94, 95
intervention, xx, 41, 48, 55, 67, 103, 104, 105, 106, 140, 195, 202, 228, 234, 235
intoxication, 64
intra-aortic balloon pump, 91
intravenous fluids, 109
intravenously, 88, 162, 222, 264
ions, 207
iron, 144, 153, 162
ischaemic heart disease, 69, 195, 196, 211
ischemia, 41, 46, 90, 115, 121, 145, 158, 159, 266, 270
isolation, 76, 203
isotope, 36, 38, 161
issues, xii, 14, 31, 33, 41, 68, 70, 194, 198, 203, 218
Italy, vii, 239

J

jaundice, 131
justification, 202

K

K^+, 184
kidney, xiii, 16, 26, 39, 46, 47, 56, 58, 60, 113, 115, 118, 119, 120, 121, 123, 131, 135, 143, 236, 237
kidney failure, 60
kidneys, xi, 1, 2, 3

L

lactate dehydrogenase, 132

L-arginine, 6, 23, 185, 191
latency, 73, 74
LDL, 237
lead, xv, xvi, 39, 51, 52, 54, 72, 109, 126, 130, 140, 141, 146, 160, 162, 169, 193, 196, 204, 210, 218, 219, 222, 224
leakage, 102, 187
left atrium, 75, 183, 212
left ventricle, 12, 72, 73, 75, 174
left ventricular outflow tract (LVOT), xiii, 99
legs, 204
lesions, xii, 31, 32, 39, 41, 67, 69, 70, 72, 79, 85, 140, 141, 197, 227
leukemia, 159
leukotrienes, 10
life expectancy, 85
lipid metabolism, 271
lipids, 160, 230, 237
lithium, 249, 250, 257
liver abscess, 187
liver cancer, 116
liver cirrhosis, xii, 23, 24, 26, 28, 29, 30, 43, 44, 45, 47, 80, 83, 84, 85, 86, 130, 134, 135, 136, 177, 185, 199, 230, 269, 270
liver disease, xi, xii, xiii, xiv, xv, xvi, xvii, xix, xx, 1, 2, 3, 6, 12, 13, 14, 16, 20, 21, 22, 23, 25, 26, 27, 28, 30, 31, 32, 33, 34, 36, 38, 39, 40, 41, 42, 43, 44, 46, 49, 52, 57, 63, 64, 68, 69, 70, 71, 73, 75, 76, 77, 80, 83, 84, 86, 93, 96, 97, 99, 104, 105, 116, 119, 125, 126, 127, 129, 130, 131, 132, 133, 134, 136, 137, 139, 140, 141, 142, 143, 144, 149, 150, 152, 177, 179, 180, 186, 187, 189, 194, 195, 202, 203, 209, 213, 217, 218, 221, 222, 224, 227, 239, 240, 251, 260, 261, 262, 266, 268, 269, 272
liver enzymes, 130
liver failure, 21, 30, 130, 141, 143, 144, 195, 212, 266, 267
liver function tests, 126, 223
liver transplant operations, xi
low risk, 38, 195, 210, 265
lumen, 241
lung disease, 18
lung function, xv, 17, 29, 179, 252
Luo, 29, 190, 191
lymph, 6
lymphoma, 158, 160, 166

M

macrophages, 184, 185
magnesium, 55, 60
magnetic resonance, 38
magnetic resonance imaging, 38

magnitude, 104, 172, 247
majority, xii, 20, 35, 40, 60, 72, 83, 127, 142, 159, 204, 206, 207, 212
malignancy, 117, 141, 209
malnutrition, 123
man, 106, 165
management, xi, xii, xiii, xiv, xv, xvii, 1, 22, 24, 31, 32, 33, 39, 40, 41, 42, 43, 45, 49, 50, 51, 52, 56, 57, 58, 59, 60, 61, 62, 64, 67, 68, 69, 70, 78, 79, 80, 87, 90, 93, 94, 95, 99, 101, 107, 108, 109, 111, 120, 125, 126, 129, 131, 133, 136, 151, 159, 160, 163, 164, 165, 169, 176, 178, 180, 185, 193, 194, 195, 196, 197, 198, 201, 214, 228, 231, 235, 236, 239, 240, 241, 253, 254, 255, 267
manipulation, 142, 240, 248
marketing, 234
Marx, 30, 232
mass, xv, 169, 174
matter, iv
mean arterial pressure, 173, 249
measurement, 26, 64, 78, 186, 195, 204, 206, 209, 214, 241, 243, 244, 249, 250, 251, 252, 253, 254, 255, 256, 257, 258
measurements, 132, 241, 242, 247, 249, 250, 251, 252, 255, 258
mechanical ventilation, 56, 90, 240
median, xiv, 114, 141, 142, 157, 163, 222, 262
mediastinitis, 70
mediastinum, 142, 160
medical, xii, xiii, 31, 40, 50, 51, 61, 64, 67, 69, 70, 75, 77, 99, 101, 102, 103, 105, 106, 107, 122, 123, 165, 185, 195, 202, 253, 267, 268, 270, 273
Medicare, 119
medication, 228, 236, 260, 263, 271
medicine, 12, 29, 80
medulla, 9
mellitus, xvii, 33, 114, 120, 121, 122, 123, 259, 263, 270
mesenteric vessels, 14, 27
meta analysis, 137
meta-analysis, 36, 44, 46, 65, 110, 119, 123, 167, 213, 235, 270
Metabolic, xx, 122, 230, 235, 237
metabolic acidosis, 143
metabolic changes, 240
metabolic disorder, xiv, 139, 143, 144, 153, 155
metabolic disorders, xiv, 139, 143, 153, 155
metabolic pathways, 221
metabolic syndrome, 33, 117, 118, 230, 237, 263, 270
metabolism, 14, 30, 70, 79, 160, 206, 207
metabolized, 173
metastatic disease, 141

methylene blue, 185, 187
Mexico, 114
Miami, 265
microcirculation, 130, 135, 184
microspheres, 163, 184
mitochondria, 160
mitogen, 231
mitral regurgitation, 75, 76, 81, 102, 104, 108, 111
mitral stenosis, 56, 75, 76
mitral valve, 69, 71, 74, 75, 95, 100, 101, 143, 152
mitral valve prolapse, 75
models, 167, 177, 202, 213
modifications, 160, 266
molecular weight, 57, 229
molecules, xii, xiv, 21, 83, 85, 134, 157
monoclonal antibody, 146, 159
morbid obesity, xiii, 113, 114, 115, 116, 117, 118, 120
morbidity, xi, xiii, xiv, xv, xvii, 31, 33, 34, 42, 43, 47, 49, 60, 61, 62, 67, 70, 104, 113, 114, 115, 118, 119, 120, 121, 122, 129, 136, 139, 140, 141, 143, 149, 150, 151, 193, 194, 198, 201, 202, 207, 209, 213, 259, 267, 268, 270
morphology, 134
mortality, xi, xiii, xv, xvii, 14, 31, 33, 34, 35, 40, 42, 43, 48, 49, 50, 52, 57, 60, 62, 63, 70, 71, 72, 74, 75, 76, 89, 102, 104, 109, 113, 114, 115, 116, 117, 118, 119, 120, 121, 122, 126, 129, 130, 136, 137, 140, 141, 142, 143, 144, 150, 151, 152, 180, 187, 188, 189, 192, 193, 194, 198, 199, 201, 202, 203, 207, 209, 210, 211, 213, 215, 219, 221, 237, 259, 263, 266, 267, 268, 269, 273
mortality rate, 70, 71, 102, 109, 116, 120, 130, 140, 144, 189, 203, 209, 211
MRI, 46, 100, 132
multivariate analysis, 35, 252, 266, 267
murmur, 105
muscarinic receptor, 24
muscle mass, 68
muscles, 161
mutation, 148, 155
mutations, 148
mycophenolate mofetil, xvi, 218, 229, 265, 272
myocardial biopsy, 158
myocardial infarction, xxi, 35, 37, 40, 41, 43, 102, 104, 117, 158, 170, 195, 228, 234, 235, 264, 267
myocardial ischemia, 50, 52, 56, 109, 158, 262
myocardial necrosis, 103
myocarditis, 265, 272
myocardium, 79, 102, 159, 160, 161, 164, 172, 203, 212, 228, 243
myocyte, 51, 159, 160, 164
myofibroblasts, 9

N

nausea, 87
nebulizer, 88, 91
necrosis, xiii, xxi, 6, 15, 125, 127, 128, 158, 163, 185
negative outcomes, 267
nephropathy, 16, 38
nerve, 161
nervous system, xxi, 27
neurohormonal, 170
neuropathy, 153, 155
neurotoxicity, 158
neurotransmitter, 8
nitrates, 9
Nitrates, xvi, 217, 224
nitric oxide, xvi, 6, 13, 15, 22, 23, 24, 26, 29, 85, 87, 88, 90, 92, 95, 184, 185, 190, 217, 224, 234
nitric oxide synthase, 23, 26, 29
nitrous oxide, 223
nodules, 9
norepinephrine, 9
North America, 55, 121
nutritional status, 141

O

obesity, xiii, 113, 114, 115, 116, 117, 118, 119, 120, 121, 122, 123, 230, 270
objective criteria, 69, 117
obstruction, xiii, 72, 84, 99, 100, 101, 103, 105, 106, 107, 108, 109, 111, 132, 170, 222
obstructive lung disease, 17, 18
occlusion, xx, 58, 65, 78, 84, 241, 248, 253
occult cardiovascular disease, xiii, 113
oedema, 2, 12, 19, 30, 74, 195, 230
oesophageal, xvii, 9, 22, 69, 70, 71, 78, 214, 239, 244, 245, 250, 252, 255, 257
OH, 121, 135, 136
opacification, 196
open heart surgery, 135
operations, 47, 134, 141, 150, 152, 214
opportunities, xvii, 239
optimization, 50, 60, 61, 93
oral anticoagulants, xvi, 217
organ, xi, xvi, 1, 2, 19, 20, 41, 69, 80, 115, 117, 119, 121, 126, 129, 130, 131, 135, 136, 137, 143, 144, 146, 152, 153, 154, 178, 186, 187, 194, 201, 204, 211, 213, 214, 217, 218, 219, 256, 261, 267, 272
orthopnea, 86
orthotopic liver transplant, xiii, 18, 42, 43, 44, 46, 47, 49, 61, 62, 65, 95, 99, 104, 111, 120, 121, 122, 150, 151, 152, 154, 155, 167, 180, 198, 199, 215, 254, 255, 267, 268, 269, 270, 272, 273
overlap, xii, xiv, 67, 68, 70, 125, 131
overproduction, 6, 184
overweight, 114, 115
oxidation, 135, 237
oxidative stress, xiii, 14, 125, 127, 134, 162, 191
oxygen, xv, xx, xxi, 11, 18, 23, 30, 72, 165, 179, 180, 183, 184, 185, 186, 203, 204, 205, 206, 210, 212, 227, 228, 241, 243, 248, 254
oxygen consumption, 204, 205, 206, 207, 243

P

pacing, 55, 58, 103, 110, 153
pain, xii, 83, 87, 105, 212, 222, 223
palpitations, xii, 51, 52, 83
pancreas, 115, 121
pancreas transplant, 121
paracentesis, 20, 25, 230
parallel, 19, 172, 189
parenchyma, 127, 170
patents, 267
pathogenesis, 29, 127, 134, 165, 178, 184, 190, 191, 223, 236
pathology, 68, 69, 74, 87, 126, 207
pathophysiological, 2, 10, 14, 22, 25, 67, 68, 75, 194
pathophysiology, xii, 2, 9, 67, 78, 79, 93, 94, 127, 162, 184
pathways, 51, 163, 167
peace, 253
peptide, xix, 6, 8, 10, 12, 13, 15, 22, 23, 24, 26, 52, 63, 86, 94, 151, 161, 164, 264
peptides, 6, 63, 141
percentile, 115
perforation, 243, 255
perfusion, xxi, 2, 12, 17, 18, 19, 28, 29, 35, 36, 38, 43, 44, 46, 73, 90, 103, 109, 135, 180, 181, 184, 197, 203, 204, 207, 212, 213, 228
pericardial effusion, 70, 141, 158, 221
pericarditis, 265, 272
perioperative arrhythmias, xii, 49, 65
peripheral neuropathy, 148
peripheral vascular disease, 37, 63
peritoneal cavity, 141
peritonitis, 17, 28, 174, 178
permeability, 129, 141
permission, 4, 92, 101, 102, 106, 107, 144, 145, 147, 148, 149, 171, 172, 175, 185, 245, 246
permit, 144, 146
peroxidation, 160
peroxide, 160
PET, 212

pharmacokinetics, 51, 71, 162, 167
pharmacological treatment, 6, 58, 185, 221
pharmacology, 163
pharmacotherapy, 88, 219
Philadelphia, 80, 109, 110
physical activity, 222
physical characteristics, 262
physicians, 50, 55
physiological factors, 206
physiology, 18
pilot study, 185, 191, 254
placebo, 95, 222, 232, 233
plaque, 32
plasma levels, 52, 177, 221, 227
plasma membrane, 11
platelets, 71, 142
playing, 6
pleural effusion, 70, 141, 262
PM, 43, 64, 80, 134, 153, 154, 234, 256
pneumonia, 187, 262
policy, 186, 188
polymorphisms, 94
polypeptide, 161
population, xi, xii, xiii, xiv, 31, 32, 33, 34, 35, 36, 38, 39, 40, 42, 43, 49, 50, 56, 57, 61, 65, 114, 115, 120, 125, 127, 129, 131, 132, 133, 139, 140, 141, 203, 208, 210, 237, 260, 261, 263, 264
portal hypertension, xi, xii, xiv, xv, 1, 2, 3, 6, 9, 12, 19, 21, 22, 23, 24, 25, 27, 28, 30, 38, 78, 83, 84, 85, 86, 91, 93, 126, 131, 133, 148, 169, 170, 173, 176, 177, 178, 179, 180, 184, 189, 221, 227
portal vein, 87, 94, 127, 134, 142, 167, 170, 240
portopulmonary hypertension, xi, xii, xv, 1, 19, 29, 30, 83, 84, 93, 94, 95, 96, 97, 141, 191, 192, 193, 196, 218, 231, 232, 233, 234, 244, 255, 269
positron, 160
positron emission tomography, 160
postoperative outcome, 192
post-transplant, xii, xiii, 31, 34, 42, 113, 114, 115, 116, 117, 119, 213, 237, 259, 260, 261, 263, 264, 265
potassium, 16, 24, 51, 55, 60, 79, 219
potential benefits, 145
predictor variables, 209
Prednisolone, xvi, 218, 229
prednisone, 146
pregnancy, 107, 111
preoperative screening, 213
preparation, iv, 79, 218, 262
preservation, 79, 153, 266
pressure gradient, xix, 26, 63, 69, 94, 110, 180, 181
prevention, 17, 20, 28, 30, 48, 56, 60, 61, 62, 64, 164, 165, 184, 235, 271

primary biliary cirrhosis, 132
primary pulmonary hypertension, 85, 88, 96, 231
principles, xii, 55, 56, 67, 68, 80
probability, xv, 145, 179, 186
probe, 244
prognosis, xiv, 11, 17, 19, 21, 27, 46, 70, 77, 125, 126, 148, 163, 164, 174, 208, 248
pro-inflammatory, xiii, 125, 127
proliferation, 19, 85, 163
prophylactic, xiv, 40, 58, 101, 153, 157
prophylaxis, 57, 65, 78, 79, 218
propranolol, 21, 22, 26, 28, 219
prostacyclins, 222, 223
prosthesis, 80, 170
protection, 146, 236
proteins, 11, 25, 148
prothrombin, 71, 130, 132
pulmonary artery pressure, xii, xx, 12, 69, 83, 84, 92, 95, 170, 171, 241, 248
pulmonary circulation, xiv, 17, 84, 85, 169, 170, 172, 173, 181, 204, 212
pulmonary diseases, xv, 179
pulmonary edema, 56, 261, 262, 266
pulmonary embolism, 148, 264, 267
pulmonary function test, 180, 202
pulmonary hypertension, xii, xiii, xiv, 18, 44, 50, 69, 74, 75, 83, 84, 85, 86, 87, 88, 91, 93, 94, 95, 96, 136, 140, 169, 173, 177, 202, 211, 213, 218, 221, 222, 227, 228, 231, 232, 233, 234, 244, 250, 261, 266
pulmonary vascular resistance, xii, xiii, xiv, 17, 18, 83, 84, 94, 169, 172, 173, 227, 248
pulmonic valve, 143
pumps, 129, 222

Q

QRS complex, 51
QT interval, xii, xx, xxi, 26, 28, 49, 50, 51, 52, 53, 54, 55, 57, 62, 63, 64, 65, 219, 260, 268
quality of life, xiv, 119, 120, 122, 157, 161, 270
quantification, 69
Queensland, viii, 179

R

radiation, 163
radical formation, 165
radicals, 160
radiotherapy, 167
reactions, 14
reactive oxygen, 159

reactivity, 2, 20, 27, 87, 94, 177, 184, 241
real time, 108, 110, 244
reality, 244
reception, 251
receptors, 9, 23, 88, 159, 163, 184, 223, 231
recognition, 108, 202, 244
recommendations, iv, 32, 38, 40, 42, 107, 140, 166, 194, 196, 197, 227, 229, 245
recovery, xv, 56, 91, 148, 158, 162, 180, 189, 218, 243, 260, 265
recurrence, 55, 56, 103, 117, 262
red blood cells, 18, 142
redistribution, 10, 248
reflexes, 60
regeneration, 9
regenerative capacity, 162
Registry, xiii, xxi, 113, 115, 116, 130, 148, 202
regression, 65, 207
regression line, 207
regulatory systems, 17
rejection, xvi, 117, 131, 137, 142, 146, 147, 217, 218, 219, 265
relaxation, 9, 11, 12, 212
relaxation times, 12
relevance, 26, 63, 73, 166, 167, 203
reliability, 241, 247, 251
relief, 219
remission, 148
renal cell carcinoma, 159
renal dysfunction, 21, 272
renal failure, xiii, 17, 113, 115, 118, 146, 148, 154, 174, 240
renal replacement therapy, 130, 142
renin, 2, 7, 9, 13, 24, 174, 178
repair, 70, 74, 76, 143, 208, 214
Reperfusion arrhythmias, xii, 49
requirements, 60, 75, 129, 136, 203, 261
researchers, 161, 263
resection, 102, 164, 209
resistance, xii, xxi, 2, 4, 6, 7, 8, 9, 14, 16, 18, 19, 58, 69, 83, 85, 86, 88, 89, 90, 107, 118, 123, 129, 141, 172, 173, 204, 219, 228, 247, 248, 250, 251, 260, 261
resolution, 17, 189, 262
resources, 114
response, xi, 1, 11, 21, 23, 25, 26, 28, 46, 56, 58, 60, 89, 103, 129, 130, 135, 160, 161, 162, 165, 166, 172, 184, 203, 204, 205, 219, 221, 227, 240, 241, 242, 251, 253, 254, 260, 267
response time, 241, 251, 254
responsiveness, xv, 11, 14, 21, 27, 29, 169, 177, 191, 247, 255
restenosis, 229

restoration, 126, 260, 261
restrictive cardiomyopathy, 131
restrictive lung disease, xiii, 113, 117
reticulum, 160, 165
rheumatic fever, 72, 74
rheumatic heart disease, 69, 72, 73, 76
rhythm, 56, 57, 64, 69, 195
right atrium, 183, 241
right ventricle, 84, 136, 160, 172, 183, 212, 241, 244
right ventricular ejection fraction (RVEF), xvii, 239, 241
right ventricular end diastolic volume (RVEDV), xvii, 239, 241
risk assessment, xvi, 46, 90, 201, 202, 207, 209, 213
risk factors, 33, 35, 36, 38, 39, 42, 49, 56, 61, 72, 80, 85, 93, 104, 114, 115, 117, 121, 122, 136, 165, 195, 196, 198, 263, 265, 267, 268, 270
risk profile, 129
risks, xii, xiii, 48, 57, 65, 67, 68, 69, 84, 88, 93, 115, 116, 117, 119, 148, 176, 227, 235, 237
RNA, 160
room temperature, 222
root, 73

S

safety, 47, 103, 148, 167, 207, 224, 233, 272
sampling error, 133
saturation, xxi, 18, 186, 204, 228, 241, 243, 248, 254
Saudi Arabia, 114
scaling, 252
schema, 194, 195
science, 47, 62
sclerosis, 127, 134
scope, 40, 244, 245
sea level, 180
second generation, 129
sensitivity, 14, 15, 16, 24, 25, 27, 28, 62, 86, 118, 132, 161, 184, 202, 212
sensitization, 145
sepsis, 35, 187, 203, 222, 236, 256, 264
septic shock, 187, 253, 256
septum, 100, 101, 102, 103, 104
serum, 26, 55, 63, 64, 70, 71, 109, 126, 130, 132, 137, 141, 148, 150, 151, 154, 161, 186, 264, 266, 267, 273
serum albumin, 132
serum cholinesterase, 71, 141, 150
services, iv
sex, 33, 85, 204, 210, 251, 266
sex ratio, 33
shape, 161, 247, 252
shear, 6, 23

shock, 143
shortness of breath, xii, xv, 83, 179, 195
showing, 18, 54, 69, 101, 132, 159, 164, 208, 209, 227
side effects, xiv, 79, 87, 157, 158, 159, 160, 163, 219, 221, 222, 224, 260, 261, 264
signalling, 231
signals, 162, 241
signs, xii, 1, 12, 16, 58, 67, 68, 70, 72, 76, 90, 149, 195, 266
Sinai, 22
sinus rhythm, 56, 57, 58, 74, 75, 76, 90
skeletal muscle, 11
skin, 1, 12, 26
smoking, 17, 266, 267
smooth muscle, 9, 15, 16, 19, 184, 223, 231
smooth muscle cells, 9, 16, 184, 223
SNS, xxi, 2, 7, 11, 13, 14, 16, 17
society, 119, 227
sodium, 6, 7, 14, 16, 20, 22, 23, 27, 75, 141, 151, 176, 177, 229, 232, 233, 266, 273
software, 251
solid tumors, 159
solution, 143, 250
South Africa, 114
species, 159, 165
spermatogenesis, 223
spinal anesthesia, 96
spindle, 158
spleen, 172, 181
splenomegaly, 87, 94, 131
squamous cell, 214
squamous cell carcinoma, 214
stability, 57, 142
stabilization, 148
stable angina, 40, 43
standard deviation, 251
stasis, 127
state, xi, xii, 1, 5, 12, 16, 22, 23, 40, 58, 83, 84, 85, 96, 129, 135, 137, 151, 152, 155, 177, 191, 195, 196
statin, 65
stenosis, xix, 37, 40, 72, 74, 75, 76, 80, 81, 143, 152, 212
stent, xiv, xvi, xix, 25, 29, 41, 43, 48, 169, 170, 176, 177, 218, 228, 229
sternum, 142
steroids, 59
stomach, 244
stratification, 35, 38, 39, 44, 50, 58, 60, 62, 118, 198, 209
stress, xii, xvi, xix, 6, 11, 20, 23, 35, 36, 37, 38, 43, 44, 45, 46, 56, 58, 62, 65, 83, 85, 118, 119, 134, 150, 152, 161, 194, 195, 197, 201, 202, 203, 204, 212, 213, 217, 219, 240, 260, 261, 267, 269, 270
stress echocardiogram, 46
stroke, xiii, 4, 11, 19, 21, 35, 56, 57, 60, 73, 100, 113, 173, 212, 241, 248, 249, 251, 255
stroke volume, 4, 21, 73, 173, 212, 241, 248, 249, 251, 255
structure, 160, 165, 174, 252
subaortic stenosis, 100
subgroups, 32, 96
success rate, 102
sulfate, 55
Sun, 80, 191
superior vena cava, 241
suppression, 17
supraventricular tachycardia, 51
surface area, 159, 252
surgical intervention, 141
surgical resection, 163
surgical technique, 59, 201, 262, 266
surveillance, xiii, 114, 119, 234
survival, xiv, xv, 3, 12, 14, 16, 28, 39, 47, 50, 52, 72, 74, 75, 85, 88, 91, 96, 102, 114, 115, 116, 117, 119, 120, 121, 123, 129, 130, 131, 132, 135, 142, 143, 144, 147, 148, 149, 152, 157, 158, 161, 163, 164, 169, 174, 175, 178, 179, 180, 187, 189, 202, 208, 210, 211, 213, 214, 215, 223, 231, 236, 248, 262, 263, 264, 266, 267, 269, 272, 273
survivors, 71, 75, 130, 202, 203, 210, 214, 263
susceptibility, 70, 131, 133, 141, 265
Swan-Ganz catheter, 253, 255
Switzerland, vii, viii, ix, 179
sympathetic nervous system, 2, 7, 13, 24
symptoms, xi, xii, 31, 51, 67, 68, 70, 72, 74, 75, 76, 83, 86, 87, 100, 101, 103, 105, 106, 107, 109, 119, 132, 148, 185, 195, 219, 221, 222, 223, 224, 230, 260, 266
syndrome, xi, xv, xx, xxi, 1, 2, 3, 5, 17, 18, 20, 29, 50, 60, 61, 62, 63, 64, 65, 68, 73, 85, 93, 96, 97, 108, 111, 117, 122, 144, 174, 179, 180, 181, 185, 186, 189, 190, 191, 192, 193, 196, 199, 202, 218, 230, 232, 237, 240, 265, 269
synthesis, 26, 185
syphilis, 73
systolic murmur, 69
systolic pressure, xiii, xxi, 84, 86, 196, 248, 255

T

tachycardia, 41, 73, 108
tacrolimus, xvi, 146, 218, 229, 230, 235, 237, 263, 264, 265, 266, 269, 270, 271
Taiwan, 61

target, 10, 38, 102, 146, 203, 227
teams, xvi, 193
technetium, 161
techniques, xvii, 3, 12, 68, 132, 140, 145, 160, 161, 164, 181, 239, 254
technologies, 249
technology, 43, 241, 247, 252
TEG, 58
temperature, 55, 60, 241, 242, 246, 249
tension, 16, 244
testicular cancer, 158
testing, xvi, xix, 35, 36, 38, 40, 46, 51, 58, 120, 161, 193, 196, 197, 198, 201, 202, 203, 204, 206, 207, 209, 210, 213, 214, 215, 252, 258
TGF, 185
Thailand, 114
thalassemia, 144, 153
thallium, 36, 213
therapeutic interventions, 53
therapeutic targets, 167, 230
therapy, xiii, xvi, xvii, 14, 20, 22, 30, 41, 47, 48, 57, 61, 64, 65, 70, 75, 78, 79, 84, 85, 87, 88, 89, 90, 91, 92, 94, 95, 101, 102, 106, 107, 108, 129, 140, 146, 152, 161, 162, 163, 164, 165, 166, 185, 191, 217, 219, 221, 222, 223, 224, 226, 227, 228, 229, 231, 232, 233, 234, 235, 236, 237, 240, 241, 244, 250, 253, 255, 259, 264, 265, 267, 271, 272
thinning, 102
thrombin, 58, 64, 71, 80
thrombocytopenia, 57, 87
thrombolytic therapy, 234
thrombomodulin, 85
thrombosis, xvi, 41, 47, 71, 93, 115, 127, 134, 167, 187, 218, 228, 235
thrombus, 57, 69, 127
thyroid, 262
time constraints, 206
tissue, 158, 163, 177, 223
TNF, xxi, 6, 15, 184, 185
tobacco, 195
tobacco smoking, 195
toxic effect, xii, 83, 158, 160, 162
toxicity, 57, 158, 160, 163, 165, 227
training, xvii, 239, 245
transaminases, 70, 142
transcatheter, 58, 152
transcranial Doppler sonography, 30
transducer, 250, 251
transformation, 249
transforming growth factor, 191
transfusion, 55, 129, 136, 194, 266
transjugular intrahepatic portosystemic stent shunt (TIPS), xiv, 169

translocation, 184, 191
Trans-oesophageal echocardiography (TEE), xvii, 239
transplant, xi, xiii, xiv, xv, xvi, 31, 32, 33, 34, 35, 36, 38, 39, 40, 41, 42, 47, 50, 52, 57, 67, 71, 76, 79, 80, 84, 85, 86, 87, 89, 91, 113, 114, 115, 116, 117, 118, 119, 120, 121, 122, 123, 129, 131, 132, 136, 140, 143, 145, 146, 152, 153, 154, 157, 180, 193, 194, 195, 196, 197, 198, 203, 209, 211, 212, 213, 217, 218, 235, 236, 237, 260, 261, 262, 263, 267, 270, 271, 272
transplant recipients, xiii, 47, 80, 113, 114, 115, 117, 119, 121, 122, 152, 154, 235, 236, 237, 260, 262, 267, 270, 271, 272
transplantation, xi, xii, xiii, xiv, xv, xx, 12, 31, 32, 33, 36, 39, 40, 41, 42, 47, 62, 67, 68, 69, 71, 73, 75, 77, 78, 79, 84, 85, 86, 87, 88, 89, 91, 92, 93, 113, 115, 116, 117, 118, 119, 120, 121, 122, 126, 129, 130, 131, 133, 135, 136, 139, 140, 143, 146, 147, 148, 149, 150, 152, 153, 154, 157, 163, 164, 192, 193, 194, 195, 196, 197, 201, 202, 203, 209, 210, 215, 229, 235, 236, 237, 240, 252, 253, 256, 260, 263, 264, 265, 267, 268, 271, 272
transport, 205
trans-thoracic, xiii, 83, 86, 100, 110
transthoracic echocardiography, 69
trauma, 254
treatment, xii, xiii, xiv, xvi, 10, 12, 21, 22, 28, 29, 40, 49, 51, 56, 58, 61, 69, 70, 72, 74, 75, 76, 80, 87, 88, 89, 90, 91, 94, 95, 96, 99, 101, 102, 103, 104, 107, 126, 127, 132, 139, 140, 143, 148, 154, 157, 158, 159, 160, 161, 162, 163, 164, 165, 166, 167, 173, 174, 185, 190, 195, 217, 218, 219, 220, 221, 222, 223, 224, 225, 227, 228, 229, 231, 233, 234, 237, 240, 244, 255, 265, 266
trial, 27, 41, 47, 48, 57, 73, 79, 87, 95, 110, 163, 167, 224, 227, 231, 232, 234, 236, 254, 269, 271
tricuspid valve, 76, 132, 143, 241
triggers, 58, 129
tumor, xiv, 127, 157, 159, 160, 162, 163, 167, 184
tumor cells, 159, 160
tumor growth, xiv, 157, 163, 167
tumor necrosis factor, 127, 184
tumor progression, 163
tumors, 158, 159, 164
turnover, 58
tyrosine, 155, 158, 159, 167

U

ultrasonography, 137
ultrasound, 132, 161, 250
uncontrolled hypertension, xiii, 113, 118

Index

United, xxi, 91, 114, 115, 120, 121, 123, 125, 131, 137, 143, 152, 186, 197, 222, 254, 255, 272, 273
United Kingdom (UK), xxi, 114, 217, 222, 239, 249, 273
United States (USA), 31, 49, 83, 99, 114, 118, 120, 121, 123, 125, 137, 139, 143, 152, 186, 193, 197, 214, 241, 254, 255, 272
unstable angina, 40
urinary tract, 148

V

validation, 44, 200, 213, 252
valuation, 12, 46, 150, 194
valve, 69, 72, 73, 74, 75, 76, 77, 78, 80, 101, 102, 143, 241, 272
valvular heart disease, xii, 55, 67, 68, 69, 70, 77, 79, 80
valvular lesion, xii, 67, 69, 70, 79
variables, xvii, 22, 115, 118, 202, 204, 205, 207, 208, 209, 211, 223, 239, 241, 242, 252, 266
variations, 114, 243, 255, 257
vascular endothelial growth factor (VEGF), 7
vascular surgery, 40, 47, 213
vascular system, 2, 13, 22, 250
vascular wall, 85
vascularization, 167
vasculature, 86, 88, 90, 162, 172, 173, 204, 224
vasoconstriction, xiv, 2, 12, 16, 85, 87, 88, 91, 169, 184, 223, 248
vasodilatatory state, xi, 1
vasodilation, 23, 190, 212, 224, 227
vasodilator, xiii, 13, 24, 84, 85, 87, 88, 89, 91, 92, 221, 233
vasodilators, xvi, 6, 7, 15, 74, 90, 184, 217, 223
vasopressin, 9, 14, 16, 17, 22
vasopressor, 240, 253
vein, 76, 127, 142, 145, 149, 160, 170
velocity, xii, xxi, 72, 83, 86, 175, 250

ventilation, xv, 17, 18, 58, 60, 180, 184, 187, 204, 207, 244, 261
ventricle, xxi, 73, 84, 161, 244
ventricular arrhythmias, xii, 49, 50, 51, 52, 58, 62, 65, 103, 254
ventricular fibrillation, 50, 55, 60, 61
ventricular septum, 102
ventricular tachycardia, 51, 60, 62, 64, 159
vessels, 12, 16, 19, 23, 244
viruses, 44
vitamin C, 14
vitamin K, 57, 71
vulnerability, 43

W

walking, 204
Washington, viii, ix, 49, 56, 113
water, xx, 6, 16, 20, 22, 27, 141, 151, 180, 247, 248, 252, 256
water vapor, 180
weakness, 86
weight gain, 265
weight loss, 123
weight management, 119, 123
windows, 251
withdrawal, 235, 272
workload, 86, 212
World Health Organisation (WHO), xxi, 114, 221, 222, 223, 227
worldwide, 163
wound dehiscence, xiii, 113
wound infection, 142

Y

yield, 251
yttrium, 163